Mental Health Disorders in Adolescents

Mental Health Disorders in Adolescents A Guide for Parents, Teachers, and Professionals

Eric P. Hazen, M.D.
Mark A. Goldstein, M.D.
Myrna Chandler Goldstein, M.A.

Foreword by
Michael S. Jellinek, M.D.

Rutgers University Press
New Brunswick, New Jersey, and London

Library of Congress Cataloging-in-Publication Data
Hazen, Eric P.
Mental health disorders in adolescents : a guide for parents, teachers, and
professionals / Eric P. Hazen, Mark A. Goldstein, Myrna Chandler Goldstein ;
foreword by Michael S. Jellinek.
p. ; cm.
Includes bibliographical references and index.
ISBN 978-0-8135-4893-7 (hardcover : alk. paper) —
ISBN 978-0-8135-4894-4 (pbk. : alk. paper)
1. Adolescent psychiatry. 2. Adolescent psychopathology. I. Goldstein,
Mark A. (Mark Allan), 1947– II. Goldstein, Myrna Chandler, 1948–
III. Title.
[DNLM: 1. Mental Disorders. 2. Adolescent. WS 463 H429m 2011]
RJ503.H29 2011
616.8900835—dc22   2010008407

A British Cataloging-in-Publication record for this book is available from the
British Library.

The information contained in this book is intended to provide helpful and
informative material on the subject addressed. It is not intended to serve as a
replacement for professional medical advice. Any use of the information in this
book is at the reader's discretion. The authors and publisher specifically disclaim
any and all liability arising directly or indirectly from the use or application of
any information contained in this book. A health care professional should be
consulted regarding your specific situation.

Visit our Web site: http://rutgerspress.rutgers.edu

Manufactured in the United States of America

I dedicate this book to my wife, Melissa, and my son, James.

—EPH

We dedicate this book with love and affection to our grandchildren:
Aidan Zev Goldstein, born February 8, 2008, and
Payton Maeve Goldstein, born December 4, 2009

—MAG and MCG

Contents

Foreword

Throughout history, adolescence has posed challenges to parents. Some of these challenges are a result of our social evolution. When we lived in primitive circumstances, adolescents—what we now think of as tenth graders in high school —were a critical resource for survival. Once physically mature, teenagers took responsibility for gathering or hunting food as well as having the children needed for family and group survival. In a less complicated world, our high schoolers, too young to drink, drive, and vote and in our view in constant need of supervision, are biologically capable of being quite productive citizens.

In modern society, adolescence is lengthened, and the issues faced during this time are complex. There is an extended period of learning, with pressure to stay in school through college and, for some, well into their twenties. Adolescents are ready to take risks, a propensity desirable when needing to leave the hut and hunt lions but undesirable with respect to drinking alcohol, using substances, and driving cars. Busy parents are conflicted by their wish for their teenager to function more autonomously and their anxiety about behavior that is irresponsible and dangerous. Therefore, a ready-to-hunt-and-procreate biology meets a world that delays autonomy and is full of opportunities requiring more learning and more judgment.

In adolescence, the prevalence of emotional disorders rises. Epidemiological studies suggest 10 to 20 percent of adolescents will develop an emotional disorder. The stakes are high, as the leading causes of death for adolescents—automobile accidents and suicide—often have emotional antecedents. Some of these disorders will be time limited; others will persist throughout life. For example, attention-deficit/hyperactivity disorder (ADHD) affects school performance, increases the chance for accidents, raises an adolescent's risk of substance abuse, and if not comprehensively and well treated, may lower self-esteem. For a third to half of teenagers with ADHD, the disorder eases or disappears in late adolescence. For others, choosing the right job that fits their skills lowers the impact of the symptoms when compared to the demands of classroom work; for a substantial minority, the disorder persists throughout adulthood, causing distress and dysfunction.

When dealing with a teenager's emotional problems, parents face many questions. How serious is the problem? What is the problem specifically? Some mental health concerns, such as depression, fit neatly into understood patterns. Others, such as a reaction to divorce or dealing with peer rejection or lying, are not diagnoses per se but cause the child and family much emotional heartache and worry. Are all lies the same? Do all teenagers who tell a lie become persistent liars or delinquents? Are some of the seemingly obvious answers, such as creating more rules, strict discipline, and limiting autonomy the best steps or possibly counterproductive? What treatments are available? How do I access the help? What is the appropriate role of medications? Are there any indicators of severity and prognosis?

When parents remember their own adolescent years or look at their own family history—depression, attention-deficit issues, anorexia—they will worry. As they hear of a teenager hurt or killed in a drunk driving accident, they will wonder if they really know what is going on at their adolescent's party or dance. As parents see a tendency in their teenager—being sad, eating less, showing anxiety, lying— they cannot help but be concerned about what the future might hold.

The first step is to learn about the diagnosis or behavior based on sound knowledge and the wisdom gained from years of experience. This information is available in the excellent chapters of this book, which has been written by a pediatrician with extensive experience treating adolescents, a sophisticated child and adolescent psychiatrist, and an independent scholar/writer. The second step is to talk to your pediatrician, who hopefully has developed a confidential relationship with your teenager and a trusted relationship to the family. A third step might be some screening tests, information gathering, and advice from the pediatrician or, if indicated, a referral to a subspecialist in mental health for a full evaluation.

Emotional disorders in adolescents are not simple problems to evaluate, diagnose, and treat. Opening up to an adult, listening to advice, and following a treatment plan are not easy for adolescents. Sometimes the problems are not clear, and at other times the treatment team and parents must share their dilemmas until there is some clarity or progress—a process that may require a considerable amount of time and resources.

As a society, we need to take adolescent emotional disorders more seriously. We must train more mental health specialists and provide adequate reimbursement for their services. We should screen children and adolescents in primary care pediatric practices to detect emotional disorders earlier. The courts must not be used as a substitute for mental health services; we need to provide mental health services to those teenagers in state care, foster care, or juvenile detention centers. We must implement the laws that require parity of treatment resources between medical and psychiatric disorders. Finally, parents and those who work and interact with adolescents should learn more about adolescent emotional disorders.

Adolescence is a time of great opportunities and great risks. Decisions, events, and emotional disorders in adolescence often have a life-long impact. This book is a significant resource to understanding adolescent emotional problems. Teenagers deserve our understanding, best efforts, and resources.

Michael S. Jellinek, M.D.
Chief, Child and Adolescent Psychiatry Service, Massachusetts General Hospital
Professor of Psychiatry, Harvard Medical School
President, Newton-Wellesley Hospital

Preface

You hear a loud and persistent knock at your front door. As you approach the door, you see a state trooper on your front step. With trepidation, you open the door. "Are you the parent of William Smith?" "I am very sorry to tell you that your son jumped in front of a truck on the interstate highway. . . ."

Suddenly awakened, you are drenched in perspiration, and your heart is pounding. You race to William's bedroom. He is safe and sound asleep.

Is this every parent's nightmare? Maybe.

Adolescence is a time of change—especially in the biological, intellectual, and social domains. Substance abuse, eating disorders, self-induced injury, and other mental health concerns emerge as teens grow physically, develop intellectually, and intensify social relationships with peers,

We have written this book to help parents and all who interact with adolescents to recognize some of the symptoms of mental illness as they emerge during this developmental period. Our perspectives are those of a child and adolescent psychiatrist, an adolescent medicine specialist, and an independent scholar/writer. After all, the medical and psychiatric aspects of illness often cannot be readily separated.

By recognizing the early symptoms of a psychiatric disorder, a teen's life may be saved. In many situations, early treatment of an adolescent's mental disorder leads to a better outcome. In addition, we have also reviewed the behaviors displayed by adolescents that do not rise to the level of a disorder but are of concern to parents.

In the foreword, Dr. Jellinek notes that up to 20 percent of adolescents will develop an emotional disorder. Accordingly, all who come into contact with adolescents will probably encounter a teen with a mental health disorder. Many of these disorders may affect the teen in his or her adult life. It is our hope that this book will answer your questions about adolescent mental health issues and adolescent behaviors and provide a guide to access the help you may need. Through a better understanding of adolescents, all of us can provide the best care and services to them.

Eric P. Hazen, M.D.
Mark A. Goldstein, M.D.
Myrna Chandler Goldstein, M.A.

Acknowledgments

I would like to thank my spouse, Melissa, for her patience and unwavering support, my son, James, for the joy that he brings, and James's grandparents for all of their help during the writing of this book. I would also like to thank Dr. Michael Jellinek and Dr. Bruce Masek for their guidance and mentorship.

—EPH

Dr. Robert Masland, Chief Emeritus of the Adolescent Unit, Boston Children's Hospital, passed away just before publication of this book. I am eternally grateful for his professional mentorship, guidance, and wisdom over the past thirty-five years. He was an outstanding role model for many physicians who have become leaders in the field of adolescent medicine.

—MAG

1 Introduction

Adolescence is a challenging time even under the best of circumstances. Overnight, a polite, happy child may appear to transform into a surly, rebellious teen. Trying as the changes that occur during adolescence may be, they serve a greater purpose: to help children who are wholly dependent on their parents for most of their needs to develop into healthy, independent adults with a secure sense of identity and the ability to think effectively through the problems that life may throw at them. The majority of adolescents manage this transition without a great deal of turmoil. However, the rapid physical, psychological, and social shifts that take place during adolescence can be quite stressful, and this stress places teens at risk of developing psychiatric difficulties. In fact, many psychiatric disorders first emerge during the adolescent years.

It is estimated that 12 percent of children and adolescents in the United States suffer from a serious psychiatric disorder that causes significant impairment in their functioning. A recent survey of U.S. high school students by the Centers for Disease Control and Prevention (CDC) has shown that over 14 percent of them have seriously considered committing suicide in the past year (down from 29 percent in the early 1990s), and approximately 7 percent of them report that they have attempted suicide in the past year. Suicide is the third leading cause of death among adolescents in the United States, led only by accidents (some of which may be related to substance abuse and other forms of mental illness) and homicide. Despite these concerning statistics, it appears that the majority of adolescents suffering from psychiatric illness do not receive the treatment that they require.

When mental illness strikes during the vulnerable adolescent period, it has the potential to cause immediate suffering but also to disrupt the critical developmental processes that are unfolding. This can cause difficulties that last a lifetime. Thus, recognizing and addressing psychiatric concerns that arise during adolescence is critical to a teen's long-term well-being. Yet, with so much change happening so quickly, it can be particularly difficult for parents to detect problems when they arise and to know what is normal and what may be the sign of a more serious concern.

In our society, these problems are compounded by not only a severe shortage of mental health services for children and adolescents that is reaching crisis proportions but also a system of psychiatric care that is frequently confusing, if not overwhelming, to negotiate. The goal of this book is to help parents and those who work with adolescents, including teachers, school counselors, coaches, and pediatricians, to recognize signs of a possible psychiatric disorder in an adolescent and to determine how to get the appropriate help. We also hope it will serve as a guide through the treatment process.

How to Use This Book

This book is divided into two parts. The first part provides an overview of mental health treatment for adolescents, including how to find help, the initial evaluation process, the roles that various providers and programs may play in a teen's treatment, and the range of treatments that are available. The second part focuses on specific psychiatric conditions. In it, we discuss the symptoms and warning signs of these conditions as they may appear in adolescence and the impact they may have on a teen's life. We cover the diagnostic evaluation for each disorder, including other possible problems that should be considered, and the major treatment options that are used to treat the condition. At the end of the book, we provide a compendium of useful resources for parents, including reliable websites that have additional information in particular areas and organizations that offer support groups and other helpful programs (Appendix A). We also provide an outline of the information that is useful to have during a psychiatric evaluation, so that parents can use the time with a mental health clinician most effectively and facilitate that clinician's thorough understanding of their teen's problem (appendix B).

Adolescent Psychological Development

Social and Emotional Development

From a developmental perspective, adolescence is something like a high-wire act. Teens must make their way from the safe platform of childhood along a sometimes scary path toward the goal of adulthood. For a teen, stepping out on the wire is anxiety provoking: What if I make a misstep? What if I choose the wrong friends? Will I be betrayed? Ridiculed? What if my girlfriend breaks up with me? What if I do not make the team?

To an adult who has already made this short but knee-shaking trip and is safely on the other side, these concerns often seem small and insignificant. Over a lifetime, there will be other friends, other girlfriends, other teams. But to teens taking those first uncertain steps, these events may feel like a jolt that might bounce them off their precarious path.

It may be tempting not to chance it but rather to stay behind among the comforts of childhood, where parents can be counted on to provide for one's emotional and physical needs and where one's identity is neatly laid out by one's role in the family. To do so, however, is to risk a lifetime of dependency and insecurity. Thus, teens may need to give themselves a psychological nudge to get started. This nudge may take the form of rejecting parents' values. This attitude may be teens' way of convincing themselves that the platform of dependency is worth leaving. The nudge may go further, from attitude to behavior, with adolescents demonstrating their rejection of a parent's worldview by actively rebelling against the rules the parent has set. Often, the very act of teenage rebellion reveals the conflict within the teen, for acting out seems to communicate "Leave me alone! I'm doing my own thing!" while, in fact, the result is usually more attention and concern from parents. Rebellious teens often end up grounded, back at home with their parents, on a temporary break from the scary new freedoms of adolescence. At a not-quite-conscious level, this may have been exactly what the teen wanted and needed.

So how do teens go about separating from their parents and developing their own sense of identity? In the middle school years, adolescents look to their peer group as a source of beliefs and values outside the family. Early adolescence is very focused on finding one's place in a group. This is the time when many adolescents are most concerned about being popular and most anxious about being an outcast. Being a proud member in a peer group early in adolescence helps provide the confidence for a teen later to move throughout different groups.

Later in adolescence, teens build their growing sense of individual identity by choosing between groups. They may try on different personas—jock, preppy, Goth, druggie, skater, and so on. This stage is a precursor to the healthy adult, secure in one's identity, a person who may be influenced by his or her culture but is nonetheless capable of making independent decisions about his or her beliefs and values.

Adolescence is also the time when interest in romantic relationships first emerges and when most people have their first experience with these relationships. For some teens, it is a period of questioning and figuring out their sexuality, which can be a stressful experience. Teens who have an attraction to members of the same sex may fear rejection or ostracism by their parents, friends, or community. These fears can make some adolescents more vulnerable to depression, suicidal thoughts, and other psychiatric difficulties. A supportive home environment can help mitigate some of this vulnerability.

As part of adolescent psychological development, most teens haves a strong drive to experiment that may take many forms, from new styles of music and clothing to risk-taking behaviors involving drugs and sex. The drive to experiment is often coupled with a sense of grandiosity and invulnerability and a limited capacity to grasp fully the potential ramifications of the risks being taken, creating a perfect storm of sorts. The adolescent's newfound physical maturity, sexual drive, intellectual advances, earning potential, and mobility may lead to trouble even in the healthiest, well-adjusted youth. New scientific findings have suggested that much of the risk-taking behavior in adolescence may be attributable to physiological changes that take place in the brain during this period. Even thoughtful, responsible teens are not always capable of making good decisions in the heat of the moment. Thus, adolescents require adequate supervision, clear expectations, and firm, caring limits from parents to keep them safe. Though they may not always like what they hear, such limits are usually perceived as signs of loving protection. While limits must be set on unsafe behaviors, parents must appreciate that experimentation is essential to the development of a sense of personal identity. By trying out different interests in everything from hairstyle to political worldview, teenagers gradually assemble a clearer picture of themselves.

Cognitive Development

Beginning in early adolescence, an individual's thinking starts to shift from the concrete, rule-oriented style of younger children to a more flexible approach. The capacity for abstract thought becomes more fully developed through the adolescent years. During this time, teens become increasingly able to think beyond their direct experience and reason about hypothetical scenarios. This allows them to think through concepts such as religion and politics and form their own opinions. Problem-solving strategies also become more logical and systematic during adolescence.

Despite the cognitive gains that occur during adolescence, teens still have limitations relative to adults in their ability to problem solve and to think through potential consequences of their actions. This aspect of adolescent cognition further fuels their tendency toward risk-taking behavior. On average, adolescents tend to have particular difficulty weighing long-term consequences, which may seem somewhat unreal to them, in their decisions. This places them at greater risk for developing problem behaviors in which the negative consequences are not experienced immediately, including smoking, unhealthy eating habits, and poor compliance with medications for chronic medical conditions such as diabetes.

Furthermore, adolescents tend to demonstrate a difference between the decisions they make in the heat of the moment, a process that cognitive scientists call "hot cognition," and the decisions they make in a less emotionally charged environment, or "cold cognition." For example, adolescents might make a different decision about driving a car with a friend who is drunk when they are at a party and surrounded by friends than they would if they were thinking through the scenario with a parent. We are all prone to letting emotion cloud our judgment, but it seems this effect is more pronounced in adolescents.

Although it was once felt that the impulsivity and risk-taking behaviors of adolescence was mostly related to social and psychological factors, recent scientific findings have indicated that these behaviors may have a large biological component. Some of the most interesting findings in human development in recent decades have emerged from studies of the changes that take place in the brain during adolescence. Until recently, it was believed that most of the major biological processes in human brain development were complete by early child-hood; thus, the brain of an early adolescent was thought not to be very different from that of a mature adult. Research over the past decade, using new brain-imaging technology, has challenged this notion.

In fact, it appears that dramatic changes in the brain continue to unfold throughout adolescence and into the early adult years. The most striking changes involve the prefrontal cortex, the area of the brain that is responsible for a group of functions that psychologists refer to as "executive function." These functions include controlling impulses, evaluating risks, and planning and making deci-sions. During adolescence, it appears that new connections between the prefron-tal cortex and other parts of the brain are formed and that existing connections are strengthened and fine-tuned. In essence, this implies that the capacity of the prefrontal cortex to regulate other areas of the brain, including centers of emotion and fight-or-flight instincts, grows stronger during adolescence. These findings fit well with the cognitive and behavioral changes that occur during adolescence. As the prefrontal cortex matures, individuals become better able to modulate their impulses and manage their emotions to make good decisions un-der a broader range of circumstances.

Physical Development

Adolescence is a time of rapid physical as well as psychological change. Because this is a book about mental health, we will not discuss the physical changes in detail here. Still, it should be noted that the physical changes of adolescence may be intertwined with the psychological ones. It is difficult to overestimate the impact that bodily changes can have on a teen's still malleable sense of self. The effect that physical changes may have can vary widely, ranging from a boost in self-esteem to significant psychological distress. The psychological impact of pubertal changes on a teen depends on many factors, including their timing and the psychological makeup of the adolescent. Gender also plays a role, as studies have shown that boys who mature physically earlier than their peers tend to be more self-confident and have a greater likelihood of academic, social, and athletic success, whereas girls who mature earlier than their peers tend to have lower self-esteem and more body-image concerns. Eating disorders (discussed in chapter 15) most frequently emerge during the adolescent years, and self-consciousness about one's body image can play a role in depression, anxiety, and the tendency toward risk-taking behavior, including sexual promiscuity.

What Is Normal?

To summarize, adolescence is a time of rapid physical and psychological change. Teens may try on different beliefs and attitudes, often borrowed from peer groups, on their way to finding their own identity. The relationship between parents and child shifts dramatically during adolescence. Teens may rebel, take risks, and act impulsively, and all of this, to some extent, is considered not only normal but a healthy part of development.

The question most parents find themselves asking is, with all of this going on, how am I supposed to realize it if there is a problem? Put another way, how can a parent tell the normal changes and behaviors of adolescence from signs of an emerging psychological problem?

It is often very difficult to distinguish healthy developmental struggles from an emerging psychiatric problem, even for mental health professionals. For some teens, the line is not always clear. Parents do not need to be correct 100 percent of the time. They should leave the diagnosis of a psychiatric problem to a professional. But they must be attuned to potential warning signs and seek further help and input when suspicion of a problem does arise. Specific warning signs for particular disorders are discussed in part 2 of this book. But a few overarching principles apply to all these trouble signals. In general, adolescent life unfolds in three main domains: home, school, and social life. It is not surprising that when a psychiatric problem emerges during adolescence, trouble in one or more of these domains is often the first sign.

Problems at home are the most obvious to parents. Although it is not unusual for there to be some friction as a teen's role within the family shifts during adolescence, dramatic changes in mood and behavior may be a sign of a psychiatric problem. Signs of trouble at home include frequent angry and explosive outbursts, extreme irritability, decreased motivation, strange and unpredictable behaviors, and persistent feelings of sadness or hopelessness. Psychiatric disorders in adolescents are often manifested through physical symptoms, including fatigue, disturbances in sleep or appetite, significant weight change, or frequent physical complaints, such as headaches and stomachaches, that do not seem to have any medical cause. Although most teens have an increasing desire for privacy and time alone, complete withdrawal from family and friends and extremely isolative behavior are often signs of a problem. Poor self-care, such as failing to bathe or wearing unclean clothes, may be a sign of psychiatric illness. Finally, but most importantly, concerns about teens' safety or the safety of those around them, including expressions of suicidal thoughts, self-injurious behavior such as cutting, and aggressive behavior are important warning signs that should never be ignored. Safety concerns are discussed in chapter 19.

In school, problems that may be signs of a psychiatric concern include a rapid drop in grades, poor attendance, frequent disciplinary troubles such as fights or acting out in class, conflict with teachers or school staff, and dropping sports or other activities in which the teen was once active. When problems start at school, parents may not always be alerted immediately. If there are concerns arising in other areas of a teen's life, it may be helpful to contact your teen's teachers or school counselor.

Certain types of social problems may indicate a psychiatric issue, such as increasing isolation and loss of interest in spending time with friends. Although interests may shift during the teen years, complete loss of interest in activities or hobbies that an adolescent once enjoyed may be a signal of trouble, especially if no new interests emerge. Changing peer groups during adolescence is quite common, but this change is of more concern when it is sudden and dramatic or when a teen begins to identify more with peers who are troubled or have problems with drug or alcohol use.

It should be noted that many of these signs may be a part of healthy adolescent development. Frequently, the difference between a normal developmental challenge and a sign of trouble is a matter of degree. For example, a teen who has a dispute with her closest friends and spends a few weekends at home moping around the house and watching TV with her younger sister before seeking new friendships is probably going through a healthy adjustment. In contrast, a girl who stops returning calls from friends for several weeks, starts spending most of her time in her room alone, does not talk with family members, and whose grades begin to slip is likely to have a larger problem for which she may well need outside help.

These examples highlight another rule that can help parents distinguish normal developmental difficulties from a possible psychiatric disorder. When a psychiatric disorder is present, it tends to cause multiple problems at the same time. An adolescent who is showing one or two warning signs, such as temporarily spending less time with friends, while otherwise doing well in other areas is less likely to have a problem than a teen who is showing several signs of distress in more than one area of his or her life.

Additionally, most developmental struggles tend to be short-lived. A healthy teen decides how to respond to a stressful situation and moves on. On the other hand, psychiatric disorders tend to persist or get worse without outside help. Thus, if a problem that has been chalked up to "typical teenage stuff" is going on for a long time and causing a lot of distress, it may be time to rethink that interpretation and get an outside opinion.

Finally, a parent's intuition is one of the most important indicators of a teen's psychological well-being. Even though adolescents may seem as if they have been beamed in from another planet, and teens may angrily assert that their parents "just don't get them," most of the time no one knows them better than their parents. Thus, parents should trust their intuition. If something does not seem right, mental health professionals should respect a parent's sense that there is a problem, even if the outward signs are initially quite subtle.

If you are unsure whether you are overreacting to "normal teenager stuff" or your child needs an evaluation for a larger problem, consider the advice that is often given to child-psychiatry trainees: Never worry alone. Talking to other parents, your pediatrician, or staff from your child's school can help you determine whether you need to pursue an issue. Pediatricians and school staff work with adolescents and see many teens. As a result, they are in a good position to help a parent decide whether a problem needs to be explored further, and if so, they may be able to help with the process of arranging an evaluation. The process of seeking a psychiatric evaluation for your child is discussed in detail in chapter 3.

Adolescence in the Internet Era

The challenges of adolescence are nothing new. Many parents have vivid recollections of their own tumultuous adolescence. Nevertheless, today's culture is quite different from that of previous generations. Perhaps the biggest cultural change affecting adolescents today is the rise of the Internet. Computers and cell phones have dramatically altered the way that teens interact with one another and with the world at large. Through e-mail, text and instant messaging, and social networking sites such as Facebook, Twitter, and MySpace, teens are able to connect with each other in a way that is at once intensely intimate and coldly impersonal, usually outside the purview of adult supervision. Adolescents frequently post online and text obsessively, sharing details of their private lives, spreading rumors, airing their grievances, pulling pranks, and sharing pictures and video of themselves, sometimes with little appreciation of the potential consequences.

The impact of the Internet and media explosion on today's youth will probably not become fully apparent until years from now. In the meantime, these changes have given rise to new problems and placed new twists on old problems. For instance, the concept of cyber-bullying has come to many parents' attention in recent years, as text messages and posts on social networking sites add another dimension of intrusiveness to the potential for teens to torment one another. As a nasty or threatening text message may find them anywhere, children are no longer safe in the confines of their own home. At the click of a button, rumors and embarrassing photos can now be shared with countless peers. Moreover, it seems that the impersonal nature of the Internet spurs some bullies to go to greater extremes. Cruelty is easier when you do not need to look your victim in the eye. Although bullying and the cruelty of an adolescent's peers have long had the potential to cause serious harm to vulnerable adolescents, new technology has seemingly upped the ante.

Bullying is just one of the concerns that the Internet raises for today's teens. The potential for Internet addiction has received a great deal of media attention in recent years. Although it remains to be seen whether certain patterns of Internet use should be viewed as an addiction, it is clear that some teens have difficulty controlling the amount of time they spend on the Internet, and this can create larger academic and social problems. Teens who are already vulnerable because of psychiatric illness or social difficulties may be at greatest risk of problematic Internet use, as it is tempting to avoid the stresses of the real world by retreating into a virtual one.

Parents should also be aware of the potential for teens to connect with sexual predators on the Internet. Adult predators may pose as teenagers in online exchanges. Just as parents advise their children never to get into a car with a stranger, teens should be advised never to arrange a meeting with someone they have met online. The FBI website has helpful information about protecting your child's safety, at www.fbi.gov/publications/pguide/pguidee.htm.

Teens with psychiatric illness may also be more susceptible to the potential negative influence of the Internet. Now teens are able to access a vast quantity of information, much of which may be inaccurate or, worse yet, accurate but dangerous. For example, countless websites provide information about committing suicide, weighing the pros and cons of various methods. Teens who cut themselves sometimes post these images on the Web. Individuals with eating disorders share information about the most effective means of losing weight and compare their extreme and dangerous dietary habits with each other. Drug information and often drugs themselves, including marijuana seeds and the potent hallucinogen salvia divinorum, are widely available over the Internet.

The Internet is not solely a bad influence on adolescents, and our intention is not to vilify it. In a sense, the Internet is a microcosm of the world at large. As such, it can serve many useful roles in adolescent development. Teens can explore their interests and connect with others who share similar interests. This can be particularly helpful for teens who have difficulty connecting with their peers. Thus, an adolescent with Asperger syndrome may have difficulty with face-to-face interactions and may have an interest, such as the workings of old computers, that is not shared by his classmates. Through the Internet, he can locate others who share this interest and can practice his social skills by interacting with them online.

Through the Internet, teens can connect with positive influences, such as community groups, volunteer organizations, and support groups for teens grappling with difficult issues, such as Alateen. Through e-mail, teens can connect more easily with their teachers and counselors. Parents can also communicate more readily with the school and check on homework assignments through schools' websites. Provided that the information is obtained from a reliable source, the Internet can also be a valuable source of information about mental illness and available resources; appendix A has a list of resources, including many trustworthy websites.

It is challenge for today's parents to manage the presence of the Internet. Many parents who would not let their child leave the house without knowing where and with whom the child is going will allow that child unlimited and unsupervised access to the Web, where he or she is at liberty to encounter more dangerous characters and to be subject to more harmful influences than many adolescents would find in their own neighborhoods.

Although there is no single solution to the challenge of supervising teens in the Internet era, the members of every family should be mindful about these issues and devise an arrangement that works for them, rather than passively settling into a pattern of behavior based on convenience. For many families, this arrangement involves limits on screen time spent in front of TV, video games, and computers. There are numerous software programs that allow parents to monitor their children's Internet use or to filter sites that are pornographic or otherwise inappropriate. Restricting computer use to a common room in the house is another way of providing an increased level of supervision. Perhaps the most effective means of protecting your adolescent from the potential risks of the Internet is an approach that is a recurring theme in this book: good communication. Discussing potential dangers of Internet use, making parental expectations about rules and behavior clear, and being open and available to discuss what teens have come across are all essential to maintaining your adolescent's safety.

Communicating with Adolescents

Connecting with adolescents can be challenging. After all, one of the primary developmental struggles they are facing is separation from their parents. This can lead them to push away parents and other adult authority figures. Unfortunately, there is no simple set of instructions that will work for connecting with all adolescents. Every teen is different, and an approach that works for one may not work for another. Still, there are a few general principles that parents can follow.

An effective approach to communicating with adolescents is similar to one you might take as a diplomat communicating with a representative from a foreign nation. As in diplomacy, respect is an essential component of a good relationship. It would be bad form for a diplomat simply to dismiss a foreign dignitary's views on an issue whenever they differ from the diplomat's own. Similarly, adolescents yearn to have their views respected by adults. It is important to maintain respect even when your child's views seem foolish or immature. That does not mean you have to agree, but parents sometimes respond to adolescents in a way that adolescents interpret as dismissive or condescending. This can be toxic to a relationship. A playful attitude is often helpful with teens, but sarcasm and teasing over an issue a teen feels strongly about can cause the teen to shut down or to go into a rage. In these situations, it is better to listen to your child, and then explain why you respectfully disagree.

When meeting people from another culture, it is quite disconcerting to assume you know more about their

---

Sidebar 1.1 | Communicating with Adolescents

- ▸ Respect the teen's point of view
- ▸ Recognize and acknowledge the limits of your understanding about how your adolescent is feeling
- ▸ Try to be open-minded about your child's culture
- ▸ Eat together
- ▸ Talk to the teen one-on-one
- ▸ Be patient

country and their customs than you really do. Thus, a second general principle in interacting with adolescents is to recognize and acknowledge the limits of your understanding about what things are like for them. It is tempting for parents to connect their adolescent's struggles with their own experiences as a teenager. It is with great empathy and the best of intentions that many parents say, "I know exactly what you're going through," in response to which their frustrated child frequently shouts, "No, you don't!" It is essential for parents to avoid acting like they have seen it all before. Your child's experience of adolescence may be different from yours. You may be missing some aspects of your child's situation by overidentifying with your own past. Adolescents often feel that their situation is unique, even when it is not.

Even if you do have the answers, they are not going to help if the adolescent is put off by feeling as if you know everything. In fact, this drives some teens to do the opposite of what their parents keep telling them just to establish their independence. This is not to say that parents should not offer their wisdom to their children or speak about their own experiences. The trick is to do so in a way that allows the teen to feel that you are not minimizing or oversimplifying the problem and that you are offering your advice and support about a challenging issue rather than telling him or her what to do.

Avoiding overconfidence in your understanding of your child's experience leads us to our next principle of adolescent diplomacy: be open-minded and curious about your child's culture. Before dismissing the music or television shows that are the object of your child's obsession as trash, ask for more information. Try to summon a genuine interest. When you approach teen culture with an open mind, it can be quite fascinating. If you are really not interested, do your best to fake it. At the very least, it will move the conversation beyond the typical "How was school?" "Fine" pattern that so many families fall into. What does your teen like about this band? Why does he or she hate that one? What's the difference between Goth and emo? Indie and punk? What is the key to beating the last level of that video game? How did he or she figure it out? Talking about a teen's interests is a method that successful adolescent therapists often use. Sometimes, directly talking about one's troubles seems too stressful. It is easier for adolescents to discuss the things they like, and these often provide a window into their inner life. Of course, parents' curiosity should not only be limited to their children's taste in popular culture. Parents should try to engage their teens to talk about every aspect of their life including their friends, activities, and social life.

In order to practice diplomacy, you must create opportunities to connect. This seems to make common sense, but too often in contemporary life family members lead parallel lives without finding time to truly interact. They may be together physically on the way to a practice or in the living room watching television, but times when they are truly together in a deeper sense are few and far between. Making time to be together as a family is one of the best activities parents can do for their children.

The simple act of sitting down to dinner together can be incredibly powerful. Sometimes it takes some advance planning and complex scheduling gymnastics to make it happen, but it is worth it. Studies have shown that teens in families that eat dinner together regularly have lower rates of substance abuse, eating disorders, and stress. In addition they achieve higher grades and maintain healthier eating habits. Parents can engage their adolescent children by making time to do activities together. Be open to trying activities that interest your child. For example, challenge them (and watch them annihilate you) in their favorite video game. Sometimes, in a two-parent household with other children, having an occasional special dinner or afternoon out with just the teen and one parent creates the right chemistry for connecting. If you want to communicate better with your child, you should make sure that there are enough opportunities for that communication to take place.

Once the opportunities for communication are in place, we come to our final principle of connecting with adolescents, and that is patience. Good relationships, whether between foreign nations or family members, take time and effort to establish and maintain. Adolescents often go through cycles of pushing away their parents and returning to them for comfort. Do not become frustrated if your attempts to connect with your child are rebuffed. Sometimes, the planets need to be aligned just right to have a moment of connection. If you keep trying, eventually the timing will be right. If you give up, with the false assumption that your child just is not interested in talking, you may miss the times when he or she wants to connect with you.

Conclusion

Adolescence is a time of rapid and often dramatic change. These changes can be stressful for teens and parents alike. Although the majority of teens negotiate the challenges of adolescence without a great deal of emotional distress, many teens need some help along the way. And, psychiatric illnesses often initially manifest themselves during the adolescent years.

Many of the critical processes in social, emotional, and cognitive development unfold during adolescence. If healthy development is disrupted by psychiatric illness, there may be negative consequences that can last a lifetime, including difficulties with a teen's self-esteem, sense of identity, and social and romantic relationships. Thus, when problems arise, it is best to address them as early as possible. This helps the teen get back on track developmentally, before any long-term harm is done.

The good news is that teens who are suffering usually want help (despite what they might say or suggest with withering eye roll). And because they are still developing, adolescents have a much greater capacity for change. Thus, treatments such as psychotherapy can be particularly powerful with adolescents. Learning about oneself and mastering effective strategies for dealing with problems can benefit teens for years to come.

Nonetheless, coping with a teen who has psychiatric difficulties is extremely stressful for the entire family, and the mental health system in the United States is sometimes confusing and difficult to negotiate. Our hope is that through this book, parents will feel better equipped to recognize potential difficulties their children might be experiencing. We hope to guide you through the process from illness to health by giving you the information you need to do what is best for your adolescent.

References and Additional Reading

Ackard, D. M., and D. Neumark-Sztainer. 2001. "Family Mealtime While Growing Up: Associations with Symptoms of Bulimia Nervosa." *Eating Disorders* 9: 239–249.

Costello, E. J., H. Egger, and A. Angold. 2005. "10 Year Research Update Review: The Epidemiology of Child and Adolescent Psychiatric Disorders: I. Methods and Public Health Burden." *Journal of the American Academy of Child and Adolescent Psychiatry* 44: 972–986.

Fulkerson, J. A., M. Story, A. Mellin, N. Leffert, D. Neumark-Sztainer, and S. A. French. 2006. "Family Dinner Meal Frequency and Adolescent Development: Relationships with Developmental Assets and High-Risk Behaviors." *Journal of Adolescent Health* 39: 337–345.

Goldstein, M. A., and M. C. Goldstein. 2000. *Boys into Men: Stay Healthy through the Teen Years.* Westport, CT: Greenwood.

Hazen, E., S. Schlozman, and E. Beresin. 2008. "Adolescent Psychological Development: A Review." *Pediatrics in Review* 29: 161–168.

Jernigan, T. L., D. A. Trauner, and J. R. Heselink. 1991. "Maturation of Human Cerebrum In Vivo during Adolescence." *Brain* 114: 2037–2049.

Larson. N. I., D. Neumark-Sztainer, P. J. Hannan, and M. Story. 2007. "Family Meals during Adolescence Are Associated with Higher Diet Quality and Healthful Meal Patterns during Young Adulthood." *Journal of the American Dietetic Association* 107: 1502–1510.

Streigel-Moore, R. H., R. P. McMahon, F. M. Biro, G. Schreiber, P. B. Crawford, and C. Voorhees. 2001. "Exploring the Relationship between Timing of Menarche and Eating Disorder Symptoms in Black and White Adolescent Girls." *International Journal of Eating Disorders* 30: 421–433.

Part I

Recognizing the Problem, Finding Help, and Negotiating the System

Introduction to Mental Health Treatment for Adolescents

Parents unfamiliar with the mental health system who are trying to find help for their child may feel that they have fallen down the rabbit hole into a strange new land filled with confusing terms and an array of seemingly well-meaning providers whose roles are not always clear. Even parents who work in the health care field are often surprised to find that in the United States in the twenty-first century mental health problems are treated quite differently than other illnesses and that the system for treating psychiatric illness can be quite confusing. This goal of this chapter is to introduce parents to some of the fundamentals of mental health care for adolescents, with the hope that this will help families find their way through the system.

Case Presentation

Anne, a seventeen-year-old high school senior, was seen by her pediatrician early in her senior year of high school for a twenty-five-pound weight loss that occurred over a period of six months. Her parents reported that she was eating very little and exercising more intensely but still doing very well in school. The pediatrician found her blood pressure and pulse to be unstable and her body mass index to be very low at 16.0, and she was admitted to the hospital for medical stabilization and treatment of an eating disorder.

At the hospital, a child psychiatrist was consulted. She agreed with the diagnosis and recommended placement for Anne in a residential treatment center for patients with eating disorders. After a ten-day hospitalization, Anne was medically stabilized, and she was transferred to the treatment center.

Anne spent six weeks at the residential treatment center, where her treatment team included a psychiatrist, a nutritionist, a psychologist, a social worker, a family therapist, and an adolescent medicine specialist. Her treatment plan included group therapy with other female teens who had eating disorders. After regaining much of the weight she had lost, Anne was discharged to intensive outpatient treatment at the same center. Her outpatient treatment team included a therapist, a nutritionist, a case manager, and an adolescent medicine specialist. She also continued in family therapy with her parents.

After two months of intensive outpatient treatment, Anne moved to a three-evening-per-week program. That enabled her to resume attending high school, and she returned to the care of her pediatrician for medical monitoring of her eating issues. During the summer prior to college entrance, Anne was discharged from the evening program; she continued outpatient treatment with weekly meetings with her therapist and monthly sessions with her nutritionist.

The Players and Their Roles

Psychiatric problems are often complex, with a basis in many different areas of a person's life (such as brain chemistry, relationships, and stressors in the environment) and potential effects in every area of a person's life, from school to family life to friendships. Psychiatric treatment is often complex as well, reflecting the multiple dynamics of the illness and its broad effects. Unlike many illnesses, which are treated by one clinician, there is often a team involved in treating mental illness. Sometimes that team is small, just two people, but frequently a bigger team is necessary to address the different aspects of the illness and treat problems in the varied settings in which they may arise. Having many people involved in the treatment has the potential to create confusion about who is serving what role and how everyone will work together. The goal of this section is to help clarify this confusion by explaining some of the mental health providers whom your family may encounter on the journey through psychiatric treatment. If it seems overwhelming to think that all these people may be involved in your life, be assured that a treatment team is designed to fit the needs of individual adolescents and families and that some of these providers may not play a role in your child's treatment. Sidebar 2.1 explains some of the issues about combining or splitting treatment roles.

The Pediatrician

For many teens, the pediatrician is the first mental health professional they will encounter, and this professional will be the point of entry into the mental health system. It may be surprising to parents (and to some pediatricians) to hear their pediatrician described as a mental health professional. However, pediatricians play a key role in psychiatric treatment. Pediatricians are essential in screening for potential problems that might need further evaluation and treatment. Increasingly, pediatricians are relying on standardized screening tools to help them with the challenging task of identifying a potential mental health problem that others may have missed. Parents may be familiar with these tools if they have found themselves filling out a symptom checklist during a pediatrician appointment.

Usually, when a potential problem is identified, the pediatrician refers families to a psychiatrist or therapist for further evaluation and treatment. In some circumstances, the pediatrician may be involved in treating a psychiatric problem on his or her own. This is more likely to be the case with a straightforward problem, such as mild attention-deficit/hyperactivity disorder (ADHD), that responds well to medication treatment. The degree to which pediatricians become involved in directly treating psychiatric problems varies somewhat and depends in part on the pediatrician's individual comfort level, training, and experience. In areas where there is a shortage of child and adolescent psychiatrists, pediatricians are often more actively involved in mental health treatment, though not

---

Sidebar 2.1 | **To Divide or Not to Divide?**

A common theme in the discussion of the various roles of members of a child's treatment team is that some roles, such as management of medications and individual psychotherapy, are sometimes performed by the same person, and sometimes the duties are divided between two people. There are advantages and disadvantages to each approach. The decision may be based on what seems as if it will work best for your child, and other times it may be constrained by the resources that are available in your area (e.g., there may not be any child and adolescent psychiatrists in your area who are available for psychotherapy). The following are some matters to consider when you are faced with this decision:

- ► Advantages to combined treatment (one clinician plays multiples roles):
  - ► The clinician managing medications gets to know your child very well, monitors very closely.
  - ► It may be easier for the teen to talk about feelings about medications and the role they are playing in his or her life and to integrate this information into therapy.
  - ► There are fewer people with whom to communicate.
  - ► You do not have to worry about lack of communication, differing ideas about what is best.

- ► Advantages to split treatment (treatment shared between two clinicians):
  - ► Two heads are better than one—one may pick up on a matter that the other has missed; there are more people thinking about the adolescent.
  - ► It allows each clinician to focus on a particular role, with fewer potential complications (e.g., a teen's refusal to take meds because he or she is mad at the therapist, time spent discussing meds or side effects does not distract or take away from issues being addressed in therapy).
  - ► There is better continuity when one clinician is away.

---

always by choice. Pediatricians may also be involved in mental health treatment by working with other professionals to address health problems associated with psychiatric illness. As seen in the case example, pediatricians play an essential role in monitoring the weight, health, and nutritional status of teens with eating disorders.

The Child and Adolescent Psychiatrist

Often, when a pediatrician decides that a mental health problem needs further evaluation, the person to whom they refer the family is a child and adolescent psychiatrist. A child and adolescent psychiatrist is a medical doctor (M.D.) who has completed a residency in general psychiatry as well as subspecialty training in the evaluation and treatment of mental health disorders in the pediatric population. In many areas of the country, where there are shortages of child and adolescent psychiatrists, adolescents may be treated by general adult psychiatrists. These physicians have not completed subspecialty training in child psychiatry, but they have some degree of comfort and experience in treating younger patients.

The role of child and adolescent psychiatrists in treating teenagers can vary somewhat. Often, they are involved in the initial evaluation, taking a detailed history and determining whether there is a role for further diagnostic workup, such as laboratory tests or neuropsychological testing. Once the initial evaluation is complete, a psychiatrist makes recommendations about an appropriate treatment plan for the adolescent. If this plan involves treatment with psychiatric medications, these will most often be prescribed by the psychiatrist, and regular appointments with the psychiatrist will be necessary to monitor and adjust the medications as needed. When psychotherapy is part of the treatment plan, the psychiatrist may perform this role directly, or your child may be referred to another therapist.

Child and adolescent psychiatrists are trained in psychotherapy, but the extent to which they practice psychotherapy varies a great deal. Although most child psychiatrists set aside at least part of their practice for psychotherapy, some psychiatrists now see patients almost exclusively for medication management, referring to a psychologist or social worker when therapy is indicated.

The role of the child and adolescent psychiatrist has been in flux in recent years, and there are pressures for psychiatrists to be less involved in therapy than they were in the past. Even when a psychiatrist is primarily managing medications, his or her role is not limited to this function, and the appointments should not simply involve discussion of dosages and side effects. A good psychiatrist functions like an architect, helping design a plan for treatment, making sure that all the parts are where they should be and that they all function well together. For example, a psychiatrist is often in regular communication with the other parts of a child's treatment, such as the therapist and the school, assuring that they are all following a plan of treatment based on the same understanding of what the problems are and what the most effective approach is.

The Individual Therapist

If a child and adolescent psychiatrist is like the architect of your child's treatment, then the individual therapist is like the foundation of the building. Not all psychiatric problems require psychotherapy, but it is an important part of the treatment of many illnesses, particularly in dealing with more severe problems. When a therapist is involved, that is generally the professional who will spend the most time with your child and get to know him or her best. *Psychotherapy* is a general term used to describe treatment centered on meeting regularly and talking through problems. The term *individual therapist* is used to indicate that the therapist is someone who meets with a patient on a one-to-one basis, as opposed to a group or family therapist. The role of therapy in treating psychiatric problems and the different types of therapy that are employed are discussed in more detail in chapter 4.

Therapists may come from a variety of backgrounds, and their training and experience can vary considerably. Some therapists are psychiatrists, as mentioned earlier, but others come from backgrounds in social work, clinical psychology, or related disciplines. There is no single educational degree or licensing program that designates someone a therapist. Furthermore, there are several different types of psychotherapy, with differing techniques and theories behind them (see chapter 4). This can all be a source of confusion for some families. If you are referred to a therapist, and you are unsure of his or her training background or experience working with teenagers, do not be afraid to ask. See chapter 3 for further tips on finding a therapist and questions that can be useful to ask a therapist to figure out if that person may be helpful in treating your child.

Parent Guidance, Family and Group Therapists

Parents struggling to help a teenage child with mental illness will need help along the way. Often, an essential part of treatment is parent guidance, or meeting with a professional who can offer useful advice. This advice may be anything from how to communicate better with your teenager to how to negotiate the mental health and educational systems to ensure your child's needs are being met. Frequently, your child's psychiatrist and/or therapist will play this role, meeting with parents on a regular basis (e.g., once a month) to address concerns. In some situations, parents need more time than the child's therapist or psychiatrist is able to provide. In these cases, parents may be referred to a separate therapist with whom they can meet more often without worrying about diverting time from their child's individual treatment.

Many psychiatric issues that affect adolescents are related to difficulties in the family as a whole. Thus, family therapy may be recommended as part of your child's treatment plan. As a general rule (though one with some exceptions), the family therapist is separate from the child's individual therapist. This allows the child to maintain a trusting, consistent relationship with the individual therapist and avoids potential problems, for example, a teen's feeling that his once-trusted therapist is siding with his parents against him in a family session.

Group therapy is another important part of the treatment of many adolescents. Meeting and talking with other kids who have similar problems can be very therapeutic. Substance abuse and social problems are among the many difficulties that groups are often used to treat (again, see chapter 4 for more discussion of group therapy and the kinds of problems it can help with). Not surprisingly, groups are run by a group leader or group therapist who directs the discussion and helps ensure that everyone in the group feels safe and maintains respect for the other members. Sometimes the group therapist will be your child's individual therapist. There tend to be fewer problems with overlap here than there are with family therapists.

The School

Schools can be valuable allies in treating mental illness in teenagers. Out of fear that a child will be stigmatized, some parents are reluctant to involve the school in addressing their child's illness. Although this concern may be legitimate, more often schools are helpful. Given that school is a place where teenagers spend a good portion of waking hours, having the school involved in the process of assessment and treatment can be very effective.

Besides students' academic needs, schools are charged with addressing their social and emotional functioning. There are several ways in which they may work toward this goal. (See chapter 10 for a more detailed discussion of schools and their role in psychiatric treatment.) Generally, schools have mental health professionals, referred to as adjustment counselors or guidance counselors, who are available to work with students with social or emotional problems. The school counselor can be an extremely useful resource in developing a relationship with your child and helping him or her face challenges at school and beyond. Counselors can also serve an essential role in communicating with other members of the treatment team. By talking with psychiatrists and therapists, they provide a window into how things are going at school, which might otherwise be a blind spot in treatment. They may also communicate with teachers and school officials to help them better understand the difficulties a student may be having and to advocate for the adolescent to receive the services he or she needs at the school.

The school's potential to play a role in your adolescent's psychological well-being goes beyond the school counselor. Teachers, coaches, and other school professionals can serve as valuable role models and sources of support and encouragement for teens. Like counselors, they can provide valuable information to psychiatrists trying to figure out the nature of the difficulties that a child is having.

Schools may offer a variety of modifications to the traditional academic program to assure that your child's social and emotional needs are being met. Some examples of modifications include extra time on tests, preferential seating in the front of the class, and study skills classes for students with ADHD. School-based social skills groups can be a useful part of treatment for teens with Asperger's disorder (see chapter 20) or other kinds of problems with social interactions. Only by talking with representatives from the school and encouraging communication between the school and the rest of the treatment team can you be certain that you are taking advantage of the potential benefit the school might provide for your child's mental health.

Agencies

Some adolescents with psychiatric illness benefit from the involvement of state agencies that offer services to families. Because many of these agencies are funded and organized by state governments, the services they offer, their criteria for eligibility, and even the names they go by may differ from state to state. Frequently, these services are available only to the most severely impaired adolescents. Some examples of agencies that may be involved in treating adolescents with mental illness include the Department of Mental Health, the Department of Mental Retardation, and the Department of Social Services (also called the Department of Children and Family Services in some areas). Usually agencies such as these will provide teens with a case manager, who is responsible for coordinating various aspects of a teen's care and helping families obtain access to the treatments and services that they need. Some agencies provide home-based services. These have a clinician come to the home to assess the problems that are happening there and offer guidance to families on possible interventions.

Agencies may also be a source of funding for services that are not covered by insurance, such as long-term residential treatment programs, which are discussed later in this chapter. The differences in the available programs from state to state make it difficult to discuss these services in a comprehensive way. If you feel that your child might benefit from having agency involvement in his or her care, discuss this with your child's psychiatrist or therapist, who should be familiar with the services available in your area.

The Legal System

At times, there is overlap between psychiatric treatment and the juvenile justice system. This most commonly occurs with adolescents who are treated for substance abuse or for behavioral problems such as conduct disorder. Although having a child involved with the juvenile justice system is many parents' worst nightmare, this system can be a useful resource in helping at-risk teens access services and in enforcing consequences on those whose behavior is difficult to manage. For example, a judge may order an adolescent who has been charged with drug possession to participate in treatment, such as a drug-treatment program or weekly therapy sessions, as a term of her probation. Adolescents may also be asked to attend school regularly and to submit to regular drug testing to prove that they are abstaining from use in order to avoid more significant consequences, such as time in a juvenile detention center. These can be powerful motivating factors for teens who do not recognize that they have a problem or who are ambivalent about treatment.

If your child is not in treatment at the time he or she is facing criminal charges or if it appears that there is a psychiatric problem related to the charges, a judge may order a psychiatric evaluation. If your child is in treatment at the time that he or she is faced with criminal charges, ask your child's psychiatrist and/or therapist to become involved in the process in order to make recommendations about how to address the teen's psychiatric problems. In short, communication between the legal system and the treatment team can help turn a potentially difficult situation to your child's therapeutic advantage.

Summary of Mental Health Providers

Ultimately, a good treatment team is like the musicians in an orchestra: listening and responding to one another, with each member having his or her own part to play. If the musicians have different ideas about the goal, the end result is disharmony. By knowing the various players in the orchestra for a child's treatment, a parent can more effectively play the role of conductor, assuring that each person is playing his or her part and that all are working with the same overall plan in mind.

Levels of Care

Depending on the needs of the adolescent and the family, mental health treatment for adolescents may take place in a variety of settings. These settings can be organized along a spectrum according to how much structure and supervision is provided in that treatment setting. Mental health professionals and insurance companies often refer to the various points on this spectrum as levels of care. On one end of this spectrum is outpatient treatment, which places very little external structure on the adolescent other than the need to show up for regular appointments. On the opposite end of the spectrum is an inpatient psychiatric hospitalization. In contrast to outpatient treatment, inpatient psychiatric units are highly structured and highly supervised. Sidebar 2.2 shows detailed information on the daily routine in an inpatient unit. Units are locked, so that patients cannot leave or have visitors without permission, and patients are very closely monitored by staff. Adolescents may move between different levels of care along the spectrum, according to their needs. This is often referred to as a step up, when an adolescent is moving to a more intensive level of care, or a step down, when an adolescent is moving to a less intensive one.

Many families are unaware that there are a number of psychiatric treatment settings available between these two extremes. The following is a brief introduction to each of these levels of care. The odds are that your child will not encounter many of these levels of care during treatment, but you should know their availability, especially if your current program does not appear to be helpful.

Outpatient Treatment

Most teenagers who enter the mental health system do so in outpatient treatment. This is where most psychiatric treatment takes place. In fact, the majority of teenagers with psychiatric problems receive only outpatient treatment and never require more intensive levels of care. Outpatient treatment involves checking in with a psychiatrist or therapist on a regular basis for outpatient appointments. There is a broad spectrum in the intensity of outpatient treatment, depending on the needs of the individual adolescent. For some teens, outpatient treatment might consist of checking with a psychiatrist once every month or so to make sure things are continuing to go well. Others require a more intensive program, with frequent meetings with individual, group, and family therapists, frequent appointments with a psychiatrist for medication management, and a specialized school program. The nuts and bolts of outpatient treatment are discussed further in later chapters, including a discussion of psychotherapy in chapter 4 and of medications in chapter 5.

Home-Based Services

Some teenagers who are struggling in outpatient treatment may benefit from home-based services, which can be considered the next level of care up from outpatient treatment. As the name implies, home-based services involve a clinician, often a social worker, coming to the house to work with the adolescent and the family. This intervention is helpful when the difficulties a teen is experiencing are related to issues within the family. Home-based services may be funded by your insurance company, but generally they are not covered by insurance and are provided instead by agencies such as the Department of Mental Health. Usually, home-based services are given on a short-term basis to achieve specific goals. The family continues to work with the outpatient treatment team while receiving home-based services and gradually transitions back to outpatient treatment alone. One example of home-based services is called a family stabilization team, or FST, which works with families in crisis by sending clinicians to the home from one to several times weekly to work with parents and teenagers until the crisis has cooled. Teens with developmental disorders may have home-based services focused on teaching applied behavioral analysis or other programs for managing problem behaviors. Families caring for children with severe disabilities, including psychiatric and developmental disorders, sometimes receive respite care, in which a temporary caregiver relieves parents for regular breaks from their caregiving responsibilities. This service has the potential to reduce parents' stress and prevent burnout.

Day Treatment Programs

The next level of care is a day treatment program, sometimes called a day hospital, a partial hospital, or an intensive outpatient program. These are short-term, intensive treatment programs in which teens attend the program during several hours of the day and return home at night.

Day treatment programs for adolescents are often generalized, treating a variety of psychiatric problems. However, some programs are more specialized, focusing on the treatment of one particular kind of problem, such as drug treatment or eating disorders. In both general and specialized programs, treatment usually takes several forms, including individual and group therapy sessions, a medication evaluation, and meetings with the family. Social workers at the program can work with families to determine whether they may benefit from additional services, such as involvement with the Department of Mental Health.

When teens first enter a day treatment program, they generally undergo an intensive initial evaluation with the staff. This evaluation involves a detailed interview with the teen and the family and discussion with outpatient providers, teachers and guidance counselors, or other important figures in the teen's life. Observation of the teen's behavior in the program and interactions with staff and fellow patients are other important components of the evaluation.

Depending on the nature of the problem, day treatment is usually fairly brief, lasting from several days to a few weeks. The goal of day treatment is to provide a period of intensive treatment and to stabilize a situation before returning the teen to outpatient treatment. Often, in the close daily observation of day treatment, the psychiatrist and other professionals in the program gain new insight into a teen's problems and make recommendations to the outpatient treatment team. For example, they may advise adding family therapy to the treatment plan after noticing that difficulties in communication within the family seem to be contributing to a teen's depression.

Day treatment generally incorporates an academic component into the program, so that teens' academic needs are met. State regulations may require programs to have certified teachers on staff. There is usually time set aside in the day for students to receive instruction from teachers and/or tutors.

Adolescents who are a good fit for a day treatment program have a significant level of impairment from their mental illness. Their illness requires more intensive treatment than can be provided on a typical outpatient basis. Still, they must be able to remain safe. Teens who are deemed to be at high risk for attempting suicide or for extreme aggression would not be good candidates for day treatment and require a level of care with closer supervision.

Acute Residential Treatment Programs

Teens who require more structure and intensive treatment than a day treatment program can offer or who are unable to return home at night are sometimes admitted to an acute residential treatment (ART) program. ART programs are similar to day programs in that they may be either general or focused on specific problems, and they provide treatment in a variety of modalities, such as group and individual therapy and medication management. Like day treatment programs, ART programs generally have an academic component as well as a therapeutic component to meet adolescents' educational needs. Patients in an ART program stay overnight at the program with staff supervision instead of returning home. The amount of time that a teen spends in an ART program varies. It is generally a short-term treatment intervention, but teens are often able to stay longer than they can in an inpatient psychiatric unit: a couple weeks would be a typical ART program stay, compared to several days for a typical inpatient admission.

Like day treatment programs, ART programs are voluntary and unlocked. This means that the adolescent must agree to attend the program (though a strong push from parents, including the threat of stiff consequences for refusing the program, is not unusual). Guidelines from state departments of mental health normally stipulate that adolescents voluntarily attending ART programs cannot be locked in, as they are in inpatient psychiatric units. This does not mean that teens are left to come and go as they please. Though a fair amount of supervision and structure is provided, it is possible for teens who really do not want to be there to run away. Thus, teens who have a high likelihood of attempting to run away may not be good candidates for ART programs. In addition, ART programs generally are not able to provide the same level of very close supervision that inpatient psychiatric units offer. For this reason, teens who are imminently at risk for attempting suicide or becoming extremely agitated can be treated more safely in an inpatient unit until they are stabilized.

So what is the advantage of an ART program over day treatment? An overnight stay at an ART program may be preferable in many situations. At times, the home environment is a source of triggers for the illness, such as conflict within the family or friends who use and provide drugs to a teen with a drug addiction. In these situations, the goal obviously cannot be to remove the teen from these triggers permanently, but through admission to an ART program the teen can be removed from the triggers long enough to gain some stability and to begin learning some skills for better managing symptoms. Other times, parents are overwhelmed or unable to provide the kind of supervision that a teen needs.

Long-Term Residential Treatment Programs

At times, teens' mental illness is so severe that they require intensive daily treatment in a highly structured environment. In these cases, adolescents can enter a long-term residential treatment program. Similar to an ART, this is a treatment setting in which patients stay overnight; during the day they attend a multidisciplinary treatment program as well as an educational program. In a long-term residential program, the goal is not to stabilize an acute situation but rather to provide ongoing treatment and maintain an adolescent's psychiatric stability while allowing him or her to progress academically and developmentally. In such long-term programs, residents may stay for a period of months to years. Families may visit at the program, and adolescents may spend time at home during evenings or on weekends.

Placement in a long-term residential program is usually a very difficult decision for families, adolescents, and mental health providers alike. It is also quite complicated to arrange. These programs are typically not covered by private insurers, so it must be determined how the program is to be funded. Often a cost-sharing arrangement must be reached among the school system, involved agencies such as the Department of Mental Health, and state-funded insurers such as Medicaid or Medicare. Once all this is arranged, there is still the matter of finding a program with availability that seems to be a good fit for the needs of the adolescent. Thus, with all these factors, long-term residential placement is not something that can be quickly arranged or decided in an acute situation, such as in an emergency room. Rather, it can take weeks or even months to arrange placement. Adolescents must be hospitalized multiple times or for prolonged periods of time before residential treatment is considered. The process of placing an adolescent in a long-term residential program can be initiated by an outpatient provider, but usually it is initiated by the treatment team in an ART program or on an inpatient psychiatric unit after consultation with the outpatient team.

Inpatient Psychiatric Units

The most intensive, highly supervised setting in the psychiatric treatment of adolescents is an inpatient psychiatric unit. These units are psychiatry's version of an intensive care unit. This is the preferred treatment setting for most adolescents whose illness has reached the level that their safety or the safety of those around them is in jeopardy. The goal of treatment in an inpatient psychiatric unit is to keep the adolescent safe while delivering intensive treatment to stabilize an acute situation. Inpatient units are generally locked for the safety of the patients, such that patients on the unit must have permission from the staff to go off the unit. Patients on such units are monitored closely by staff. Patients are frequently placed on "checks" in which a staff person checks patients at specified intervals, such as every fifteen minutes, to assure that they are safe. Patients face restrictions on inpatient units, such as being unable to wear clothes with a drawstring or being allowed use of razors or other "sharps" only under direct supervision. Even when individual patients on the unit do not appear to be in any danger of harming themselves or others, they may be asked to adhere to the same strict safety measures for the safety of the other patients. All these safety measures may be frightening for teens and families at first, but it is important to remember that these measures allow the unit to remain a safe and stable therapeutic environment.

The treatment in an inpatient unit is similar to that for day treatment and residential programs. There is a thorough initial assessment and multidisciplinary treatment involving individual and group therapy, family meetings, academics, and, when appropriate, initiation or adjustment of medications. Yet treatment on an inpatient unit can be more intensive and move a bit faster than in other settings, in part due to the acute nature of the problems being addressed and also due to the relatively brief length of stay for most patients. There may be

Sidebar 2.2	**A Typical Day in an Inpatient Psychiatric Unit**
7–8 a.m.	Wake up, shower, and get ready
8–8:45 a.m.	Breakfast
8:45–9:30 a.m.	Morning group: patients check in with each other, identify their goals for the day
9:30–10:15 a.m.	Individual meeting(s) with psychiatrist, therapist, and/or social worker
10:15–12 p.m.	School work
12–12:45 p.m.	Lunch
12:45–2:45 p.m.	School work
2:45–3:30 p.m.	Activity group, e.g., art therapy
3:30–4:15 p.m.	Individual meetings with psychiatrist, therapist, and/or social worker
4:15–5 p.m.	Community meeting: check in as a group about issues affecting the whole unit
5–6 p.m.	Family meeting: discussion of issues with patient and parents, with guidance from therapist or case manager
6–7 p.m.	Dinner
7–8:30 p.m.	Free time, homework, activities in the psychiatric unit
8:30–9:15 p.m.	Evening wrap-up group
9:15–10:30 p.m.	Free time, getting ready for bed
10:30 p.m.	Lights out for bedtime

more frequent contact with the psychiatrist and meetings with the family. In addition, the ratio of staff to patients tends to be greater on inpatient units compared to lower levels of care, with more direct staff involvement in patients' daily activities.

Years ago, it was not unusual for adolescents admitted to inpatient psychiatric units to remain in treatment for several weeks or even months. In recent years, the average length of stay on inpatient units has declined dramatically. This is due, in part, to pressure from insurance companies; they prefer to keep costly inpatient treatment to a minimum and may refuse coverage if they feel it is not absolutely necessary. Now, one week would be a more typical length of stay for many kinds of problems, and some patients now remain on inpatient units for only a few days before being discharged or stepped down to a lower level of care, such as an ART or day program.

Emergency Department

In times of crisis, many families rely on the emergency department. Although the emergency department can play a useful role in the mental health system, it is important to recognize the limitations of emergency departments in delivering psychiatric care. Staff are seeing a teen at one moment in time, often a difficult time, and they do not have the ability to get to know the teen. Depending on when and where the teen is being seen, the evaluating physician may not have access to all the sources of information, such as the school, that would be part of a thorough evaluation. Furthermore, the training and experience of the physician or mental health professional who is conducting the evaluation may widely vary. Most hospitals do not have a child and adolescent psychiatrist available at all times, and the evaluator may have very limited experience in working with adolescents. For all these reasons, emergency departments are very limited in their ability to address longer-term problems and to develop appropriate treatment plans. Rather, they are most useful, as the name implies, in emergency situations, such as when parents are uncertain if their child is safe. Under these circumstances, the emergency department can keep your child safe while evaluating what level of care is appropriate.

As the shortage of child and adolescent psychiatrists and other mental resources has grown in recent years, families and schools are increasingly turning to emergency departments for help. You should realize that the emergency department visit can be a frustrating experience. Emergency departments can be crowded and hectic, with long waits to be seen and even longer waits to find the appropriate placement. Still, there are some things parents can do to make the process go more smoothly:

▸ If your child has a psychiatrist and a therapist, before going to the emergency department, contact that professional to discuss the situation. Ask whether an emergency department visit is warranted. Also, have the professionals' emergency contact numbers so both the staff and treaters can communicate and be involved in any decisions that are made.

▸ Be prepared for a possible wait. Bring snacks and distractions for your child, such as hand-held video games, books, or magazines, as well as for yourself. Hunger and boredom can aggravate an already difficult situation.

▸ Bring a cell phone or change for a public phone so that you will be able to contact your spouse, your other children, your child's outpatient treatment team, and so on.

▸ If you have other children, do not forget to make appropriate arrangements for them. You may need to ask your spouse or a friend to pick them up from school and stay with them if needed. Be proactive. The emergency department visit will probably take longer than expected.

▸ Bring a list of your child's medications to provide the physician. If you do not have a list and it is difficult to remember, bring the pill bottles themselves. Be sure to inform the physician of any allergies or adverse reactions your child has had to medications.

▸ Sometimes, in emergency situations, teens need a dose of medication to help them remain calm, safe, and in control. Let the doctor know if there are medications that have helped in this way in the past.

▸ Come with appropriate expectations. Psychiatric problems rarely have a quick fix, and emergency departments have significant limitations in their ability to treat them. The emergency department should help you figure out how to deal with the immediate situation and give you a clear idea of what steps to take next. A definitive diagnosis and a long-term treatment plan, including initiation or adjustment of medications, are usually best made in other settings.

Other Programs

The treatment programs described here are meant to provide a general outline of the main settings in which adolescent mental health treatment takes place. The list is by no means comprehensive, as there are a number of other programs including therapeutic summer camps for children with developmental disorders and wilderness programs for children with behavioral or disciplinary problems. Available treatment options may vary depending on where you live. Your child's outpatient treatment team will know more about the resources available in your area. Parent support groups can also be useful sources of information and can help parents find the services and programs that may benefit their children.

Insurance and Level of Care

It is important to note that insurance plays a different role in mental health than it does in other forms of health care. This can affect treatment in many ways, from the number of psychotherapy visits an adolescent is able to receive to the amount of time spent waiting in an emergency room in an urgent situation.

Mental health providers usually do not have a free hand in deciding what level of care is appropriate for an adolescent. Before treatment can begin, the mental health provider must obtain authorization from the patient's insurance company. For example, if a patient is seen in an emergency room and the psychiatrist who is evaluating the patient determines that the patient needs to be admitted to an inpatient psychiatric unit, the psychiatrist is frequently required to contact the patient's insurance company to review the case and gain the insurer's approval before admitting the patient to a unit. Different insurance companies have different requirements and procedures for gaining this approval, which can be confusing for patients and physicians alike.

At times, the insurance company representative who is reviewing the case will disagree with the physician who is seeing the patient and deny coverage for a particular service, such as inpatient psychiatric hospitalization. When this happens, the physician must reevaluate the situation and determine whether the patient truly requires the level of care that he or she was seeking. If not, the physician can request a lower level of care, such as a day treatment program, from the insurance company. If the physician continues to feel strongly that the patient

> **Sidebar 2.3 | Questions to Ask about Treatment Costs**
>
> ▶ What are the reasons for the clinician's wanting to continue with the recommended treatment despite the disagreement of the insurance company?
> ▶ What risks are involved in not continuing with the recommended treatment?
> ▶ What steps have been taken so far to appeal the insurance company's decision? What further recourse is available? What role can the parents play in contesting the decision?
> ▶ If it is necessary to pay for the recommended treatment out of pocket, can the hospital make any accommodations to help the family afford it (e.g., payment plans or a reduced fee program)?

requires the level of care that was initially requested, he or she can appeal the insurance company's denial, which can be a time-consuming process.

When an insurance company has approved a particular treatment, such as inpatient care, it is usually for a limited period of time, just a few days and sometimes as little as one day. Following this period, the facility where the patient is being treated must review the case to request additional days of treatment. As in the case of the initial treatment decision, insurance companies may refuse to continue covering a particular treatment if they feel that it is no longer necessary, even if the physician caring for the patient believes that it is. This decision can also be appealed with insurance companies. Parents can play an important role in this process by contacting their insurance company directly and advocating for their child to get the recommended treatment. Under rare circumstances, the insurance company refuses to continue coverage. If this happens, parents may be placed in a very difficult position. They may be forced to decide whether they want to continue the recommended treatment despite knowing that it might not be covered and that they may be responsible for a sizable hospital bill. If this should happen to you, there are some important questions to discuss with your child's treatment team, as noted in sidebar 2.3.

These situations are certainly not the norm, and in the majority of instances, insurance companies are willing to cover the treatment that is recommended. When there is disagreement, it is important to understand the reasons why a noncovered treatment is being advised.

Confidentiality

Confidentiality is an important but often tricky issue in adolescent psychiatric treatment. In order for treatment to be effective, the adolescent must be open and honest. So it is essential that teens trust their psychiatrist or therapist. For a number of reasons, however, teens may be reluctant to share information with providers. Teens may fear that information they tell clinicians will then be told to their parents, leading to disapproval or punishment. For example, a teen may not mention that she is using marijuana every day. Without this information, the provider may make an inaccurate diagnosis of the problem and devise a treatment plan that is not as effective as it could be.

Early in the treatment, mental health providers, teens, and parents should establish confidentiality ground rules. Teens need to know what information will be shared with whom and under what circumstances. The most common, and usually most effective, confidentiality arrangement is for the mental health provider to promise not to reveal any information noted during the therapy sessions. The therapist will only discuss an issue with the parents if there is concern for the safety of the adolescent. Parents should also be informed about this arrangement, as it attempts to strike a balance between allowing open communication with an adolescent and protecting the adolescent from harm. Sometimes, parents feel that their child's providers should share all important information with them. But a teen who feels that his or her therapist or psychiatrist is an "informant" will quickly shut down, keeping secrets or often refusing to talk or to go to appointments.

What constitutes a safety risk that will lead a provider to break a teen's confidentiality is often a gray area. Clearly, suicidal plans or attempts pose a serious safety risk and require a clinician to inform a teen's parents. Behaviors such as superficial cutting, substance abuse, or risk-taking are less clear. Whether these behaviors constitute a serious safety risk may depend on the role they play in the teen's life. In these gray areas, the clinician must make a judgment call as to when parents should be notified, taking into account the importance of maintaining a helpful therapeutic relationship with the teen, the teen's well-being, and the parents' right to know important information about their child. When a clinician does break a teen's confidentiality, he or she will do so only after discussing it with the teen, reminding him or her of the original confidentiality arrangement and explaining the clinician's reasons for doing so. On occasion, the clinician will offer the adolescent the opportunity to inform his or her parents. Measures such as these are not always possible, particularly when there is an emergency situation threatening a teen's safety, but they can help to mitigate the damage that can be done to a trusting treatment relationship when confidentiality must be broken.

Confidentiality with respect to sharing information with people other than an adolescent's parents or legal guardians is stricter, and it is protected by federal privacy laws. In general, for adolescents under age eighteen, a clinician must have permission from the adolescent's legal guardian in order to communicate information with outside parties. It is usually a good practice to discuss such third-party communication with the teen. Parents or guardians may be asked to sign written consent forms to confirm their approval for a clinician to share information.

Table 2.1 | **Summary of Levels of Care**

Program	Features	Typical Length of Stay	Clinical Examples
Outpatient	Regular meetings with psychiatrist, therapist, and/or other professional	Ongoing	Teen with an anxiety disorder who is distressed by symptoms but continues to function fairly well, spending time with friends and attending school
Home-Based Services	Clinicians come to the house from once to several times per week to provide treatment and/or respite for parents	2–8 weeks (may be longer in some situations)	Teen with conduct disorder, substance abuse, and/or ADHD who is getting in frequent, often often heated arguments with parents; parents having difficulty managing teen's behavior with outpatient treatment alone
Day Treatment	Intensive daily treatment at a program Patient goes for several hours and returns home at night May be general or focused on specific problem (e.g., drug treatment, eating disorders)	1–2 weeks	Teen with depression worsening in outpatient treatment who has started missing school and with-drawing from friends and family but for whom there are no concerns about safety OR Teen with psychotic disorder stepped down from an inpatient unit after being acutely stabilized but still having some symptoms, with medications being adjusted and family in need of support and education
Acute Residential Treatment (ART)	Similar to day treatment, but patient stays overnight at the program Unlocked and voluntary	2–4 weeks	Teen with poor functioning due to severe mood disorder and drug abuse with problems exacerbated by conflict at home; parents feel unable to manage teen's risky behaviors, but there are no concerns about suicide
Long-Term Residential	Patient lives and attends school long term in a therapeutic setting Usually requires funding agreement from involvement agencies, such as school system and Department of Mental Health	Months to years	Teen with severe mood and behavioral problems who is unable to be safely cared for at home despite attempts at intensive outpatient services; often patient has had several inpatient hospitalizations

Program	Features	Typical Length of Stay	Clinical Examples
Inpatient Psychiatric Unit	Locked and either voluntary or involuntary Highest level of supervision for patients who may be unsafe Tends to be short term	1 week	Teen who is at high risk for harming him- or herself or someone else related to his or her psychiatric symptoms, e.g., a teen with a psychotic disorder who is hearing voices telling her to kill herself and has attempted suicide by overdosing on pills but has been medically treated and stabilized

Table 2.1 | **Summary of Levels of Care** (continued)

Evidence-Based Medicine

Evidence-based medicine (EBM) is a term that is used in health care, and it is important for parents to understand its meaning. EBM is an approach to care that includes scientific evidence based on published medical literature, the clinician's expertise, and the patient's and parents' choice. A detailed explanation of EBM is available at http://www.teenmentalhealth.org/images/pages/EBM_Guide_Patients.pdf.

Practice parameters for clinicians, such as one on the treatment of anxiety disorder in adolescents (Connolly and Bernstein 2007), frequently list the quality of the evidence supporting treatment recommendations. That said, there is a limited evidence base in adolescent psychiatry. Lack of funding for strong research studies coupled with an unwillingness of many parents to enroll their teens in such studies are barriers. Some evidence is extrapolated from adult studies, case reports, chart reviews, and the experience of the clinician.

Conclusion

In this chapter, we have described a variety of settings in which psychiatric care for adolescents is delivered, which are shown in table 2.1. The message for parents is that psychiatric care takes place on a spectrum, with a range of possible programs that should be matched to an adolescent's needs at any particular time. As the adolescent's needs change, he or she may move from one place on the spectrum to another. By knowing a bit about the kinds of programs that make up this spectrum, parents can feel better prepared to manage a system that can otherwise seem confusing and to advocate for their child to receive the best possible care.

References and Additional Reading

Connolly, S. D., and G. A. Bernstein. 2007. "Work Group on Quality Issues: Practice Parameter for the Assessment and Treatment of Children and Adolescents with Anxiety Disorders." *Journal of the American Academy of Child and Adolescent Psychiatry* 46: 267–283.

Mangione-Smith, R., A. H. DeCristofaro, C. M. Setodji, J. Keesey, D. J. Klein, J. L. Adams, M A. Schuster, and E. A. McGlynn. 2007. "The Quality of Ambulatory Care Delivered to Children in the United States." *New England Journal of Medicine* 357: 1515–1523.

"Practice Parameter on Child and Adolescent Mental Health Care in Community Systems of Care." 2007. *Journal of the American Academy of Child and Adolescent Psychiatry* 46: 284–299.

Shepperd, S., H. Doll, S. Gowers, A. James, M. Fazel, R. Fitzpatrick, and J. Pollock. 2009. "Alternative to Inpatient Mental Health Care for Children and Young People." *Evidence Based Mental Health* 12: 117.

3 Finding Treatment

It is often difficult for parents to know when to seek a psychiatric evaluation for children with problems that arise during adolescence. The normal adolescent developmental process typically involves rapid and dramatic changes in behavior. Your once pleasant, mild-mannered child may seem to turn surly and withdrawn overnight. The bodily changes of puberty and shifting social pressures of adolescence are common stressors for teens. Parents of adolescents may feel surprised when their children discuss their problems with their peers and rely less on adults for support. This is all part of natural development and identity formation. So with all these changes taking place, how is a parent to know when to suspect a mental health problem and when to reach out for help?

When to Consider Evaluation

There are a few basic, commonsense principles to follow to help guide parents in determining when to consider an evaluation for a problem.

- The problem causes a significant disruption in one or more of the three major areas of a teenager's life: home, school, and social life. These areas are the cornerstones of an adolescent's life, and if a problem has reached the level that it causes a major disturbance in one of these areas, the teen should be evaluated.
- Your child asks for outside help. This may not always be explicit but may be expressed in statements such as "Maybe I need to talk to someone" or "I wish somebody could help me with this." Even if your child seems to be doing fine, asking for outside help may be a sign that he or she is struggling with a problem. Obviously, this does not mean that you should drag your teenager to a psychiatrist if he or she is merely seeking parental advice or support. Still, if there is a problem for which your child is repeatedly asking for your assistance but seems frustrated or unsatisfied with what you as a parent can provide, then it is worth asking, "Would you like to talk to someone about this?"

> **Sidebar 3.1 | When to Seek an Evaluation**
>
> - The behavior is causing a significant disruption in the adolescent's life
> - The adolescent is asking for help
> - You are worried there is a problem
> - Safety is a concern

▶ When in doubt, ask an expert. Your pediatrician and your adolescent's teachers are experts on adolescent behavior. They will help to determine if your teen's behavior is "normal." Pediatricians are trained to recognize the warning signs of psychiatric illness and may be able to diagnose and manage some problems. When they are not sure what the problem is, they can help parents decide when to seek an opinion from a specialist in mental health.

▶ When safety is a concern, get help. This includes the safety of parents and other children in the household. If your child is engaging in a pattern of behavior that feels unsafe, including physical aggression, self-harm, or threats of suicide, see a mental health clinician as soon as possible. If you are uncertain as to whether your child will remain safe while you are waiting for an evaluation, then an emergency evaluation is warranted, either at an emergency room or through a crisis team at a mental health center.

Obtaining an Evaluation

Once you have decided to seek an evaluation by a psychiatrist or other mental health professional, you may face a new set of challenges. Throughout the United States, there are shortages of child and adolescent psychiatrists. In some areas the shortage is critical. This can translate into long wait times and difficulty finding a psychiatrist or psychologist who is taking new patients.

By providing you with a referral to psychiatrist or clinic, your child's pediatrician is a valuable resource to help you obtain an evaluation. Often the pediatrician has referred adolescents to some of the mental health providers in the area

---

Case Presentation

Robert, a sixteen-year-old boy, came to an adolescent medicine specialist as a new patient thirteen months after his father died suddenly from a heart attack. During the intervening year, the adolescent reported that he had periods of sadness and even some thoughts of suicide. The teen's father had been depressed, and his mother was taking an antidepressant medication.

On further questioning, the teen reported low energy, problems falling asleep, and lack of interest in his academic work. He felt totally bored by life. In addition, he participated in minimal activities outside school; he primarily occupied himself at home by playing video games. The teen had few friends and a history of being bullied.

The adolescent also reported that he had begun to smoke marijuana up to three times a week to feel better. He denied any other drug usage including alcohol.

Two incidents prompted the visit to the adolescent specialist. The adolescent sustained a significant hand injury after fighting with another teen. In a separate incident, the teen was caught brandishing a toy gun at a student who reportedly had bullied him in the past. The adolescent medicine specialist referred him to a psychiatrist.

and will be able to help you choose an appropriate clinician. If you are given a referral by your pediatrician, it is important to check if the provider is covered under your insurance plan. If your pediatrician's practice is affiliated with a hospital that has a child psychiatry department, you may be referred to the hospital clinic. When there is a wait to be seen, hospitals often give preference on the waiting list to patients whose pediatricians are affiliated with the hospital.

Your insurance company can also assist you in finding a provider who is covered under your plan. By calling the customer service number on your insurance card or checking the company's website, you can obtain a list of mental health providers enrolled in your plan. Share these names with your pediatrician. Together you can select an appropriate clinician.

All too often, none of the mental health professionals is able to take on your child. It may be necessary to determine other resources available in your area. Local hospitals and community mental health centers may be able to arrange for an evaluation with one of their clinicians or at least to point you in the right direction. Consider asking your child's school for help, particularly if some of the problems are occurring there. Some school systems have contracts with child psychiatrists or other mental health professionals who may be able to evaluate your child as a consultation and make recommendations for further treatment. Even if this option is not available, school staff are likely to be familiar with providers in the area and may be able to offer some recommendations.

If you continue to experience difficulty in arranging a psychiatric evaluation for your adolescent, here are a few more suggestions:

- *Be persistent.* Clinics and private practitioners are sometimes overwhelmed by the number of referrals. Keep track of whom you have called and when. If you left a message and have not heard back, try again after a few days. Your message may have gotten lost in the shuffle. If there is a waiting list, place your name on it. Call back periodically to make sure that your name is still on the list and to inquire whether there have been any cancellations. Because waits are sometimes long, it is not unusual for other patients to cancel once a crisis has passed.
- *Explore your options.* Many parents will try calling one or two referrals that they have been given and end up settling for an appointment six months away. If the first few places you try do not have availability, try some other options. When asking your pediatrician, insurance company, or other sources for referrals, try to obtain a list of several options rather than just one or two, and try all the names on the list. It is fine to put your name on more than one waiting list. Just be sure to cancel any appointments that you do not intend to keep.
- *Be courteous.* This process can be extremely frustrating. It is very upsetting to be unable to obtain the help your adolescent needs. However, anger is not helpful in this situation.

The Initial Evaluation

What to Expect

The first step in diagnosing and treating mental health problems is a thorough initial mental health evaluation. Although other mental health professionals including a psychologist or social worker may be the first clinician to evaluate your teen, as outlined in chapter 2, this chapter reviews the mental health evaluation when your adolescent is seen initially by a psychiatrist. In addition, a psychiatrist may ask a psychologist, neuropsychologist, or social worker to see the adolescent and be a member of the treatment team.

Parents may arrive with a sense of mystery about what the evaluation session will involve. Essentially, the initial evaluation is a detailed gathering of information from both the adolescent and the parent or parents. The exact nature of the evaluation may vary depending on the type of problem for which you are seeking help and the style of the clinician performing the evaluation. The evaluation may occur in one or more sessions. Some practitioners have a loose, open-ended approach to gathering information, whereas others are more structured and regimented. Regardless of these differences in approach, a good evaluation will usually include the following:

▸ Detailed information about the primary problem that led you to seek treatment
▸ Questions about risky behaviors or dangerous situations, including drug use, self-harm, and suicidal thoughts
▸ Screening questions about symptoms of common psychiatric disorders that may be involved in your child's difficulties
▸ A review of past psychiatric problems and treatment, including any previous trials of medication or psychotherapy or admissions to hospitals or other treatment programs
▸ A medical history, including current and past medical problems, medications, allergies, and information about your child's pediatrician and any other involved medical providers
▸ Questions about your family and home life
▸ Information about important aspects of your child's life, including school, activities, and friends
▸ Queries about a family history of major psychiatric or medical problems
▸ Time spent talking with your teen to get his or her perspective and allow him or her to discuss issues that might be difficult to discuss in front of parents
▸ Feedback to you and your adolescent about the clinician's understanding of the difficulties and the best approach for managing them
▸ Time for questions from parents and the teen

In addition, the clinician performing the evaluation may employ other means of gathering information. It is common to ask for parents' permission to speak to other people who know your child. The clinician may ask you to sign "release of information" forms to document that this permission has been granted. Communication with your child's pediatrician is important both during the initial evaluation and during active treatment. The evaluator may also ask to speak with teachers or other school staff, coaches, involved agencies, other mental health providers, or anyone else who plays an important role in your child's life. Parents have the right to refuse to give permission for the evaluating clinician to contact particular people. For example, some parents are wary of having a psychiatrist contact their child's school, out of concern that their child will then be labeled as "crazy" and stigmatized by teachers. These are valid concerns, but they should be weighed against the value that information from these sources can have in guiding the clinician to a thorough understanding of your child, making an accurate diagnosis, and formulating a comprehensive plan for treatment. If this is a concern for you, it is worth discussing the issue further with the clinician.

Laboratory Tests and Other Studies

At times the evaluation process may involve laboratory tests or other medical studies, such as blood pressure, an electrocardiogram (ECG or EKG), or, rarely, imaging studies of the brain. These are not a standard part of every evaluation. Rather, the need for them is based on the particulars of the situation and is guided by the information that the clinician gathers during the evaluation. Diagnosis and treatment of most psychiatric disorders can be made without obtaining lab tests or other studies. When lab tests are ordered, it is often for one of two reasons. The first is to make sure that the teen's symptoms are not caused by a medical problem masquerading as a psychiatric problem (for example, depression being caused by hypothyroidism). Laboratory tests may also be ordered to monitor medication and to look for possible adverse effects of treatment, such as changes in measures of liver or kidney function.

Sometimes, the initial evaluation involves the use of symptom checklists or standardized screening tools to be filled out by the adolescents, parents, or teachers. These tools can be useful in identifying a problem as well as monitoring treatment. For example, in the diagnosis of attention-deficit/hyperactivity disorder (ADHD), asking parents and teachers to fill out checklists, such as the Conners Rating Scale, can help a psychiatrist determine the severity of symptoms at home and at school. Repeating this scale during treatment can help determine how the teen is responding to treatment.

The Role of Neuropsychological Testing

At times, even after a thorough initial evaluation, an adolescent's diagnosis may remain unclear. There are a number of reasons why this might be the case. The occurrence of more than one psychiatric disorder at a time can confuse the picture and make it difficult to determine a correct diagnosis. The presence of a learning or communication disorder can also complicate matters. For a variety of reasons, some teenagers have difficulty recognizing and describing aspects of their inner experience, and this can make diagnosis challenging as well.

To help with this process a psychiatrist may recommend neuropsychological testing. Neuropsychological testing is generally performed by a psychologist with specialized training in administering and interpreting the tests. Testing can provide valuable information about a teenager, opening a window into the teen's inner life, including cognitive functioning and prominent emotional states. In this way, testing can identify learning or cognitive difficulties and guide psychiatric diagnosis. Yet test results must be interpreted in the context of the teen's actual experiences and symptoms, and diagnoses should not be made on the test results alone.

Preparation for the Initial Evaluation

Ideally, the psychiatrist and parents function as a team, working together toward the common goal of understanding your child's problems and developing an effective plan to address them. A team works best when there is good communication in both directions. By coming prepared for the evaluation, you can make the process more efficient, which can enable you to save time and money and to obtain more immediate relief for your child. Good preparation can also allow for more accurate diagnosis and effective treatment. For example, if your child has been treated with medications in the past, providing the psychiatrist with detailed information about the medications, the doses, and the efficacy better equips him or her to determine which medication will most likely help.

The following steps will help you to prepare for the initial evaluation and to assist the psychiatrist or other mental health professional:

- Spend some time reviewing your primary concerns. Think about when the problem began, how it has changed over time, and factors that seem to be exacerbating or relieving the issues.
- Try to provide a detailed description of the problem. Think of specific examples that illustrate the problem. For example, if you are concerned that your child is explosive, describe some times when the teen lost his or her temper. Be as specific as possible.
- Get the perspective of important people in your adolescent's life. If only one parent is able to go to the initial evaluation, talk to your spouse beforehand to see if there are concerns that he or she has that should be mentioned in the evaluation. Consider touching base with teachers, coaches, or other caretakers to obtain their perspective on your teen's difficulties.
- Gather important contact information for people in your child's life. This may include the pediatrician, teachers, school counselors, and other mental health professionals your child is seeing or has seen in the past.

▸ Review details of past treatment. If your adolescent has received any form of mental health treatment in the past, share as much information as you can. If your child has been on medication in the past, useful information would include when it was started, how long it was tried, dosage, effects (for example, was there any benefit?), side effects, and why it was stopped. If you do not recall what medications your child has tried, consider contacting your pharmacy.

▸ List details about your teen's medical history, including any medical conditions, current medications, and allergies or adverse reactions to medications.

The Follow-Up Appointment

After the initial evaluation, the psychiatrist will want to meet with you and consider the evaluation of your teen. The psychiatrist will also present a therapeutic plan. In the case of Robert, the sixteen-year-old boy with sadness and low energy described at the beginning of this chapter, evaluations were completed by an adolescent medicine specialist, child psychiatrist, social worker, and nutritionist. With these consultations in hand, the psychiatrist confirmed the diagnosis of depression and recommended therapy and medication.

In your discussion with the psychiatrist or other clinician, you should discuss the most likely diagnosis and other possible diagnoses. Any further blood or psychological testing should be reviewed. It is important for parents to know what symptoms would signal worsening of the illness. For anorexia, this could be further weight loss, decreased pulse and blood pressure, or increased obsessive activities including inappropriate levels of exercise. For depression, this could be increasing somatic symptoms such as sleep, appetite, or activity changes.

The clinician will note treatment options. For example, for anorexia, this could be immediate hospital admission for medical stabilization, referral to a residential treatment center for eating disorders, an intensive day program, or weekly visits with mental health clinicians, nutrition and adolescent medicine specialists, or your child's pediatrician. The psychiatrist may prescribe medication, and it is important to understand the risks and benefits of these medications.

What If Your Child Does Not Want to Go?

It is not unusual for a teen to put up some degree of resistance to going to a psychiatric evaluation. Frequently, this resistance masks a deeper ambivalence toward getting help. When there is a serious problem, most teens realize they are ill and want to get better. Still, the desire to fix the problem may be mixed with anxiety about seeing a psychiatrist. Obtaining an evaluation can be scary to adolescents for many different reasons. What will their peers think? Will they be stigmatized? In a time of life when one's identity is being established, the notion of being scrutinized by a professional in search of a problem can be frightening.

If your child is resisting an evaluation, the first step, as is often the case with such problems, is to talk to your adolescent. Try to do so in a calm, open, non-judgmental way. The goal, at least initially, is not to force your teen into going to the evaluation but rather to understand his or her feelings about it. Ask your child what concerns him or her. After you have listened, calmly explain why the evaluation is important. Try to address the concerns your child has raised. For example, some adolescents fear that going to a psychiatrist may lead them to taking medications or engaging in treatments against their will. If this is the case, you should reassure your teen that he or she will have some say in the process. You should suggest to your adolescent that you are bringing him or her to an evaluation because recent behaviors have you concerned that there is a fixable problem that is getting in the way of your child's well-being.

If all else fails, a little coercion may be necessary. Some parents offer a reasonable reward, such as a trip to the mall or tickets to a ball game. Less desirable is posing consequences, such as grounding or restricting privileges for a period of time, for a teen's refusal to participate.

As a last resort, parents can go without their teen to the initial meeting with a psychiatrist. Under these circumstances, the psychiatrist will be limited in his or her ability to make a definitive diagnosis or to determine a specific treatment plan. However, in meeting only with the parent or parents, a psychiatrist can begin to gather information about the problem and may be able to offer some advice on how best to proceed.

How Do You Know If a Therapist Is a Good Fit for Your Child?

Often insurance companies will provide a list of therapists available in their plans. The therapist needs to have sufficient training and experience in working with adolescents and in treating the types of problems your child is experiencing. The therapist should be able to describe a plan for treatment. Sidebar 3.2 lists some questions you can consider asking a potential therapist during the initial meeting.

Once a prospective therapist has been selected and before the first meeting, ask your teen whether he or she has a preference for a male or female therapist or for a youthful or older person. Revisit the discussion after meeting with the therapist. After the first visit with a therapist, the best a parent can hope for is a child's grudging agreement to return for a second appointment. Early on, it is most important to make sure there no major barriers to the potential for building a helpful relationship. A therapist whose style is intimidating to a teenager or who reminds the teen of someone with whom he or she has had a difficult relationship, such as a despised teacher or coach, may not be the best option.

Sidebar 3.2 | Some Questions to Consider Asking a Therapist

► What kind of training and education have you had? (e.g., Licensed Independent Clinical Social Worker [LICSW], Ph.D. in clinical psychology, M.D.)

► How would you describe your approach? (e.g., psychodynamic, cognitive behavioral therapy, supportive, mixed)

► How much experience do you have in treating adolescents?

► Do you treat adults also? How much of your practice is devoted to adolescent patients?

► Will you be in touch with the other people involved in my child's care? (e.g., psychiatrist, pediatrician)

► How often do you like to meet with parents?

► How much of what my child tells you is confidential? Under what circumstances will you discuss it with me?

► How can we communicate with you between appointments to update you and/or ask you questions? (e.g., Do you use e-mail, voicemail?)

► How can we reach you if there is an emergency?

Other aspects of the fit are harder to define and are a matter of the chemistry between the individual personalities of the therapist and the adolescent. A skilled and experienced therapist may be able to establish a wonderful therapeutic relationship with one patient while having a great deal of difficulty in clicking with another patient with similar problems.

Different patients have different needs. Some feel more comfortable talking with a male therapist, and others feel more comfortable with a female therapist. Some patients do well when the discussion is quite targeted and directive, whereas others do best with a more open-ended approach. Good therapists can adapt their style somewhat to the needs of the individual teen. Ultimately, however, the chemistry just may not be there in some therapeutic relationships.

Once the relationship has been established, your teen probably will not rave about the therapist. Many teens have a healthy skepticism of adults in general and therapists in particular. It is not unusual for an adolescent to grumble a little about a therapist or point out the therapist's shortcomings. These are not necessarily signs of a poor fit, particularly if the same teen goes willingly to appointments most of the time and seems to be making progress. Therapy is hard work and can be uncomfortable at times. Both positive and negative feelings toward the therapist are a normal part of the process, and sorting through these feelings can lead to great progress, as issues that come up with a therapist often parallel issues that come up in other relationships in a teen's life.

If your teen is continually complaining about the therapist, try to determine the source of the problem. Often a teen will say, "I'm sick of going!" Try to get a more specific response such as "I don't feel like he realizes how hard things are for me at school."

If you and your child have concerns about the fit, it is important to share this with the therapist. If your child is reluctant to do so or if the concern is yours, then it may be best to request a separate parent meeting with the therapist to discuss the issue. Often the problems that arise can be fixed with good communication, and working through problems with the therapist can be an essential component of the treatment. Parents who shy away from raising concerns with the therapist due to fear of offending the therapist or stirring up conflict may miss an opportunity to help their child make an important step in therapy and may unwittingly model for their children a pattern of avoiding problems rather than talking about them.

If it still seems that a therapeutic relationship is not working despite an open discussion about the concerns, then it may be time to look for another therapist. If possible, try to allow your child and your child's therapist to be a part of this decision. The therapist may agree that there is not a good fit and be able to recommend someone whose style may be a better match for your child's needs.

Conclusion

Finding psychiatric treatment for your teenager can be challenging. A shortage of providers in the United States means that parents must be resourceful and persistent in order to obtain the help they need for their child. Enlisting existing resources in your child's life, such as your pediatrician, your insurance company, the school system, a community mental health center, or a local hospital, will help set your family on the right path toward treatment. Once you have arranged for an evaluation with a child and adolescent psychiatrist or other mental health professional, good preparation can help assure that the process goes smoothly and efficiently and that the clinician is able to develop a complete and accurate picture of the difficulties your child is experiencing. Finally, if psychotherapy is recommended for your child, it is important to find a suitable therapist who is likely to be a good fit for your child.

References and Additional Reading

Lemmon, K. M., and M. M. Chartrand. 2009. "Caring for America's Children: Military Youth in Time of War." *Pediatrics in Review* 30: e42–e48.

Levitt, J. M. 2009. "Identification of Mental Health Service Need among Youth in Child Welfare." *Child Welfare* 88: 27–48.

Pecora, P. J., P. S. Jensen, L. H. Romanelli, L. J. Jackson, and A. Ortiz. 2009. "Mental Health Services for Children Placed in Foster Care: An Overview of Current Challenges." *Child Welfare* 88: 5–26.

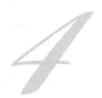

Psychotherapy

One of the oldest forms of psychiatric treatment is psychotherapy, and it remains one of the most powerful tools available for treating mental illness and promoting psychological health. *Psychotherapy* is a general term that encompasses a broad variety of treatments for individuals, families, and groups. The common thread of these treatments is that they are primarily talk based and the changes that occur through them are brought about by the interaction between the patient and the therapist. In the preceding chapter, we discussed the process of obtaining an initial evaluation and finding a therapist who is a good fit for an adolescent. In this chapter, we provide an overview of the more commonly used methods in psychotherapy and the conditions that they can help.

When Should Therapy Be Considered?

Psychotherapy can be helpful for a broad range of psychiatric problems including anxiety, depression, bipolar disorder, substance abuse, psychosis, obsessive-compulsive disorder, and attention-deficit/hyperactivity disorder. It should at least be considered as part of the treatment for any adolescent with mental illness. Psychotherapy can also be useful for teens without a diagnosed psychiatric disorder. It can help adolescents develop a secure sense of self, become more psychologically resilient, learn ways of managing stress, and improve their ability to communicate and interact with others. Teens dealing with stressors, such as the loss of a loved one, parental divorce, or a chronic illness, can benefit from psychotherapy. Changes made in psychotherapy may last a lifetime and place adolescents on the track of psychological health at a critical point in their development.

Who Can Perform Psychotherapy?

Mental health clinicians from a variety of different professional backgrounds practice psychotherapy. Most therapists who work with adolescents are social workers, licensed professional counselors, nurse practitioners, clinical psychologists (who generally have a Ph.D. degree in psychology), or psychiatrists (who have a medical degree and are also able to prescribe medication). Generally, there are no strict guidelines or licensing processes for an individual who wishes to call him- or herself a therapist. Moreover, even a licensed mental health professional, such as a board-certified psychiatrist or a licensed clinical social worker, may have had training primarily in working with adults and may not be a good match for adolescents. Thus, in searching for a potential therapist, it is important to review the therapist's education, credentials, and experience. Because working with adolescents in psychotherapy presents unique challenges, it is important to find a therapist who has had formalized training and practical experience working with teens.

When medications and psychotherapy are both indicated for treatment of an adolescent, some parents ask if it is preferable to have combined treatment, in which the teen takes part in therapy with the same clinician who is managing the medication, usually a child and adolescent psychiatrist. Or should the teen should have split treatment, in which there are separate clinicians providing therapy and medication management? As is so often the case in adolescent mental health, the answer is not clear-cut, as there are advantages and disadvantages to both approaches.

With combined treatment, the clinician who is prescribing the medication will know the teen very well through the course of therapy and will be able to monitor symptoms and the effects of the medication. By lowering the number of office visits, combined treatment can also be more convenient for parents. That said, split treatment has its benefits as well, particularly when the psychiatrist managing the medications has good communication with the therapist. Splitting treatment frees the therapist from having to focus on medications, which can be a distraction from the issues that need to be addressed. As a tactic to avoid discussing difficult issues, some teens may even focus on medication side effects rather than touching on emotionally laden feelings. Splitting treatment also has the advantage of two heads being better than one. Having two clinicians involved can provide a broader perspective on your child's difficulties and help make up for any potential blind spots that either clinician might have in missing certain aspects of a problem. Having two clinicians is also particularly helpful when one of the clinicians is away from the office. With split treatment, usually one of the clinicians involved in your teen's care will be available should a crisis develop.

What Type of Therapy Is Best for Your Child?

Deciding which type of psychotherapy will be most helpful for an adolescent can be challenging. The factors to be considered include the nature and severity of the illness. For example, teens with psychotic disorders often do better with supportive or problem-solving approaches and may respond poorly to the intense emotion and loose structure of a psychodynamic approach.

The adolescent's personality and unique characteristics are an important consideration. Teens who are more concrete in their thinking and have trouble expressing their feelings may do better with a structured treatment such as cognitive behavioral therapy, whereas patients who are introspective and verbal may do well with psychodynamic psychotherapy.

In practice, the decision of what approach to take for a particular adolescent is often more complicated and may be influenced by the intuition or by the theoretical biases of the clinician. The choice may be further influenced by what types of treatment are locally available. A particular psychotherapeutic approach may be based on the knowledge that is gained through a thorough evaluation. Parents should feel comfortable asking why a particular approach is being recommended and whether there are other methods that may also be effective. Frequently, the therapist's qualities and abilities to connect with the adolescent are more important than the specific type of therapy that is used.

> **Sidebar 4.1 | Questions to Ask a Potential Therapist**
>
> ► What is your educational background?
> ► What training have you had in psychotherapy?
> ► How much experience do you have working with adolescents?
> ► Do you have experience treating my teen's problem?
> ► What theoretical approach do you use?
> ► Do you combine different techniques, or do you generally stick to one approach?
> ► How do you think therapy may help my child?

Individual Psychotherapy

Psychodynamic Psychotherapy

One of the most common forms of psychotherapy used to treat adolescents is psychodynamic psychotherapy. The theory behind psychodynamic psychotherapy can be traced back to Sigmund Freud in the early twentieth century, although the practice has evolved considerably since then. The fundamental idea behind psychodynamic psychotherapy is that symptoms are produced by the interactions among various forces at work in a person's mind. These forces may be unconscious and have a basis in early experiences and relationships. Through an adolescent's talking with a therapist and the relationship that is formed, some of these unconscious forces can be brought to awareness and changed.

Psychodynamic psychotherapy tends to be less structured than other forms of therapy. It is usually open-ended, without the predetermined number of sessions that characterize other types of psychotherapy. It may continue for a few weeks or a few years depending on the problem being addressed and the goals of the patient.

During psychodynamic psychotherapy, teens may be asked to talk about whatever is on their mind. The therapist usually plays a somewhat passive role, following the adolescent's lead but asking questions to help clarify or further explore matters under discussion. Allowing the adolescent to direct the discussion gives the therapist a better understanding of the kinds of feelings and conflicts that are at work. Therapists often pay close attention to the associations between ideas or feelings that the adolescent discusses. For example, it may be relevant that an adolescent switches the subject from talking about feeling angry at a teacher to mentioning that he visited his father, with whom he has not been getting along.

In a purely psychodynamic approach, the therapist rarely, if ever, gives the adolescent direct advice on what to do. At times, the therapist may offer an interpretation of a possible deeper psychological significance behind something the adolescent has experienced. Thus, a therapist may say, "I wonder if part of the reason you're having so much trouble with this teacher is that he reminds you of your father, who can also be strict and demanding with you." However, in working with adolescents, many psychodynamic therapists do not strictly follow this traditional approach and will occasionally offer advice and guidance.

With time, psychodynamic psychotherapy can help adolescents have a greater understanding of themselves and their relationships. They may be able to identify patterns of thinking and behavior that contribute to their difficulties and to learn better ways to respond to the stresses in their lives. Psychodynamic psychotherapy can also help teens build a secure sense of self and develop healthier relationships with others.

At times, it may seem to teens and parents that this treatment has no clear agenda, particularly at the beginning, when the therapist is trying to build an understanding of the teen, and the teen is still trying to feel at ease. Teenagers may complain, "I just go in there and talk about random stuff. I don't know how that's supposed to help." For parents who are desperate for assistance and wondering what is happening in the therapist's office, this can be upsetting. Despite seeming loose and open-ended, psychodynamic psychotherapy is a remarkably powerful tool for many teens, with benefits that can last a lifetime. No form of therapy is a quick fix. A therapist needs time to establish a relationship with the teen, which can take longer for some teens than for others. Problems that have been building over many years take time to unravel, and unhealthy patterns that have developed over a lifetime take time to break. Even if you are not seeing immediate results, it is important not to give up on therapy or a particular therapist too quickly.

If you have doubts about your child's therapy, bring them up with the therapist. You may consider scheduling a separate session to talk about your concerns. Similarly, if your child has doubts, encourage him or her to discuss these concerns with the therapist. Because patterns of feelings and behavior from other areas of life (such as children's interaction with parents) are often played out with the therapist during treatment, working through concerns about therapy can be an important part of the process itself. Giving up on a therapist at the first sign of resistance or discontent on your child's part can result in missing an opportunity for positive change.

There are many problems for which psychodynamic psychotherapy may be particularly helpful. Some of these include depression, anxiety, low self-esteem, difficulties with interpersonal relationships, and coping with a loss, a chronic illness, or a stressful situation. There is no condition in which it should never be used. But adolescents who are more concrete in their thinking, those who have difficulty and become frustrated when expressing themselves in words, those with significant cognitive or developmental delay, and those with psychotic disorders may have more difficulty with psychodynamic psychotherapy. Many of these patients would do better with a different approach.

Cognitive Behavioral Therapy

Cognitive behavioral therapy (CBT) is one of the most common forms of psychotherapy used to treat adolescents, and it has been shown to be effective for a number of psychiatric disorders. CBT is based on the theory that many psychiatric problems are rooted in unhealthy, distorted thoughts, or cognitions, and patterns of behavior that may be based on these unhealthy cognitions. To break this cycle, CBT aims to challenge these thoughts and alter patterns of behavior. In depression, one example of a distorted cognition is for a depressed teen to think, "I am not a likable person." This may cause the teen to avoid social situations and opportunities to make new friends in order to escape the rejection that the unhealthy cognition leads him or her to anticipate. This avoidance, in turn, causes greater social isolation and, in the distorted logic of depression, lead the teen to think, "See, I have no friends. I must not be likable." In CBT, the therapist helps the teen identify these thoughts, challenges them in discussion, and encourages the teen to test them out by changing behaviors. A similar approach may be taken for anxiety disorders, in which distorted thoughts can cause an exaggeration of the risk involved in a particular situation. An example is an adolescent believing that he will make a fool of himself during a school speech and that his friends will ridicule him for months.

The behavioral component in CBT may involve breaking unhealthy, self-perpetuating cycles of behavior and learning new strategies for managing symptoms or triggers that bring out symptoms. Thus, relaxation exercises, such as deep breathing, may be incorporated into the treatment of anxiety to help teens deal with stressful situations. In the treatment of phobias, teens may be encouraged to stop avoidance behaviors and increase their exposure to an object or situation that typically triggers anxiety and then use relaxation techniques to manage their response to it. For example, for a teen afraid to fly, this exposure would be done in a graded fashion. It could begin with a less anxiety-provoking situation (such as looking at a picture of an airplane) and build up to more anxiety-provoking situations (such as visiting the airport and, ultimately, getting on a plane). Through repeated exposure, the fear associated with a previously avoided situation typically diminishes.

CBT tends to be a highly structured treatment. Some therapists follow a manual that outlines the steps taken in each session. Usually there is a prescribed duration of treatment, often on the order of eight to twelve weeks, although refresher sessions or additional treatment may be necessary once the initial course of treatment is completed. During the treatment, teens may be asked to keep a journal to record activities and thoughts to help them identify patterns that are contributing to their problem. They may be given homework assignments between sessions. These assignments may be aimed at testing out inaccurate negative thoughts. One such assignment may be, "Start a conversation with the kid whom you sit next to in art class and who always seems to laugh at your jokes." Or the assignments may be aimed at breaking up negative patterns of behavior, such as by starting an exercise program or scheduling rewarding activities into the adolescent's routine or overcoming avoidance behaviors.

Because CBT is so structured, it is easier to examine in research studies than other forms of therapy, such as psychodynamic psychotherapy. Thus, CBT has a great deal of evidence to support its use in the treatment of psychiatric disorders including mood disorders, anxiety disorders, posttraumatic stress disorder, and attention-deficit/hyperactivity disorder. It is generally viewed as the preferred form of therapy for obsessive-compulsive disorder. Whether CBT is superior to psychodynamic psychotherapy in treating mood and anxiety disorders is not clear and is a difficult question to answer scientifically given individual differences in how psychodynamic psychotherapy is performed. It appears that both treatments are effective for these disorders, and the characteristics of the adolescent plays an important role in determining which approach is preferable.

Biofeedback

Biofeedback is tool that is often combined with CBT to help individuals become attuned to their body's physical responses to problems such as stress and, ultimately, to teach them to modify these responses. In biofeedback, the adolescent may be attached to monitors that measure how the respiratory system, heart rate, perspiration, and skin temperature and react to stress. By being able to observe these parameters, teens may be better able to use relaxation techniques to reduce their body's physiologic stress reactions. Biofeedback may be used to treat physical symptoms such as recurrent headaches.

Dialectical Behavioral Therapy

Dialectical behavioral therapy (DBT), a newer form of psychotherapy, is growing in popularity for the treatment of adolescents. DBT is closely related to CBT, as it involves a structured approach and an emphasis on teaching coping skills. But DBT also incorporates ideas from Zen Buddhism, such as learning to observe one's emotions and developing the ability to accept and tolerate strong feelings.

DBT was initially developed for the treatment of adults with borderline personality disorder (see chapter 13), a condition that involves dramatic mood swings and problems with interpersonal relationships. With some modifications, DBT has been used to treat adolescents with similar difficulties and may be useful in the treatment of other disorders including mood disorders. DBT is particularly helpful in treating adolescents who engage in self-injurious behavior, such as cutting themselves, and it may be more successful in reducing these behaviors than other forms of therapy are.

In addition to individual therapy, DBT includes group therapy. During group sessions, teens learn to become mindful of their feelings, have more effective interactions with others, regulate their emotions, and tolerate strong, negative feelings without resorting to unhealthy coping mechanisms such as cutting. In individual therapy sessions, the therapist helps the teen learn to apply these skills to his or her own difficulties.

Neurofeedback

Neurofeedback is a recently developed, controversial form of biofeedback treatment that has been used primarily in the treatment of ADHD. Some studies have shown that individuals with ADHD have more slow brainwave activity and less fast wave activity than patients who do not have ADHD. Using an electroencephalogram (EEG) to document brainwave activities, neurofeedback trains teens to normalize their abnormal EEG frequencies as well as understand how the normalized EEG pattern feels. At present, there is very limited evidence to support the efficacy of this treatment, and it is not covered by most insurance plans. Nevertheless, it may be helpful for some teens when used in conjunction with more validated treatments.

Interpersonal Psychotherapy

Interpersonal psychotherapy (IPT) is a form of therapy that addresses psychological symptoms by focusing on improving and strengthening the adolescent's interpersonal relationships. Similar to CBT, IPT involves a structured, time-limited approach. Typically, a course of treatment lasts between twelve and sixteen weeks. In adolescents, IPT is used most frequently to treat depression. But it may have a role in the treatment of other psychiatric disorders including eating disorders and substance abuse. IPT may also be useful for teens who are struggling with a loss or a difficult life adjustment.

Supportive and Psychoeducational Therapies

Supportive psychotherapy involves helping a teen manage an illness or cope with a stressful life event by bolstering existing psychological defenses, offering emotional support, and encouraging use of existing supports. The aim in supportive psychotherapy is not to guide the teen to deep psychological insight or bring about dramatic changes in the way he or she responds to problems. Rather, the therapist takes a practical, problem-solving approach to help the teen address day-to-day challenges.

Usually supportive psychotherapy is the preferred approach for the most severe forms of psychiatric illness, such as schizophrenia, in which a deep exploration of the teen's inner life may be frustrating or destabilizing, and the teen may be unable to engage in the behavioral changes involved in CBT (though studies have shown CBT to be effective for some patients with schizophrenia). Supportive psychotherapy is also useful in relatively mild forms of psychological distress, such as difficulty adjusting to a stressful situation.

Psychoeducational psychotherapy, which is often incorporated into supportive therapy and other forms of treatment, involves teaching the adolescent and family about the illness that is under treatment. By learning about their illness, teens can come to better understand the warning signs of impending relapse and learn what they can do when these signs occur. They may be better able to develop a collaborative relationship with their treatment team and feel more empowered to express concerns and ask questions. As adolescents learn to connect inconsistencies in their compliance with medication treatment and appointment keeping to worsening symptoms, psychoeducation can improve that compliance.

Combined and Eclectic Approaches

Although the foregoing treatments are presented as distinct approaches, in practice elements from several different approaches are often combined to tailor the treatment to the individual needs of the teen. For example, a therapist may educate the adolescent about his or her illness, as in psychoeducational therapy, and incorporate teaching of some CBT skills into a course of therapy that is psychodynamic in its overall approach. Therapists may refer to this combination of different techniques as an eclectic approach to psychotherapy. While some theoretical purists object to this mix-and-match approach, this is a common practice and can provide a more flexible way of meeting the needs of the teen.

Group Therapy

As most parents attest, adolescents have a remarkable capacity to tune out adults. Though this can be frustrating for parents, it is a healthy developmental task for adolescents to establish an individual identity distinct from their parents. Part of this process involves looking to one's peers as role models for what to think and how to behave. Thus, group therapy, which is shown to be a useful tool in the treatment of adults, can be a particularly powerful tool in the treatment of adolescents.

Because struggling with mental illness during adolescence can be lonely, groups are helpful in breaking down this sense of isolation. Teens in a group realize that they are not alone and that other kids are wrestling with similar problems. By allowing teens to interact with peers in a safe and supportive environment under the guidance of a group therapist, group therapy can help improve self-esteem, social skills, and interpersonal relationships. In addition, group therapy can give adolescents a place to explore their problems and get support and reassurance from their peers.

Adolescents are often much more receptive to feedback that they receive from their peers, particularly those who have dealt with the same issues, than they are to adults giving the same message. For example, a parent's concerns about a certain peer group may be ignored, but when a teen in the early stages of recovery from substance abuse hears from a fellow group member, "Why do you keep hanging out with those kids when you know you're just going to want to use when you're with them?" it may have a significant impact.

Group therapy is commonly used to treat adolescents with mood disorders, anxiety disorders, eating disorders, and substance abuse. The approach taken depends in part on the disorder being treated. Some groups take an open-ended, teen-directed approach similar to that of individual psychodynamic psychotherapy. Other groups take a focused, educational approach. For example, DBT groups teach the core skills that make up the treatment. Social skills groups, which may be used to help adolescents with Asperger's or other developmental disorders, focus on teaching and practicing principles of interpersonal interaction that may seem second nature to those who do not have these difficulties. Self-help groups, such as Alateen or Alcoholics Anonymous, focus on encouraging change through a stepwise process of self-discovery and through sharing one's story with others.

Most therapy groups have one or two clinicians who serve as the group leaders. Their role varies somewhat according to the nature of the group, but in general the leaders guide the discussion and help maintain the group as a therapeutic environment. The group leaders determine which teens will be invited to join the group. They usually meet with a prospective member once or twice to review the teen's history and determine whether the teen seems as if he or she would be a good fit for the group. Often groups will have ground rules. A common ground rule for groups is to insist that the members not develop relationships or seek out contact with one another outside the group. Such contact has the potential to interfere with the therapeutic atmosphere of the group.

Group therapy is less expensive than individual therapy. Sessions typically last ninety minutes and cost between thirty-five and eighty dollars per person; they usually meet once a week. Insurers often cover the sessions. You should check with your psychiatrist, therapist, primary care physician, or insurer for help in finding a group. Listings can also be checked at the website for the American Group Psychotherapy Association.

Family Therapy

Many problems that emerge in adolescents are related to issues affecting the family as a whole, and an adolescent's psychiatric illness is likely to have a huge impact on a family. As a result, family therapy can be an important treatment option for adolescents. Depending on the nature of the problem and the theoretical background of the therapist, family therapy may take a variety of forms. In general, the goals of family therapy are to provide education and support to parents and siblings of an adolescent with mental illness and to identify and correct problems within the family system that may be affecting the well-being of each of its members. Family therapists frequently work to improve communication, to decrease conflict, and to enable families to talk about issues they may be avoiding.

An adolescent's symptoms may be an expression of an issue that has been festering in the family. Psychiatric symptoms may serve as a teenager's desperate attempt, which may be conscious or unconscious, to obtain outside help for the family. In this situation, therapists sometimes speak of the adolescent as the identified patient, meaning that he or she is the one who is acknowledged by the family as having a problem, when in fact the problems involve others in the family as well. There are many different scenarios in which this can happen: for example, a parent's drinking problem that is being ignored may cause a teen to develop psychiatric symptoms.

Marital problems that are not explicitly acknowledged may be manifested through a teen's distress. Secrets held within a family, such as sexual or physical abuse, may cause tension that may be expressed by anxiety, depression, or other problems in one or more of the children. Although any family member may express family problems through mental health symptoms or behaviors, adolescents are often the ones most likely to do so.

Family therapy need not involve the entire family. Often, the therapist will want to meet with the family as a whole at some point early in the process, but at different times during the treatment, the therapist may meet separately with different groupings: the parents, a parent and a child, or a pair of siblings. Some degree of family work, including meetings with the parents to discuss treatment and offer advice, are typically part of individual therapy for children and adolescents. Still, when major family issues are being addressed and family therapy sessions are frequent, it is often better to have a separate therapist devoted to the family therapy. Having an individual therapist helps a teen maintain a good, trusting relationship with his or her own clinician; the teen need not worry about confidential information coming out in a family therapy session.

What If Therapy Is Not Working?

Since unhealthy patterns of thinking and behavior have developed over several years, psychotherapy takes time to have an effect. However, if your child has been in therapy for some time and you do not feel that there has been any improvement, it is important to address your concern with the therapist. It is best to meet with the therapist separately to discuss the therapist's understanding of your child's difficulties, the progress that has been made, and the roadblocks that are impeding progress. Consider the following questions at this meeting:

▸ Does the teen have a good connection with the therapist? Although occasional negative feelings toward the therapist are a normal part of the process, an adolescent should feel some sense of connection to the therapist and feel that the therapist is listening. A good connection takes time to develop. If a teen and therapist just are not clicking after a reasonable amount of time, a switch to another therapist should be considered.

▸ Can the communication between the parents and the therapist be improved? Sometimes therapy is not moving forward because the therapist does not have a good sense of the issues. Teens frequently minimize or avoid talking about their most difficult problems. Establishing a pattern of good, regular communication with the therapist can help address this problem.

▸ Should the frequency of therapy visits be increased? Seeing a therapist once per week is often the norm, but treatment every seven days has more to do with the calendar than it does with the needs of your child. If therapy is not progressing, increasing the frequency of visits is often a good way to move it along. The results can be dramatic, and each session may have a greater impact as the treatment gains momentum.

▸ Are there other approaches to therapy that may be more effective for your child? For example, some teens may feel that cognitive behavioral therapy is more helpful for them than psychodynamic psychotherapy.

▸ Should other therapeutic interventions be added? Sometimes adding family therapy or group therapy in addition to individual therapy has a tremendous benefit.

▸ Would it be useful to involve the school or other resources in the treatment? Schools can build on gains being made in therapy, add additional supports or services, or extend and reinforce a behavioral plan that is being used at home (see chapter 10 for a discussion of the role of schools in psychiatric treatment). Involvement of the legal system or social services agencies is necessary in some cases. Thus, a probation officer can mandate drug screens for adolescents with a history of substance abuse and can enforce serious consequences for those with risky and defiant behavior.

▸ Should treatment with medications be considered? If therapy alone is not helping, referral for a medication evaluation may be indicated. For some disorders, combined treatment with therapy and medications is the most effective treatment. Medications not only work directly on psychiatric symptoms, but they can also help some teens make better use of therapy. For teens who are so depressed that they cannot engage with the therapist or so anxious that they are overwhelmed by the thought of trying the interventions a therapist has suggested, medication can relieve symptoms so that therapy is successful.

Conclusion

Psychotherapy is one of the most common and effective treatments for psychiatric problems in adolescents. Even in the absence of a clearly defined disorder, psychotherapy can help teens build a firm foundation of psychological health by developing healthy ways of dealing with stress, learning to manage interpersonal relationships, and firming up self-esteem. A number of different clinicians including social workers, clinical psychologists, nurse practitioners, and psychiatrists may have training in psychotherapy. Because adolescents can present unique challenges for clinicians trained primarily in working with adults, it is preferable to find a therapist who has experience in working with this age group.

There are a number of theoretical approaches to psychotherapy. The best approach for a particular adolescent depends on the nature of the problem and the characteristics and personality of the teen. Ultimately, finding a therapist who is knowledgeable, experienced, and a good fit with your child may be more important than the particular theoretical approach that is used. Many therapists take an eclectic approach, blending techniques from various approaches according to the needs of the teen. For some teens, it may be helpful to combine individual therapy, group therapy, and family therapy.

References and Additional Reading

Eisenberg, L. 1986. "Mindlessness and Brainlessness in Psychiatry." *British Journal of Psychiatry* 148: 497–508.

Leichsenring, F., and S. Rabung. 2008. "Effectiveness of Long-Term Psychodynamic Psychotherapy." *JAMA* 300: 1551–1565.

Paris, J. 2008. *Prescriptions for the Mind: A Critical View of Contemporary Psychiatry.* New York: Oxford University Press.

Terr, L. 2003. "'Wild Child': How Three Principles of Healing Organized 12 Years of Psychotherapy." *Journal of the American Academy of Child and Adolescent Psychiatry* 142: 1401–1409.

5 Psychiatric Medications

Medications are one of the most effective tools available for the treatment of mental illness. Compared to the previous generation of medications, many newer medications have been shown to be useful for the treatment of mental issues in adolescents, and increasing numbers of teens are prescribed these agents. However, parents are frightened by the idea of giving psychiatric medication to their teenage child, and many questions arise: When should medication be considered? What risks does it carry? Will it work, and if so, how long will my child need to continue taking it?

This chapter presents an overview of commonly prescribed psychiatric medications for adolescents, including their indications for use, risks, side effects, and length of treatment. If you are considering medications for your child, the information provided here should not replace an in-depth conversation with your child's doctor.

When Should Medication Be Considered?

Initiating medication for an adolescent's psychiatric disorder can be one of the hardest decisions a parent may need to consider. How do you know if medication is the right choice, or should you explore other treatment options? There is no simple answer. Some illnesses, such as psychotic disorders, are very difficult to treat without medication. However, anxiety may respond well to psychotherapy alone, and it is reasonable in many cases to try this form of treatment first. During the initial evaluation and feedback process, talk with your child's doctor about the treatment options and their relative effectiveness in addressing your teen's problem.

Another factor to consider is the severity of your child's symptoms. ADHD is a disorder that responds better to medications than to psychotherapy, even though in mild cases the symptoms can often be managed through a combination of school-based interventions and behavioral strategies. On the other hand, mild depression often responds to psychotherapy, and parents may opt to try a course of psychotherapy alone before starting medication. When the symptoms of depression are so debilitating that a teenager is barely able to

> **Sidebar 5.1 | Factors to Consider before Starting Medication**
>
> - Type of mental disorder
> - Severity of symptoms
> - Preferences of adolescent, family, and clinician

function or his or her safety is at risk because of intense suicidal thoughts, then medications should be considered earlier in the course of treatment. Psychiatrists will be more likely to recommend medication when symptoms are severe enough to threaten the safety of the child or those around him or her, to impair the teen's ability to function on a daily basis (e.g., getting out of bed, bathing, going to school), or to significantly interfere with the adolescent's psychological development.

The beliefs and preferences of the family and the adolescent are an essential part of the decision to treat a psychiatric disorder with medication. Although it is important not to let personal bias interfere with making a decision that will be in the best interests of your child, the family's attitudes toward medication may be the deciding factor when choosing between similarly safe and effective treatments. While your child's psychiatrist may not always agree with your personal beliefs, he or she should respect them. Just as some families are less inclined to try medication treatment, some psychiatrists are more likely than others to recommend medication. If you feel that your doctor is not providing a balanced perspective, it is reasonable to seek a second opinion.

Who Can Prescribe Medication?

Medications can be prescribed by a licensed medical doctor (M.D.) or by a nurse practitioner (N.P.) who is working in collaboration with a medical doctor. For straightforward problems, such as uncomplicated cases of ADHD or mild depression, pediatricians may feel comfortable starting and managing psychiatric medications. For more complicated issues, pediatricians usually make a referral to a psychiatrist.

Some general psychiatrists, who have training in the treatment of adults but less formal training in the treatment of adolescents, are comfortable managing medications for adolescents, particularly older adolescents. Other medical specialists, including neurologists and developmental pediatricians, also have training and experience in managing psychiatric medications. If your teen is being seen in an academic medical center, he or she may receive treatment from a resident in general psychiatry or a fellow in child and adolescent psychiatry who practices under the supervision of more experienced specialists.

With the array of clinicians that is often involved, psychiatric treatment can be confusing. When discussing medication with a physician or nurse practitioner, parents should not be embarrassed to ask about the training and experience of their clinician. Some questions to ask include the following:

▸ What training have you received? Have you received specific training in prescribing medications for adolescents (for example, a child and adolescent psychiatry fellowship)? Are you board certified?

▶ Do you treat many adolescents, or do you treat mostly adults, mostly children and adolescents, or a mix? How long have you been in practice? Have you treated many patients with my child's condition?

▶ For nurse practitioners and physicians in training: Who is your supervisor, and what is his or her training and experience? How often do you meet with your supervisor, and how often will you discuss my child's case? If I have a concern at some point, is it possible for me to meet with your supervisor in person? Is he or she available in emergencies?

How Is a Medication Chosen?

Many different factors are considered before deciding on a medication. Parents should participate in this process and discuss why a particular medication has been chosen. Compared to other forms of medication, such as antibiotics, adolescents have a great deal of variability in their response to psychiatric medications. This variability is due to differences in an individual's brain chemistry and genetic makeup. At the outset, it is difficult to know which medication is the best choice for your teen. For example, given two patients with similar depressive symptoms, one may respond well to the antidepressant citalopram but have minimal response to fluoxetine, a similar antidepressant in the same class of medications, while the other patient may have no response to citalopram but have a good response to fluoxetine. Although in the future genetic markers may help guide initial treatment choices, currently prescribing psychiatric medication is an imperfect science, and there is some degree of trial and error involved in finding the right match.

The medication's safety profile (the degree of risk of serious side effects) and its efficacy (how good it is at treating the patient's condition) are the most important factors to consider for medication selection. Medications within a particular class that have a more proven track record in adolescents with respect to safety and efficacy should be preferred over brand-new medications. Older medications have been used more often in clinical practice and examined in more scientific studies. For example, because of the degree of clinical experience and scientific data that supports the use of fluoxetine, one of the first selective serotonin reuptake inhibitors (SSRIs) to become available on the market, it is still a popular choice in treating adolescents.

The tolerability of a medication, or the degree to which a patient suffers annoying but otherwise harmless side effects such as drowsiness or headaches, is another consideration. Tolerability is closely related to patients' adherence, sometimes called compliance, which refers to the degree to which a person takes a medication as prescribed. A medication will not work well if it is not taken as directed. Unpleasant side effects, when and how frequently the medication is taken, and the need to undergo blood-monitoring tests can affect adolescents' medication compliance.

The side effect profiles may dictate a choice between similar medications. Thus, a medication known to cause drowsiness may be chosen and given at bedtime for a patient with insomnia, for example. When medications are equally safe and effective, cost to the family and the health care system is another important consideration.

There are many factors that are taken into account when choosing a medication for the treatment of a psychiatric disorder. Although parents need not weigh all these factors themselves, it is helpful to understand the prescribing clinician's thought process. It is also reasonable to ask your teen's clinician why he or she is recommending a particular medication over the other treatment options. The discussion that follows often helps parents learn more about their child's condition and treatment.

General Principles of Adolescent Psychopharmacology

It is important for parents to understand how physicians manage psychiatric medications since the process of medication prescribing can be confusing. The following are a few general principles:

- *Start low, go slow.* Medications are often started at a very low dose in the pediatric population to help ensure that they will be safe and well tolerated. The dose is then slowly increased until the effective dose is found.
- *Be patient.* Many psychiatric medications work slowly, over a period of weeks, not days. It will probably take some time to reach the desired effects and appropriate dose for your child.
- *Take one step at a time.* Prescribers should avoid making too many changes, such as starting, stopping, or changing doses of medication all at once. In general, only one change should be made at a time. Otherwise, if there is a problem, such as a significant side effect, one will not know which change caused it. In addition, if the teen feels a lot better after two medications were started together, one will not know which of the medications led to the improvement, or if it was due to the combination of the two.
- *Be systematic.* Prescribers who are inexperienced or uncomfortable with managing psychiatric medications may have a disorganized approach to medication prescription. They may try one medication, give up on it too soon, try two medications at once, switch to something else because of side effects, then go back to the first medication but at a higher dose. This approach is not only messy, but it is potentially harmful. It may take longer to find an effective medication regimen and increase the likelihood of side effects. Good prescribers take a more scientific, methodical approach. Parents can help this process by keeping accurate records of medications prescribed for their adolescent, the

doses used, and the results. This is particularly helpful if you switch doctors but useful even if you do not.

Tips for Parents

▸ *Establish good communication with the prescriber.* In the first meeting, get your doctor's contact information including after-hours phone or pager numbers, and keep this information in a convenient location. Do not be afraid to contact the prescriber if something seems wrong. Teenagers may respond to medications in many different ways. If you are unsure, it is always appropriate to check.

▸ *Stick to your doctor's recommendations.* Doctors may ask you to come in for frequent appointments, particularly when a medication is started or adjusted. The doctor may be able to pick up a subtle change in behavior that you have missed. Some medications require laboratory studies. It is important to be clear about what testing is required and to be diligent about following through. Clarify with your doctor whether there are any special instructions for blood draws, such as just before a medication dose, first thing in the morning, or after fasting.

▸ *Do not adjust medications on your own.* This could be very dangerous. Adjustments include stopping medication. Some medications need to be tapered gradually. If your teen refuses to take a medication as prescribed, notify the doctor as soon as possible. Although a face-to-face appointment is not necessary for all adjustments, some discussion with the doctor should take place to ensure your child's safety.

▸ *Maintain consistency with the medication.* Be sure your teenager is taking medications as prescribed, and try to avoid missed doses. This may sound obvious, but it proves to be a challenge for many families. Make one family member responsible for ensuring that the medication is administered. For younger adolescents, a parent is usually the best person to do this. Older teens may be able to assume this responsibility for themselves. Even then, parents should act as a safeguard, keeping track to make sure the teen is taking the medication as prescribed. Well-intended adolescents are often forgetful. A day-of-the-week pill box can help parents and teens keep track of medication. Working the medication into the daily routine, such as taking it at the same time every day, can reduce the number of missed pills.

▸ *Keep medications secure.* Medications are safest if they are kept in a locked area. This is particularly important if there are young children in the house or if your teenager may be at risk for suicide or prescription drug abuse. If your teenager is learning to manage his or her own medications, he or she may be given a small amount at a time, such as a week's supply in a day-of-the-week pill box.

► *Keep track of your child's medication supply.* Although it is probably not possible or in most cases helpful to know the exact number of pills remaining, it is important to keep track of the medication supply. This allows for timely refills. In addition, it can help you learn if your teenager is not taking the medication as directed. In the unfortunate event that your child overdoses on medication, your knowledge of how many pills were in the bottle can help doctors estimate the amount of medication that was taken.

How Long Does Your Child Need to Continue on Medication?

Once the decision has been made to start a medication, the next question that concerns parents is, "How long does my child need to take this?" The answer is, it depends. Several factors are considered when deciding on the length of medication treatment, and this topic should be discussed early in the course of treatment and revisited when your child's symptoms have improved.

Some psychiatric conditions, such as ADHD, are chronic, with symptoms that, when untreated, are constant over a period of several years and sometimes persist throughout a person's life. For chronic conditions, medication is generally continued for as long the underlying condition persists. In contrast, some conditions, such as depression, tend to be episodic. Symptoms occur over a discrete period of time before going into remission. For an episodic condition, stopping medication may be considered sometime after the episode has resolved. Nevertheless, many episodic psychiatric conditions, including depression, have high rates of relapse. The risk of relapse is usually highest in the interval immediately following the previous episode, so stopping medication too soon after symptoms have resolved places a teen at risk. Therefore, it is generally best to wait until the teen has been symptom free for some time before stopping the medication. After the first episode of depression, it is generally recommended that medication be continued at least nine months to a year after the teen has been in remission.

The length of medication administration should be customized to the particular teen. For example, in the case of depression, an adolescent's risk for future recurrences increases with the number of past depressive episodes. Thus, teens who have had multiple episodes of depression are at very high risk of having further episodes. For these teens, it is often recommended that they continue taking medication for a longer period of time to help prevent relapse. Similarly, symptoms from an illness that were particularly severe (such as depression leading to a serious suicide attempt) or particularly difficult to manage (those requiring multiple medication trials before achieving remission) may warrant a longer course of medication.

Before stopping mediation, look at the events in your teen's life. A symptom-free year may have passed since your teen started taking medication for depression, but if he has experienced a traumatic event such as breaking up with his girlfriend and has midterm exams, then it may be best to wait a bit longer before lowering the dose. Common sense dictates that times of low stress are best for tapering medications. Summer vacations are often a good time, though not when your child is away at camp or a trip abroad. Close supervision is also essential.

When you do decide to stop your child's medication, this should always be done under the doctor's supervision and guidance. Many medications need to be tapered gradually. If SSRIs are stopped suddenly, there is the potential for unpleasant side effects. A serious and fatal withdrawal can result from suddenly stopping benzodiazepines. In addition, as the medication dosage is lowered, monitoring is important to detect early symptoms that the illness is relapsing.

Major Classes of Medication

Selective Serotonin Reuptake Inhibitors

Some of the most commonly used medications for the treatment of psychiatric disorders in adolescents are the selective serotonin reuptake inhibitors (SSRIs). Although classified as antidepressants, SSRIs are also very effective in the treatment of several other conditions, including certain forms of eating disorders, anxiety disorders, obsessive-compulsive disorder, and panic disorder. Commonly used SSRIs include fluoxetine (Prozac), sertraline (Zoloft), citalopram (Celexa), escitalopram (Lexapro), and paroxetine (Paxil).

SSRIs seem to work by increasing the amount of serotonin, an important chemical messenger thought to be involved in mood regulation. The increase of serotonin occurs in the synapses, which are the small spaces between brain cells through which they communicate. After the cellular release of serotonin, it is normally absorbed back into the cell very quickly. SSRIs partially block this process, leaving more serotonin in the synapse to act on the receiving brain cell. Improvement of mood and reduction of anxiety are believed not to be a direct result of the increase in serotonin in the synapses but rather a consequence of a cascade of indirect effects set in motion by this increase. This theory is based on the finding that the beneficial effects of SSRIs usually begin a few weeks after the medication is started, even though the synaptic serotonin increase is rather immediate.

Because SSRIs are relatively safe, are well tolerated, and have minimal potential for abuse or dependence, over the past two decades they have emerged as a first-line treatment for depression and anxiety. It does not appear that SSRIs are significantly more effective in the treatment of depression than were older antidepressant medications, such as tricyclics or monoamine-oxidase inhibitors (MAOIs), which are now used very rarely in adolescents. However, the risks from overdose and side effects and, in the case of MAOIs, the need for dietary restrictions make use of SSRIs more desirable for both patients and prescribers.

Common side effects with SSRIs include headache, dizziness, upset stomach, changes in appetite, dry mouth, and constipation. Effects may vary between individuals. As a result, some people experience drowsiness, whereas others feel an energy boost or restlessness. These medications generally reduce anxiety, but some adolescents report a worsening of their anxiety. SSRIs can cause a variety of sexual side effects, including decreased sex drive, erectile dysfunction, and difficulty having an orgasm. These side effects can be very distressing to adolescents and difficult for them to talk about with their parents or prescriber.

In rare cases, SSRIs can cause dramatic changes in mood or behavior, such as inducing a manic episode. It is thought that this occurs mostly in people who have an underlying biological predisposition toward bipolar disorder, though it can be difficult to predict. Another downside of SSRI treatment is that it usually takes up to four weeks before there is a significant reduction in the symptoms from a mood or anxiety disorder. And it can take up to six weeks for the medication to reach its full effect.

Antidepressants and Suicidality. When SSRIs first emerged as a treatment for depression about twenty years ago, they were hailed as wonder drugs for their safety and efficacy. Recently concerns have been raised about evidence that suggests SSRIs may increase the risk of suicidal thoughts or attempts in younger people.

Because some children being prescribed SSRIs are already at risk of having suicidal thoughts, the relationship between suicidal thoughts and antidepressant treatment is challenging to study. Furthermore, the increase in risk appears to be small, so large numbers of subjects are needed in order to detect the effect. To address this issue, the U.S. Food and Drug Administration (FDA) conducted an analysis in 2004 of suicidal thoughts and behaviors (such as attempts). Using data pooled together from multiple individual studies of SSRIs and similar antidepressants involving over forty-four hundred children, it was shown that children treated with antidepressants had slightly higher rates of suicidal thoughts and behaviors than those treated with placebo. In this analysis, which is discussed on the FDA website, www.fda.gov, 4 percent of children treated with antidepressants had suicidal thoughts or behaviors, compared to 2 percent of those given the placebo. Based on this finding, the FDA issued a black box warning, which is printed on the labels of SSRIs and some related medications, indicating the possible suicidal risk associated with these medications.

It is not fully understood why SSRIs may be linked to an increased risk of suicidal thoughts. Many psychiatrists suspect that it could be related to the small number of individuals who become activated, feeling restless, anxious, or even manic, when started on SSRIs. Some of these individuals may have a biological predisposition toward bipolar disorder.

Parents may be dismayed to think that the medication they are giving to their child for depression could make things worse. But it is important to realize that the percentage of patients who appeared to experience suicidal thoughts while on antidepressants was relatively small (four out of one hundred in the FDA analysis). Furthermore, there is no evidence that these medications actually increased the risk of a child's committing suicide, as none of the forty-four hundred children studied in the FDA review committed suicide. In fact, more-recent studies have shown that even though SSRI treatment may increase the risk of suicidal thoughts in the few weeks after they are started, their use may decrease the risk of completed suicide over the longer term (Gibbons, Brown, et al., 2007; Gibbons, Hur, et al., 2006).

The risks associated with antidepressants should be taken seriously, but they must be weighed against the significant risks associated with having a serious psychiatric problem that is undertreated. If SSRIs are appropriate for treating your teen's condition, it is important to be certain that your child is closely monitored by the doctor to assess his or her safety and evaluate for adverse effects. After a teen starts an SSRI, parents should observe for dramatic changes in their teen's behavior and know how to reach the doctor in the event of an urgent concern.

Buproprion

Although SSRIs are the most commonly used medications to treat depression in adolescents, there are other medications available that may be used. Buproprion (Wellbutrin) is an antidepressant that is thought to work by inhibiting the reuptake of the neurotransmitters dopamine and norepinephrine into brain cells. Although approved by the FDA for use only in adults, it is frequently prescribed off label for adolescents. There is evidence to support that buproprion is safe and effective for teenagers. Unlike SSRIs, buproprion does not appear to help anxiety disorders and, in some cases, may worsen anxiety.

Buproprion has some similarities to the stimulant medications in its mechanism of action, and like stimulants, buproprion appears to have some benefit in treating symptoms of attention-deficit/hyperactivity disorder (ADHD). However, it appears that it is not as effective as other medications, and it is not usually viewed as a first-choice medication for treating ADHD.

In contrast to SSRIs, buproprion does not seem to cause sexual side effects and, when given with an SSRI, may ameliorate some of these effects. Similar to other antidepressants, buproprion may induce mania or rapid switching between depressed and manic states in people with bipolar disorder. However, in studies of adults this risk appears to be much lower with buproprion than it is for other antidepressants. For this reason, buproprion may be used to treat depressive episodes in teens with bipolar disorder.

Mirtazapine

Mirtazapine (Remeron) is an antidepressant with a unique mechanism of action that indirectly leads to an increase in the transmission of serotonin and norepinephrine in the brain. Similar to buproprion, mirtazapine is FDA approved only for adults, but it is occasionally used to treat adolescents. It is also used to treat anxiety disorders.

The most common side effect of mirtazapine is drowsiness. Psychiatrists may take advantage of this side effect by giving the medication at bedtime for teens who have difficulty sleeping. Weight gain is also common with mirtazapine, and teens taking it should have their weight and body mass index (BMI) monitored. Other side effects include dry mouth, constipation, dizziness, and decreased blood pressure.

Tricyclic Antidepressants

Tricyclic antidepressants are an older class of medications that have been used much less commonly since SSRIs became available. They include amitriptyline, nortriptyline, desipramine, and imipramine. These medications share a similar chemical structure, from which they take their name, and work in a similar way by inhibiting the reuptake of the neurotransmitters norepinephrine and serotonin. They have been used to treat depression, anxiety, obsessive-compulsive disorder, and bedwetting in children and adolescents. Occasionally tricyclics are used to treat certain kinds of pain-related conditions, including fibromyalgia, neuropathic (nerve) pain, and chronic headaches.

The tricyclic antidepressants appear to be as effective as SSRIs in treating depression and anxiety. The biggest concern with tricyclic antidepressants is that they increase the risk for disturbances of the heart rhythm. This risk makes these medications very dangerous when taken in an overdose, when they are much more likely than SSRIs to be fatal. Checking an ECG before and after starting a tricyclic medication may help identify patients at high risk of having cardiac side effects.

Other side effects from tricyclic antidepressants may include dry mouth, constipation, weight gain, dizziness, sedation, upset stomach, and blurry vision. They may also increase risk of seizures, particularly in people who have had seizures in the past. Some side effects are similar to those of SSRIs, including the sexual side effects and the risk of inducing mania in people with bipolar disorder. Although the side effects of tricyclic antidepressants limit their use, they may be quite useful for those teens for whom other medications have not worked or who would benefit from the pain-reducing properties of these medications.

Serotonin-Norepinephrine Reuptake Inhibitors

One of the newest classes of medications, the serotonin-norepinephrine reuptake inhibitors (SNRIs) work in a similar fashion to the tricyclic antidepressants in that they inhibit reuptake of serotonin and norepinephrine into brain cells. Moreover, they avoid some of the more concerning side effects of tricyclics medications. The two SNRIs currently available in the United States—venlafaxine (Effexor) and duloxetine (Cymbalta)—are used to treat depression and anxiety. Side effects are similar to those of SSRIs, including potential for developing suicidal thoughts in a small percentage of patients. While these medications appear to be safe and effective in adolescents, they are relatively new and have not been as well studied as other antidepressant medications.

Benzodiazepines

Benzodiazepines are a group of medications used primarily to treat anxiety disorders. Medications in this class include lorazepam (Ativan), clonazepam (Klonopin), diazepam (Valium), and alprazolam (Xanax). These medications are very effective in reducing anxiety, and unlike many psychiatric medications, benzodiazepines have the advantage of having an immediate effect within minutes to hours.

Despite these advantages, there are a number of potential problems that may arise from the use of benzodiazepines in adolescent patients. Over time, teens who take them regularly may develop a tolerance that requires higher and higher doses to achieve the same effects. In addition, benzodiazepines have the potential for abuse, since doses above the prescribed level can lead to a high similar to alcohol intoxication. Benzodiazepines may be lethal at elevated doses, and they can be habit forming. In addition, since an individual can develop a physiological dependence on benzodiazepine, these medications must be tapered gradually before they are stopped.

Benzodiazepines have several potential side effects. The most common side effect is sedation; difficulties with concentration and learning may also occur. Rarely, benzodiazepines cause a paradoxical reaction in some teenagers, in which the effects of the medication are the opposite of what is usually seen. Instead of relaxation and sedation, patients may become extremely anxious, agitated, or out of control. Some patients may experience brief hallucinations. If this occurs, notify your doctor immediately. This effect is fortunately transient, lasting only as long as the medication remains in the system. Until the medication wears off, be certain to keep your child safe. Avoid giving another dose of the medication until consulting with the doctor.

Stimulant Medications

The stimulant class of medications is a very effective and the first-line treatment for attention-deficit/hyperactivity disorder (ADHD). Stimulants work by increasing levels of dopamine and norepinephrine in the synapses between brain cells. The activity of these two chemicals in specific brain regions appears to play a major role in the modulation of attention and impulse control. Stimulants may dramatically improve focus and reduce impulsivity and hyperactivity, helping teens to feel more in control in their activities. When stimulants are effective, they usually reduce the symptoms of ADHD quickly, even after the first dose. However, the beneficial effects of stimulants last only as long as the medication remains in the system.

Two stimulants are used most often: methylphenidate and amphetamine salts. These medications are available in a variety of formulations, usually varying according to their time-release properties. Formulations of methylphenidate include Ritalin, Ritalin LA, Metadate ER, Concerta, and, most recently, the Daytrana patch. Amphetamine salts are available as Adderall, Adderall XR, and Dexedrine. The goal of the controlled-release formulations is to allow for less-frequent, more-convenient dosing while providing optimal levels of medication in the person's system throughout the day.

The common side effects from stimulant medications include headache, stomachache, decreased appetite, and difficulty with sleep. Problems with sleeping can often be addressed by switching to a different time-release formulation or by changing the timing of the doses. Occasionally teens may become more irritable or moody when taking stimulants, and this frequently occurs as the medication is wearing off late in the day. This side effect also can be addressed by changing to a different formulation.

There is some concern and controversy that stimulants may slow the rate of growth for some adolescents. The results of studies are mixed. Some suggest that stimulants do not significantly affect growth, but other studies indicate that there are small growth differences in a small number of patients. It is recommended that while adolescents are taking stimulants, they should have their height and weight monitored.

Stimulants may also cause increases in blood pressure and heart rate. These increases are usually very small and do not have any significant medical implications in an otherwise healthy teenager. Still, blood pressure and pulse should also be monitored by the prescribing doctor.

The most serious concern about stimulant medications are rare cases of sudden death due to cardiovascular problems such as arrhythmias. These events have been reported in a small number of adolescents who were taking stimulants. This issue is discussed in greater detail in chapter 11. Since stimulant medications are helpful for such problems as attention-deficit disorder, what should parents do about this concern? As always, it is important to talk with your child's doctor to weigh the potential benefits of a medication against the risks associated with it. In general, it is advised that stimulant medications be used with caution in those adolescents whose medical history suggests that they may be at increased risk for a cardiac problem. In addition to a known history of heart malformation or heart-rhythm disturbance, symptoms that may suggest such a risk include a history of unexplained fainting spells, heart palpitations, or shortness of breath with minimal exertion. Teens with a family member who has a known heart-rhythm disturbance or a close relative who has died suddenly from a heart problem at a young age may be at increased risk as well. For some teens, prior to starting a stimulant medication, an electrocardiogram (ECG or EKG) or a consultation with the pediatrician or a cardiologist may be recommended. Before taking a stimulant, all teens should have a physical exam and a detailed review of their medical history.

There is also a risk of abuse of stimulants by adolescents. Inappropriate use of stimulants, including taking excessive doses or snorting or smoking them, may cause a high with feelings of euphoria and a surge of energy. The appetite-suppressing qualities of these medications lead some teens, including those with eating disorders, to use them in an effort to lose weight. Stimulant abuse may lead to severe problems, including physiological and psychological dependence on the medication, extreme mood swings or irritability, and even paranoia and psychosis. For this reason, parents and physicians should give careful consideration to the risk of abuse before giving stimulants to teens who have a history of substance abuse. That said, a history of substance abuse does not mean that stimulants should never be used. Parents should closely supervise medication administration, or the physician should use a stimulant formulation with chemical properties that makes it more difficult to abuse.

Other ADHD Medications: Atomoxetine and Clonidine

A commonly used nonstimulant alternative in the treatment of ADHD is a medication called atomoxetine (Strattera). This medication has a unique mechanism of action, blocking the reuptake of the neurotransmitter norepinephrine after it is released by brain cells. Blocking reuptake of norepinephrine increases its transmission between cells and indirectly increases levels of dopamine in certain parts of the brain. Atomoxetine has been shown to be effective in treating both the inattentive and hyperactive symptoms of ADHD. Unlike stimulants, atomoxetine may take some time to reach its full therapeutic effect. Though there may be some benefit after a single dose, with daily use there may be continued gradual improvement in symptoms over a period of four to eight weeks.

While most teens tolerate atomoxetine, it does have potential for side effects, some of which are similar to those seen with stimulants. Common side effects include decreased appetite, upset stomach, dry mouth, constipation, fatigue, and difficulty sleeping. As with stimulants, atomoxetine may cause small increases in heart rate and blood pressure, and it is advised that these signs be monitored when the medication is first started.

Some people may experience irritability or anxiety. Very rarely, a person may have onset of manic episodes following initiation of treatment with atomoxetine (see chapter 7 for a description of manic symptoms). Atomoxetine may cause a small increase in risk of suicidal thoughts or gestures, and adolescents taking it should be closely monitored by the prescribing doctor.

Clonidine is a medication that was originally used to treat high blood pressure, but it is occasionally used to treat ADHD and other psychiatric disorders in children and adolescents. For ADHD, clonidine appears to have greater efficacy in reducing the hyperactive symptoms. It is less useful in addressing cognitive symptoms of inattention and disorganization. As a result, clonidine tends to be a second-line medication in ADHD treatment.

Since sedation from clonidine is a potential and significant side effect, its usefulness may be limited in adolescents. Other side effects include decreased blood pressure, dizziness or lightheadedness, dry mouth, and depressed mood. Clonidine may also increase risk for a cardiac arrhythmia in people who have an underlying heart condition. Adolescents should have a detailed medical history and recent physical exam before starting clonidine. In some cases, the doctor will also order an ECG. During treatment, teens taking clonidine should have their blood pressure monitored.

Antipsychotics

Antipsychotics are a group of medications that were originally used to treat psychotic disorders such as schizophrenia. Yet, many of these medications have also been shown to be effective in treating other forms of psychiatric illness. Some of the older antipsychotics, called typical antipsychotics, have been used to treat patients for more than fifty years and are quite effective in treating psychotic symptoms such as hallucinations and delusions. These medications, which include haloperidol (Haldol) and chlorpromazine (Thorazine), may have dangerous side effects. These side effects include muscle stiffness and slowed movements similar to those seen in Parkinson's disease, involuntary movements termed tardive dyskinesia, and severe uncomfortable muscle spasms in the head or neck. For this reason, the typical antipsychotic medications are rarely used in the treatment of adolescents.

Over the past decade, a newer generation of antipsychotics, called atypical antipsychotics, has been used with increasing frequency. These medications appear to be equally effective in the treatment of psychosis, but they are much less likely to cause some of the more severe side effects noted for typical antipsychotic medications. It is also believed that atypical antipsychotics may be more effective than typical in treating the negative symptoms of schizophrenia, such as lack of motivation and emotional flattening. Commonly used antipsychotics include risperidone (Risperdal), aripiprazole (Abilify), olanzapine (Zyprexa), quetiapine (Seroquel), and ziprasidone (Geodon).

Antipsychotics have also been shown to be useful in the treatment of other psychiatric illnesses, especially adolescent mood disorders. These medications have been shown to help stabilize mood and reduce the symptoms of bipolar disorder and may be particularly effective in the treatment of juvenile-onset bipolar disorder (see chapter 7 for further discussion of bipolar disorder in adolescents). For this reason, atypical antipsychotics are now used by many psychiatrists as the first line of treatment for children and adolescents with bipolar disorder. When added to an antidepressant, atypical antipsychotics are also used to treat depression that is resistant to the usual treatments.

Atypical antipsychotics may also reduce some of the most troubling symptoms related to developmental disorders such as autism, though they do not address the underlying problem. In particular, in autistic adolescents, these medications have been shown to reduce aggression and self-injurious behaviors, such as head banging (see chapter 18 for further information).

Despite the many uses of atypical antipsychotics and their advantages over older antipsychotics, these medications are also associated with a number of potential adverse effects. Among these, weight gain is the most problematic for teenagers. A substantial proportion of people treated with atypical antipsychotics will experience some degree of weight gain. When weight gain occurs, the degree may be relatively small, on the order of a few pounds, and it may be addressed by eating a healthier diet and exercising. But some patients gain a great deal of weight. When weight gain is substantial, parents should explore the management options with the psychiatrist. Some atypical antipsychotics have greater potential to cause weight gain than others, so switching to a different medication may solve the situation. If there are strong reasons not to switch medications, then the psychiatrist could consider adding an additional medication to help suppress appetite.

When atypical antipsychotics are used for prolonged periods, teens are at increased risk for developing medical problems related to metabolic changes in the body, including elevated cholesterol and type 2 diabetes mellitus. These problems may place adolescents at risk for further medical illness, including heart disease, later in life. Monitoring of cholesterol and blood sugar may help to detect early signs of metabolic changes related to atypical antipsychotic usage. Adolescents who develop elevated blood cholesterol or sugar may need to change medications, although the relative risk of the side effects must be weighed against the risk of the return of symptoms from the underlying disorder. This may be a particularly difficult decision for adolescents whose symptoms were severe and difficult to control, as is often the case with psychotic disorders. In these circumstances, a psychiatrist can help parents weigh both sides of this decision and make an informed choice.

Other common side effects of atypical antipsychotics include drowsiness, dizziness, restlessness, dry mouth, upset stomach, and constipation. Some teens may have a decrease in blood pressure resulting in lightheadedness, particularly when getting up from sitting or lying down. Though less common, there may be muscle stiffness or tremor. In extremely rare cases, people may experience the kinds of problems associated with the older typical antipsychotics such as painful muscle stiffness.

Atypical antipsychotics are fairly similar to each other in both their efficacy and their side effects. Nevertheless, there are some differences between them in the specific brain receptors targeted and in the side effects that are most likely to occur. Among the notable differences in the atypical antipsychotics, clozapine has been associated with a rare but potentially serious drop in white blood cells, which fight infection. Because of this concern, clozapine use is restricted to people whose symptoms have been resistant to other medications. People taking clozapine are required to enter a program of regular blood tests involving close monitoring of drug levels and white blood cell counts. Adolescents are not commonly prescribed clozapine.

In a small number of people, it appears that ziprasidone, another atypical antipsychotic, may increase the risk of a potentially fatal cardiac arrhythmia. The risk of this side effect is so low that it is difficult to estimate its frequency; nonetheless, it is generally recommended that people taking ziprasidone be monitored with an ECG before and during treatment.

Risperidone, which is one of the more commonly used medications in treating adolescents with psychosis, may lead to an elevation in the blood level of a naturally occurring hormone called prolactin. This hormone is involved in menstrual regulation and lactation in females; it plays an unclear role in males. While prolactin elevation is usually benign, high levels of prolactin may lead to lactation in adolescent girls, particularly when risperidone is used at higher doses. Elevated prolactin levels can also lead to menstrual irregularities. In males, an elevated prolactin level may lead to development of breast tissue, called gynecomastia. These effects are harmless and reversible when the dose is lowered or the medication is stopped. But they may be alarming and embarrassing for teens. Before adolescents start treatment with risperidone, it is advisable for the psychiatrist to warn them and their parents of these possible side effects.

Mood Stabilizers

Mood stabilizers are a group of medications used to treat bipolar disorder. As the name implies, mood stabilizers reduce symptoms of both mania and depression and help to maintain the teen's mood in a stable state between these dangerous extremes. Lithium (Eskalith, Lithobid) was the first mood stabilizer identified, and it is still commonly used. Most other mood stabilizers are anticonvulsant medications, meaning they are also used to treat seizures. These medications include valproic acid (Depakote), carbemazepine (Tegretol), oxcarbazepine (Trileptal), and lamotrigine (Lamictal). Atypical antipsychotics are occasionally called mood stabilizers because of their efficacy in bipolar disorder.

Lithium has been effective in treating bipolar disorder for over sixty years, but the mechanism of action is still not well understood. It is believed to modify complex biochemical pathways that take place inside brain cells, which, in turn, alter the flow of electrically charged ions into the cells. As one of the most effective mood stabilizers available, lithium can help bring episodes of mania and depression into remission and prevent future occurrences. In cases of depression in adults that are difficult to treat, lithium is occasionally added to an antidepressant medication. Still, the use of lithium is limited by potentially serious side effects and the need to monitor blood tests during treatment. Common side effects include frequent urination, increased thirst, skin rash, acne, hair thinning, tremor, sedation, and weight gain. Less common but potentially serious side effects include cardiac arrhythmias and damage to the kidneys and thyroid gland. This damage is more likely to occur at blood levels above the typical therapeutic range. Very high levels of lithium, as might be seen in an overdose, can cause seizures, confusion, and even death.

Lithium has a relatively narrow therapeutic window, meaning that the blood level at which it has its beneficial effects is not far from the level at which serious side effects can occur. For this reason, lithium levels must be checked during treatment to assure that the level is high enough to have an effect but not so high as to be dangerous. Levels are checked more frequently when the medication is first started until the appropriate dose for an individual is determined. The lithium level is usually checked as a trough level, meaning that the blood is drawn immediately before a scheduled dose, when the blood level is at its lowest point. Once the patient is on a stable dose, levels may be checked less frequently to make sure the level stays within the therapeutic range.

When your teen is prescribed lithium, it is important to talk with the doctor before starting any new medication. Lithium is metabolized by the kidneys, and other medications that affect the kidneys, including diuretics and nonsteroidal anti-inflammatory drugs (NSAIDs) such as ibuprofen, may affect lithium levels. Also, lithium levels may increase if your child becomes dehydrated. If your child is unable to take in fluids or has excessive vomiting or diarrhea, you should contact your child's doctor to discuss whether it is necessary to reduce the lithium dose temporarily.

In addition to lithium levels, several other laboratory tests must be monitored. Because lithium has the potential to be harmful to the kidneys and the thyroid gland, blood tests measuring kidney and thyroid function are checked before and during the course of treatment. To assess a teen's risk for developing an arrhythmia on the medication, some doctors also check an ECG before treatment. To assess for excessive weight gain, height and weight should be measured during treatment. Teens who do gain weight on the medication may need additional monitoring to check for onset of diabetes or other metabolic problems associated with excess weight.

Some anticonvulsants have been found to be effective in stabilizing mood in bipolar disorder. Valproic acid is an effective and commonly used mood stabilizer that is thought to be more effective than lithium in treating rapid cycling or mixed mood episodes of bipolar disorder. Although it may be very helpful to many people, valproic acid use is limited by side effects and the need for monitoring with blood testing. Sedation, weight gain, stomach upset, constipation, tremor, dizziness, unsteadiness when walking, and headache are the most common side effects from valproic acid. Use of valproic acid during pregnancy has been linked to serious birth defects including abnormal development of the nervous system. Thus, it is essential to warn adolescent girls about this risk and to ensure that they are taking appropriate measures to protect against an unwanted pregnancy. In very rare circumstances, valproic acid may cause significant liver damage. Other possible but rare side effects include decreased blood cell counts and irritation of the pancreas.

Blood levels of valproic acid should be monitored to be certain they are within a range that is safe and effective, These levels are checked more frequently when the medication is first started and when the dose is adjusted; generally the level is drawn just before a scheduled dose. Regular monitoring of liver functions and blood cell counts is also required. If these tests remain normal, they can be checked every six months. Adolescents should also have their height and weight monitored during treatment to assess for excessive weight gain.

Valproic acid has the potential to interact with many other medications that are also metabolized by the liver. Thus, it is particularly important that your doctor knows of all medications prescribed for your teen. For teens taking valproic acid, before starting any new medications, potential medication interactions need to be considered.

Lamotrigine (Lamictal) is a newer anticonvulsant that has been gaining increased favor for the treatment of bipolar disorder. Because blood levels are not required, lamotrigine has an advantage over lithium and valproic acid. However, treatment with lamotrigine does carry some risks including, in extremely rare cases, a potentially life-threatening rash called Stevens-Johnson syndrome. Stevens-Johnson syndrome symptoms include a rapidly spreading rash that may involve the eyes, lips, mouth, or palms of the hands and may be associated with fever, malaise, abdominal pain, and swollen lymph nodes. If your child experiences any of these symptoms while taking lamotrigine, contact the doctor immediately. Stevens-Johnson syndrome tends to occur early in the course of treatment and when the dose is increased. To minimize risk, the medication is started at a low dose and increased gradually. Thus, it often takes several weeks to get the dose of lamotrigine up to a therapeutic range. If your child has missed his or her dose of lamotrigine for a few days in a row, contact your doctor before restarting it, as restarting at a high dose can also increase your child's risk of Stevens-Johnson syndrome.

Although Stevens-Johnson syndrome is rare, rashes that are mild and benign are fairly commonly seen with lamotrigine administration. It is best to alert your doctor if you notice any skin changes in an adolescent taking lamotrigine. Other common side effects of lamotrigine include sedation, headache, dizziness, insomnia, and upset stomach. Lamotrigine may interact with other medications metabolized by the liver, including valproic acid, so as always it is important to inform your child's doctor about any other medications your child is taking.

Two other anticonvulsant medications used to treat adolescents with bipolar disorder are carbamazepine (Tegretol) and a similar medication, oxcarbazepine (Trileptal). Because these medications on their own do not appear to be as effective as other medications such as lithium and valproic acid, they are often used either as a second-line agent or to augment another mood stabilizer. Side effects of these two medications are similar and may include sedation, upset stomach, diarrhea, dizziness, headache, blurry vision, and rash. An uncommon but more serious side effect of carbamazepine is a reduction in the body's infection-fighting white blood cells. Cases of liver damage and Stevens-Johnson syndrome have been reported in association with carbemazepine treatment, but they are exceedingly rare. Carbamazepine blood levels are monitored during treatment to assure the medication is in a therapeutic range, and liver function tests and white blood cell counts are also administered. Blood levels are not routinely monitored for oxcarbazepine, yet it may cause a potentially dangerous drop in the blood sodium level. For this reason, sodium levels are usually checked during treatment, particularly when the medication is first started.

Conclusion

Medications may be a very effective treatment option for many adolescents struggling with psychiatric disorders. An essential component for the safe use of medications is establishing good communication and a trusting relationship with your child's doctor or nurse practitioner. As part of good communication, parents should provide a detailed medical history during the first visit, including current and past medications, and they should notify the doctor of any changes in their child's condition. Parents should feel comfortable asking the doctor questions about the medications.

When you are considering medication, it is important to talk with your child's doctor about the medication's efficacy for the teen's condition. There are some conditions, such as ADHD, that respond very well to medications, whereas others, such as learning disabilities, respond very little or not at all. The expected benefit from a medication must be weighed carefully against its potential risks and side effects. Adolescents taking medications should be monitored closely for problems associated with the medications as well as for exacerbations in the underlying illness. Some medications require monitoring of blood tests, weight, blood pressure, or other parameters to help assure the teen's safety. By working together with a child's doctor,

> **Sidebar 5.2 | Medication Tips for Parents**
>
> ▶ Establish good communications with the prescriber
> ▶ Stick to the monitoring recommendations
> ▶ Do not adjust medications without consultation
> ▶ Maintain consistent medication administration
> ▶ Secure medications
> ▶ Keep track of the medication supply

parents will help to maximize the benefits and minimize the risks associated with medication treatment.

References and Additional Reading

Gibbons, R. D., K. Hur, D. K. Bhaumik, and J. J. Mann. 2006. "The Relationship between Antidepressant Prescription Rates and Rate of Early Adolescent Suicide." *American Journal of Psychiatry* 163: 1898–1904.

Gibbons, R. D., C. H. Brown, K. Hur, S. M. Marcus, D. K. Bhaumik, J. A. Erkens, R. M. Herings, and J. J. Mann. 2007. "Early Evidence on the Effects of Regulators' Suicidality Warnings on SSRI Prescriptions and Suicide in Children and Adolescents." *American Journal of Psychiatry* 164: 1356–1363.

Gould, M. S, B. T. Walsh, J. L. Munfakh, M. Kleinman, N. Duan, M. Olfson, L. Greenhill, and T. Cooper. 2009. "Sudden Death and Use of Stimulant Medications in Youths." *American Journal of Psychiatry* 166: 992–1001.

Perrin, J. M, R. A. Friedman, and T. K. Knilans. 2008. "Black Box Working Group; Section on Cardiology and Cardiac Surgery: Cardiovascular Monitoring and Stimulant Drugs for Attention-Deficit/Hyperactivity Disorder." *Pediatrics* 122: 451–453.

Wilens, T. E. 2009. *Straight Talk about Psychiatric Medications for Kids.* 3rd ed. New York: Guilford.

Part II

Common Psychiatric Problems in Adolescence

Major Depressive Disorder

Depression is one of the most common psychiatric conditions affecting adolescents and may be one of the most devastating. It is estimated that 4 to 8 percent of adolescents are suffering from major depressive disorder at any given time, and by the age of eighteen, about 20 percent of adolescents will have experienced the symptoms of clinical depression. Unfortunately, as common as depression is, it frequently goes unrecognized. Many of the symptoms of depression make it more likely for depressed teens to keep their suffering to themselves. A sense of guilt or worthlessness may make teenagers feel that telling others about their suffering will make them a burden or reveal to others that there is something "wrong" with them. Thus, the outward signs of depression may be subtler than those of many other mental health problems and are often mistaken for the moodiness and behavioral changes that are part of normal adolescent development.

To complicate matters further, depression in adolescents may appear very different from the picture of adult depression that is portrayed in the media. Although teenagers with depression, like adults with the same illness, may seem sad and tearful much of the time, often this sadness is less apparent. Instead, the depressed adolescent may appear more withdrawn, irritable, angry, or easily frustrated.

If depression is so common yet often so hard to identify, how can a parent know if a teen is at risk? As always, do your best to keep lines of communication open with your child. It is essential to recognize a problem. Even when attempts at communication are rejected, which is not unusual at a time when teenagers are struggling to find their independence, the effort is worthwhile. It lets your child know that you are concerned and available. In addition to good communication, it is important for parents as well as those who regularly work with adolescents, such as teachers and coaches, to be familiar with the warning signs of depression so that they may seek help as early as possible.

What Causes Depression?

The causes of depression are complex and not fully understood. Still, there are a number of factors that psychiatrists often classify into three major categories: biological, psychological, and social.

There is strong evidence that depression is in part a biological illness involving abnormal brain functioning. Depression tends to run in families. Your child's

Case Presentation

Melissa was a thin, pale fourteen-year-old girl whose mother brought her to her pediatrician for a routine checkup. During the visit, the pediatrician noticed that Melissa seemed different than he remembered from her last visit. She did not have her usual warm, friendly smile but rather wore a blank look and did not show much expression. For most of the visit, she looked down at the floor and spoke in a soft, barely intelligible voice. When he asked her how she was doing, she muttered "OK, I guess," which was about as long a response as he was able to elicit.

Melissa's mother expressed frustration over her daughter's recent behavior, saying, "She spends all her time in her room. I don't know what she's doing up there." Melissa had always been exceedingly polite and respectful to her parents, but lately she had been snapping angrily over minor things including her mother's gentle request that she pick up her increasingly cluttered room. Melissa's mother reported that she heard Melissa arise in the middle of the night and walk around the house, but during the day she looked tired, with dark circles under her eyes.

When Melissa's mother was asked what she thought could be wrong, she was at a loss. She said, "She might be worried about her grades, which have really taken a hit since she started high school. She was always on the honor roll in junior high. Sometimes I worry about how the divorce affected her, but that was so long ago, and she seemed fine at the time."

After a thorough medical evaluation, the pediatrician found no evidence of a medical problem. Concerned about how Melissa was doing, the pediatrician referred her to a therapist who worked with his practice. After reviewing Melissa's history, the therapist established a diagnosis of major depressive disorder and recommended that Melissa meet with her weekly for psychotherapy. Initially, Melissa resisted. However, she liked the therapist, and with time she felt more comfortable. The therapist helped Melissa negotiate the difficulty of adjusting to a new school and cope with the stress she had about her schoolwork. After several weeks of therapy, Melissa felt less depressed, and she was more hopeful about the future. Her mother reported to her pediatrician, "I feel like I have my daughter back."

risk of developing depression at some point in life is much greater if he or she has a close relative with depression. Researchers studying the genetics of depression have identified several genes that, when present in an abnormal form, appear to predispose an individual to developing depression, particularly when the individual is faced with stressful life events.

The biology of depression seems to involve abnormalities in the functioning of certain neurotransmitters, which are chemical messengers in the brain. The two neurotransmitters with the most evidence for a role in depression are serotonin and norepinephrine. Many of the medications used to treat depression affect these neurotransmitters.

There are a number of psychological factors that may predispose an adolescent to developing depression. These factors include patterns of thinking and behavior that have developed over a person's lifetime. Self-esteem is a psychological factor closely related to depression, with low self-esteem increasing a teen's risk of developing depression. Another psychological factor is called attributional style.

This term refers to how a person tends to view events in his or her life. Someone with a negative attributional style may blame himself when bad things happen in his life, even when those events were out of his control. Over time, this pattern may contribute to depression. But having healthy psychological defenses and good coping skills for dealing with life's inevitable stresses and conflicts may help protect against depression. A goal for psychotherapy in treating depression is to identify whether psychological factors may have played a role in a patient's depression and, if so, to work toward correcting them.

Social factors may also play a critical role in the development of depression. Good relationships with family and friends and a social environment in which a teenager feels appreciated and connected may help protect against depression. Conversely, difficulties in relationships, including a family relationship with a lot of hostility and conflict, may contribute to depression. In those who are at risk, feeling isolated from peers may contribute to depression. Stressful social environments may play a major role in the development of depression. It is not unusual for depression to first strike a teenager following a transition to a new school where he or she does not know anyone. Teens who are struggling with issues related to their sexual identity, such as homosexuality, are also at increased risk for depression, particularly when they fear that their family or their peers may not be accepting of them. Recognizing the social factors that contribute to a teen's depression is important in order to develop an appropriate treatment plan.

Symptoms and Warnings Signs

When psychiatrists and other mental health professionals talk about depression, they are generally referring to the diagnosis of major depressive disorder. This diagnosis is defined according the presence of certain core symptoms (see sidebar 6.1). The *Diagnostic and Statistical Manual of Mental Disorders*, fourth

---

Sidebar 6.1 | Symptoms of Depression

The following are the symptoms that mental health professionals look for to diagnose major depressive disorder. In order to make the diagnosis, these symptoms must be present for at least two weeks and must be causing significant distress or impairment of functioning.

- Depressed or irritable mood most of the time
- Sleep disturbance
- Loss of interest in activities
- Feelings of guilt or worthlessness

- Decrease or increase of energy
- Loss of concentration
- Change in appetite
- Agitation or lethargy
- Suicidal thinking

edition, text revision (DSM-IV-TR) is the most recent edition of the guide that mental health professionals use to agree on the criteria that define a particular illness. The core symptoms of depression, as defined by DSM-IV-TR, are either a depressed or irritable mood most of the time or a loss of interest in or a loss of the ability to get pleasure out of things that a person once enjoyed. Professionals refer to this condition as anhedonia.

In addition to one of the symptoms listed in sidebar 6.1, in order to be diagnosed with depression, the adolescent should demonstrate at least four of the following symptoms (or three if both depressed mood and lack of interest are present): change in appetite; change in sleep patterns; feeling slowed down in either movements, speech, or thoughts or feeling excitable, restless, or agitated; decreased energy; feelings of guilt or worthlessness; difficulty concentrating; or persistent thoughts about death or suicide.

To establish a diagnosis of depression, these symptoms must be present for at least two weeks and cause the teen a significant amount of distress or impairment in functioning, such as dropping grades in school or losing friends. Additionally, the symptoms must not be a result of other factors such as substance abuse, a medical condition, or bereavement after loss of a loved one. (This is not to say that teenagers mourning the loss of a loved one cannot become depressed. See chapter 17 for more discussion of how adolescents handle losses in their lives.)

Although these are the symptoms that psychiatrists and other clinicians use to make the diagnosis of depression, there are other symptoms and warning signs that are associated with depression. These are listed in sidebar 6.2.

Similarly, communication with parents often dramatically changes during the teenage years. The chatty sixth-grader eager to give you a detailed recap of the kickball game at recess may appear to undergo a sudden transformation into a moody middle school student who meets a parent's attempts at conversation

---

Sidebar 6.2 | Warning Signs of Depression

In addition to the core symptoms that make up depression, there are a number of warning signs that should alert adults that an adolescent may be depressed.

- Hypersensitivity to rejection or failure
- Decline in school performance or attendance
- Ceasing to participate in sports, art, or other previously enjoyed activities
- Social isolation
- Frequent physical complaints such as headaches or stomachaches
- Frequent negative statements about oneself (e.g., "I'm worthless")
- Pessimism or frequent expressions of hopelessness
- Talk about or attempts to run away from home
- Self-destructive behavior including cutting or talk about suicide

with grunts and shrugs. Still, this teen is usually interested in talking with someone, even if it is not a parent. Talking less with parents and more with peers, like it or not, is often a normal part of adolescence. But cutting off ties with friends and family alike is usually a warning sign.

How is a parent to know if the symptom their child is experiencing is truly a warning sign of depression or if it is just a part of normal development? Unfortunately, there is no easy formula. Often, it is a matter of the degree and persistence of symptoms. A teenager who displays one or two of the symptoms of depression but appears to be doing well socially and academically is less likely to be depressed than one who has several of the symptoms in a pattern that seems to be worsening and causing increasing difficulty. Ultimately, it is safer to err on the side of caution. It is better to seek advice from a professional only to learn that your child appears to be going through a normal adjustment process than it is to let a problem as potentially severe as depression go unrecognized and untreated.

Getting Help: What to Do If You Are Worried

Talking about the Problem

Suppose your teenager has been showing several of the warning signs: she has been irritable and withdrawn, spending most of her time in her room, and she does not return calls from her friends. She cries easily over little things and complains that she cannot sleep. During the day she is sapped of energy, with dark circles under her eyes. She has gone from a B+ student to getting Cs and Ds. What should you do?

Frequently, the first step toward understanding the problem and obtaining help is to try to communicate with your teen. The feelings of guilt and worthlessness that are part of depression make it difficult to ask for help, but your child may be quietly suffering and hoping that someone will take notice. Parental silence may confirm in the child's mind the thought that nobody really cares.

There is no single approach that works for every teen, but usually it helps to be empathetic and to remove any hint of judgment from your voice. Your child may think that the conversation is really just another attempt to get her to clean up her room or to scare her into getting back on the honor roll. She is more likely to open up if she sees that you are genuinely concerned about her.

In a nonjudgmental way, point out the changes that you have noticed. Ask if she also has noticed these changes. If she has, ask what she thinks is wrong. Be curious. Ask questions. Listen and try not to interrupt. Before speaking again, leave time for silences. Depression may slow down thoughts and speech, and your child may still be trying to answer your questions. If your first attempt at communication has minimal success, do not give up.

If you are able to talk with your child about what is wrong, you have made a big step toward addressing the problem. Determine what your adolescent feels is happening and what he or she thinks would help. Explain your concerns, and discuss your own plan for helping, such as seeking advice from a professional. However, it is not unusual for a teenager to deny that there is a problem, even when it is clear to everyone else that there is one.

Evaluating Depression

It is time to get help if you are concerned that your teenager is depressed. You should seek an evaluation from a clinician who is experienced in diagnosing and treating depression. This may be a pediatrician, a psychiatrist, a clinical psychologist, or a licensed social worker. Ideally, you will have discussed your concerns with your child and explained why you are seeking help, and your child will be open to it. Still, there may be times when your child resists. Do not let this resistance stop you from seeking help. Your child's life may be at stake. (See chapter 3 for advice about how to handle a teenager's resistance to an evaluation.)

How does a clinician evaluate for depression? Depression, like most psychiatric illnesses, is primarily a clinical diagnosis based on symptoms. These symptoms are revealed through a detailed interview with the teen and from information gathered from the important people in the youth's life.

The diagnosis of depression may be made after a single visit, particularly in mild and straightforward cases. Or the initial evaluation may occur over two or more visits. Besides information obtained from the questions, the assessment is also based on the behavior of the teen during the interview. Thus, a psychiatrist might note that the patient speaks very softly and slowly, looks at the floor most of the time, never laughs or smiles, and looks disheveled. Observations such as these may help experienced clinicians confirm the suspected diagnosis.

There is no blood test or brain scan that makes the diagnosis of depression. Still, research has demonstrated certain findings on biological tests that tend to be seen in patients with depression. Studies have shown that depressed patients have lower levels of certain chemicals related to brain function in cerebrospinal fluid (CSF) that surrounds the brain and spinal cord. Other studies using new brain imaging techniques have determined that subjects with depression tend to have different patterns of brain activity. At present, none of these tests is used for the diagnosis of depression.

Testing

When the diagnosis of depression is particularly challenging, psychological testing may be useful. This may occur when other problems, such as a language disorder or another severe psychiatric problem, cloud the picture. Performed by a psychologist with specialized training, testing may involve the use of symptom checklists to inquire about a number of possible symptoms for depression and related problems. The responses of an individual may be compared to a large number of previous test subjects with and without depression. In addition, projective tests may be useful in diagnosing depression. In this type of testing, the teen is asked to give an active answer to a test question or situation, such as completing a sentence or making up a story to go along with a picture. The famous Rorschach inkblot test is one example of a projective test that is still used.

Psychological tests may be very useful in some circumstances, but ultimately they are only a tool. By themselves they cannot make a diagnosis. The results must be analyzed and interpreted by a properly trained professional, and the results must then be understood in the context of the adolescent's life.

Other Problems to Consider

Differential Diagnosis: What Else Might Be Wrong?

A number of other psychological and behavioral problems may look similar to depression, and a thorough evaluation will explore other possible causes for a teen's symptoms before settling on the diagnosis of depression. Correctly identifying the problem is essential to outlining the treatment. Sidebar 6.3 lists conditions that may resemble depression.

There are many sources of stress in the life of an adolescent. At times, dealing with these may feel overwhelming. Teens who are having difficulty adjusting to a change or major stressor in their life may react by showing many of the symptoms of depression. They may have trouble sleeping, difficulty concentrating in school, and appear tearful and sad much of the time. When these symptoms occur in reaction to some identifiable problem in an adolescent's life and the symptoms seem out of proportion to what one may expect in the situation or are causing significant problems, a psychiatrist might make the diagnosis of adjustment disorder. To make this diagnosis, the symptoms must not be so severe that they meet the full criteria for major depressive disorder or any other major psychiatric problem, such as an anxiety disorder. Suicidal thoughts are an indication that the problem is more severe than depression. The symptoms of adjustment disorder begin shortly after the stressor first appears, and unlike depression, they generally resolve within six months after it is gone. (See chapter 17 for discussion of adolescents' reactions to stress and loss.)

> **Sidebar 6.3 | Problems That May Look like Depression**
>
> ► Medical conditions
> ► Reaction to medication
> ► Drug abuse
> ► Dysthymia
> ► Adjustment disorder: difficulty coping with stressors or transitions in one's life
> ► Reaction to loss
> ► Bipolar disorder

Depression in adolescence must also be distinguished from normal bereavement after the loss of a close friend or loved one. Usually these symptoms are part of the normal grieving process. Yet significant losses may trigger an episode of major depression in susceptible individuals. There is a great deal of variability in how people react to a loss, but signs that your teenager could be experiencing more than typical grief and may be depressed include thoughts about death or suicide, excessive and unrelenting feelings of guilt or worthlessness, or major problems that persist for more than two months after the loss.

Medical illnesses, as noted in sidebar 6.4, may cause mood problems and a similar pattern of symptoms that is seen in depression. When symptoms of depression are present but are due to a medical problem, psychiatrists do not give the diagnosis of major depressive disorder. Instead, the condition is given the descriptive label of "mood disorder due to a general medical condition." In this case, the treatment approach may overlap with that used in major depression but should also focus on treating the underlying medical problem. For example, in the case of hypothyroidism, mood symptoms and energy levels usually improve once a regimen of thyroid medication is initiated.

Similarly, as noted in sidebar 6.5, some medications used to treat medical conditions may trigger a depression or cause similar symptoms. For example, corticosteroids, such as prednisone, which are used to treat a number of different inflammatory illnesses, may have dramatic effects on mood and thinking in some people, including symptoms of depression. A detailed medical history including a review of any medications being used should be part of an evaluation for depression.

Whenever an adolescent appears depressed, drug abuse should also be considered. As noted in sidebar 6.6, some commonly abused substances can have a significant impact on mood and behavior, and these effects may mimic depression. Marijuana use may cause drowsiness, poor concentration, and lack of motivation. Repeated use of a substance, such as a steroid to build muscles, may induce a depressed state that persists for weeks or even months after use of the substance is stopped.

A psychiatrist may consider a teen with symptoms of depression as having dysthymia, a term that refers to a less intense but more chronic, smoldering

---

Sidebar 6.4 | Medical Illnesses That May Mimic Symptoms of Depression

▶ Hypothyroidism, hyperthyroidism
▶ Addison's disease
▶ Lyme disease (late phase)
▶ Mononucleosis
▶ Anemia
▶ Lupus

Sidebar 6.5 | Medications That May Trigger an Underlying Depression

▶ Corticosteroids
▶ Interferon alpha
▶ GNRH agonists
▶ Mefloquine
▶ Propranolol and other beta blockers
▶ Isotretinoin (Accutane)

form of depression than major depressive disorder. In dysthymia, there are fewer or less severe symptoms than in major depression, but the symptoms last longer; they must be present for at least one year.

Though bipolar disorder is less common than depression, whenever symptoms of depression are present, it must also be considered as a possible diagnosis, especially when the symptoms are not responding well to treatment. In adults with bipolar disorder, periods of depression alternate with episodes of mania, which include an abnormally

> ### Sidebar 6.6 | Drugs of Abuse Associated with Depression
>
> ▸ Opiates (illicit drugs including heroin and prescription pain medications such as oxycodone)
> ▸ Alcohol
> ▸ Anabolic steroids (used to build muscles by bodybuilders)
> ▸ Cocaine
> ▸ Amphetamines
> ▸ Benzodiazepines (prescription medications such as lorazepam, diazepam, or alprazolam)

high, euphoric mood, a decreased need for sleep, a dramatic increase in energy and activity, very fast thoughts or speech that may be hard to follow, and impulsive or risky behavior with little thought about the consequences. However, teenagers with bipolar disorder do not always follow this pattern. They may not have euphoric mood. Moreover, they may have symptoms of depression and mania that take place at the same time or that alternate more rapidly than in adults.

Comorbidities

Psychiatric illnesses tend to appear in groups. The term *comorbidity* refers to the presence of more than one psychiatric illness at a time. It is important to recognize a comorbid illness when it is present along with depression. An untreated comorbid disorder is one of the most common reasons for the failure of treatment for depression.

Anxiety is among the most common comorbid disorders seen with depression. In fact, the combination of anxiety and depression is so common that some psychiatrists have suggested that anxiety should be included in the criteria for depression, though this has not been done in part to avoid confusing the two distinct (but often overlapping) disorders. If your child has been diagnosed with depression, be on the lookout for symptoms of anxiety (discussed in chapter 8). If you are concerned that your child may have an anxiety disorder, discuss these concerns with your child's psychiatrist or therapist. If possible, provide specific examples of symptoms or problems that you think may be related to your child's anxiety. Addressing anxiety helps to improve depression.

The abuse of alcohol and other drugs is another problem commonly seen in adolescents with depression. This may be a two-way street: adolescents may turn to drugs when they are depressed in a desperate attempt to numb their suffering or self-medicate their symptoms. But many substances may exacerbate depression. Alcohol, among other substances, may interact with psychiatric medications, increasing the risks of adverse effects and preventing a beneficial response. Although it is always important to talk with your teenager about substance use and to look for signs of a problem, recognition and treatment of substance abuse is even more critical with a depressed teen. (See chapter 12 for further discussion).

Treatment

The first steps to helping a teen with depression are to recognize that there is a problem and seek professional help. Generally, the treatment for depression includes psychotherapy and medication. Each of these approaches is effective; there is evidence to suggest that using both medication and therapy together may be more effective than using either alone.

Psychotherapy

There are several different types of psychotherapy that appear to be effective in treating depression. Understanding which kind of psychotherapy is most useful is challenging and a source of some controversy in the field. Many therapists do not stick to one particular model. Rather, they use an eclectic approach, borrowing techniques from a few different schools of psychotherapy and attempting to tailor the treatment according to what works best for an individual. These issues are discussed in chapter 4. But the characteristics of a particular therapist are at least as important, and often much more so, than the type of therapy being performed. The therapy stands the best chance of working if the therapist has a good connection with the teen, listens well to the adolescent and the parents, and communicates clearly.

At times, a very good therapist will not be a good fit for a particular teenager. The therapist's style may clash with the teen's personality, or the teen may have so much trouble feeling comfortable that he or she is unable to move forward with treatment. These issues may be worked through and even be an important part of the treatment. It is not unusual for a teenager to feel at first uncomfortable about participating in therapy. It may take some time to settle into the process. If your teen is unable to become comfortable in therapy after several sessions, it is best to discuss your concerns with the therapist. The therapist may have some thoughts about what is causing the difficulty and suggest how to address it, or the therapist may feel that changing to another therapist is appropriate.

Cognitive Behavioral Therapy. One of the common and effective forms of therapy used to treat depression in adolescents is cognitive behavioral therapy (CBT), which is described in more detail in chapter 4. CBT therapists may work on overly pessimistic thinking about the future, such as "Nothing I try seems to work out, so there's no point in putting any effort into anything," or feeling an excessive sense of personal responsibility for negative events, such as "If I hadn't been such a screw up, my parents wouldn't argue so much."

Because CBT is a highly structured treatment, adolescents may be asked to record activities and thoughts in a journal to help them identify patterns that are contributing to their problems. They may be given homework assignments between sessions. These assignments are aimed at testing out inaccurate negative thoughts, with such assignments as "Start a conversation with the kid whom you sit next to in art class and who always seems to laugh at your jokes." Or they may be aimed at breaking up depressive patterns of behavior, such as by starting an exercise program or scheduling rewarding, pleasurable activities into the teen's routine.

Psychodynamic Psychotherapy. Psychodynamic psychotherapy is a general term used to describe a form of treatment based on the idea that symptoms are produced by the interactions among various forces at work in the mind of the adolescent, many of which may be unconscious (see chapter 4). By talking with the therapist and through the ensuing relationship that is formed, the teen may bring some of these unconscious forces to awareness, opening the door for change.

"Anger turned inward" is one way of understanding depression in the model of psychodynamic psychotherapy. The model suggests that in some cases of depression, the teen has unconscious anger about something but is unable to express this anger toward its original source because of other psychiatric forces at work. For example, an adolescent might harbor anger toward her parents for divorcing when she was a little girl. However, since it has long been important for her to have her parents see her as a good, well-behaved child, it makes it difficult for her to express her angry feelings. So the girl's desire to be seen as good and well behaved comes into conflict with the anger that she is feeling toward her parents. This conflict between unconscious forces may result in her anger being ignored and repressed. But the anger does not disappear. Rather, it remains in the girl's unconscious mind searching for an outlet. If it finds an outlet by the girl's turning her angry feelings toward herself and feeling that she is a bad and worthless person, then depression may be the result. Through psychodynamic therapy, the therapist helps the youth identify how these forces have been at work inside of her and helps her understand a new way to resolve the tension between them.

Psychodynamic psychotherapy is less structured, at least on the surface, than some other therapy, such as CBT. Adolescents may be asked to talk about whatever is on their mind. This, in turn, gives the therapist a better understanding of the teen's feelings and conflicts. It may seem to adolescents and their parents that the treatment has no clear agenda, particularly in the beginning, when the therapist is trying to build an understanding of the teen and the teen is trying to feel comfortable. Teenagers may complain that they do not understand how the talking they do in therapy is supposed to help. Given time, psychodynamic psychotherapy may be a powerful tool with lifelong benefits.

Other Therapies for Depression. Interpersonal psychotherapy (IPT) focuses on improving teens' symptoms by improving and strengthening their relationships. Supportive psychotherapy bolsters their defenses, encourages the use of existing supports, and takes a practical, problem-solving approach to negotiate day-to-day challenges.

Although therapists may identify themselves as belonging primarily to one school or another, in practice they may take a more eclectic approach, borrowing techniques from different schools at various times in the treatment according to the needs of the child. Furthermore, the distinctions between different forms of therapy are often not as clear-cut in the real world as they appear in the textbooks.

Medication

One of the most difficult decisions that parents of a depressed teenager must face is whether to use medication as part of their child's treatment. Medication may be a very effective weapon in the fight against depression. Yet, many parents are concerned about possible side effects or are uncomfortable with the idea of having their child take medication for a psychiatric problem. So how do you know if medication is the right choice for your child?

There is no clear checklist of symptoms that can determine when a particular adolescent should take medication for depression. For mild to moderate cases of depression, in which a teenager is suffering but the symptoms are not so severe that they are having a dramatic impact on the teen's ability to function, many psychiatrists would suggest first trying a course of psychotherapy. If it seems that therapy alone is not working, medication may be added to the treatment. In more severe cases of depression, medication should be considered earlier in the treatment. Signs that treatment with medication may be indicated are noted in sidebar 6.7.

Medications used to treat depression are discussed in chapter 5. Most often, the first-line medication for depression in adolescents is a group of drugs called selective serotonin reuptake inhibitors (SSRIs). These medications are generally quite effective for depression and are usually well tolerated with few side effects. Compared to older medications, such as tricyclic antidepressants, they are safer when taken in large amounts, such as in a suicide attempt.

Any medication can have side effects, and the most common side effects that occur with SSRIs are gastrointestinal complaints including upset stomach, decreased appetite, dry mouth, or constipation. Headache and dizziness are also frequently reported. Some teens taking SSRIs complain of feeling drowsy, whereas

---

Sidebar 6.7 | Indications That Medication May Be Helpful for Depression

▶ Symptoms of depression are so severe that they are significantly interfering with the teen's functioning and healthy development

▶ The adolescent's safety is threatened as a result of depression, which includes thoughts of suicide or acts of self-harm

▶ The child continues to be depressed despite a good attempt at treatment with psychotherapy

▶ The teen is becoming depressed again after having past episodes of severe depression, requiring hospitalization or resulting in a suicide attempt

---

others may experience restlessness, nervousness, or difficulty sleeping. If the teen experiences drowsiness, then the medication can be taken before bedtime; conversely, if the teen experiences insomnia, then the medication can be taken in the morning.

In some teens, a rare but serious concern in using SSRIs is the risk of activation, a term used by psychiatrists to describe a pattern of extreme restlessness, acute anxiety, agitation, and/or insomnia that occurs in rare cases when an adolescent begins taking an SSRI. Activation has the potential to trigger a depressed adolescent to attempt suicide or to act impulsively or dangerously. Adolescents with undiagnosed bipolar disorder are particularly at risk for becoming activated by SSRIs. In these patients, SSRIs may cause a manic episode or rapid switching between mood states. Inform your doctor right away if your child experiences dramatic behavioral changes after starting an SSRI, including insomnia, significantly increased energy or activity, restlessness (such as pacing or an inability to sit still), rapid and excessive talking, or increased impulsivity.

Media attention recently has focused on the controversy surrounding the use of SSRIs and other antidepressants in adolescents and concerns about suicidal ideation (see chapter 5 for additional information). Several studies have shown that there appears to be a small but significant increase in risk for having suicidal thoughts while on antidepressants. Why antidepressants may cause a small number of adolescents to be more likely to have these thoughts is unclear and is the subject of some debate. It is possible that some of these youth were experiencing the kind of activation just described. Because these effects are relatively rare and some teens with depression experience suicidal thoughts as part of their illness, this issue is difficult to study and remains the subject of some controversy.

It appears that the overall number of adolescents who have suicidal thoughts related to antidepressant use is small. When investigators reviewed information from many studies of antidepressant use in adolescents, they found that patients treated with one of these medications had a 4 percent risk of having suicidal thoughts, compared to 2 percent of patients who received a placebo. In this analysis, there did not appear to be any increased risk of attempting suicide in patients treated with antidepressants, but whether there is a small increase in the risk of suicide attempts after starting an antidepressant remains a question that is being examined. Because of the concerns about these findings, in 2004, the Food and Drug Administration issued a black box warning for SSRIs and some related medications to warn patients and parents about this issue.

So how is a parent to interpret these concerns about antidepressants? Parents should understand that antidepressants may be very effective in treating depression, but like most medications, they carry some degree of risk and should be used with caution. The best way to manage this risk is by close monitoring. When adverse reactions do occur, they usually occur early in treatment. To assess for problems, adolescents who are started on an antidepressant should be seen by their doctor frequently. Parents should closely monitor their children for any changes in behavior and notify the doctor immediately if there are concerns.

Other Treatments: Groups, Family Therapy, Activities

Although psychotherapy and medication are the cornerstones of treatment for depression in adolescents, there are other options. In many cases, problems within the family play a big role in the development of a teenager's depression. When this is true, family therapy is often an essential part of treatment, leading not only to improvement of the teen's depression but also to improved relationships in the family.

By recognizing that there are other kids with similar problems, group therapy may help depressed teens feel less isolated. Teenagers may learn how their peers worked through similar problems. For adolescents with social difficulties, a group gives them a safe place to improve their social skills and build their confidence in interacting with their peers.

Since teenagers spend much of their time in school, to determine whether issues at school are contributing to the depression, it is important to assess the child's school environment. If the school environment is an issue, interventions may range from the relatively minor, such as having your child meet a counselor at the school, to major changes, such as placement in a therapeutic school for adolescents with severe emotional problems. (See chapter 10 for further discussion of the role of schools in psychiatric treatment.)

For every depressed teen, psychological education is an essential part of treatment. Teenagers who understand their illness are more likely to comply with treatment and to seek help. In addition, family members should educate themselves about depression and its treatment. Parents are then better equipped to assist their children through the challenges they face together and may be able to recognize warning signs of a relapse. Also, having a depressed brother or sister may be a scary and overwhelming experience. Teaching your other children about depression in a way that is appropriate for their developmental level may relieve their anxiety, assist them in understanding what is happening, and reduce possible resentment toward a sibling who is receiving extra attention.

To learn about depression, read books such as this one and have a discussion with your child's therapist. Family support groups are another valuable resource. Some Internet resources are a great source of information, but be careful to check the source. Appendix A of this book provides a list of useful resources.

Electroconvulsive Therapy

Electroconvulsive therapy (ECT) involves the induction of a seizure for therapeutic reasons and under controlled circumstances. Although it is not commonly used in adolescents, it is sometimes considered in cases of severe depression that have not responded to other treatments.

Commonly called shock therapy, this therapy is imagined by many people as a brutal, extreme form of treatment. This view is partly based on dramatized portrayals of the procedure in books, movies, and television shows. However, use of modern anesthesia techniques, including medications that temporarily paralyze the patient to prevent the limbs from convulsing as they typically do in a generalized seizure, have made this procedure much easier on patients.

In adults, ECT has been demonstrated to be a highly effective treatment for depression and some other psychiatric disorders. Use of ECT in adolescents has not been studied as extensively. Still, it is sometimes used to treat adolescents under unusual circumstances, such as when an adolescent's symptoms have not responded to multiple medication trials or when an adolescent is unable to take medications. Although use of ECT is not the draconian procedure that many people imagine, it carries significant risks and side effects. These include memory loss for events around the time of the procedure and a brief period of confusion after the procedure. If considering ECT, parents should have a detailed discussion with their psychiatrist including the risks and benefits of ECT and other available treatment options for their adolescent. All teens should have a thorough medical evaluation before undergoing ECT to rule out medical conditions such as a bleeding disorder or a cardiac arrhythmia that would place them at greater risk for complications.

Prognosis

With proper treatment, nearly all adolescents with depression will recover. Still, you should realize that treatment of depression takes time, regardless of whether the treatment involves medication, therapy, or both. Progress is usually measured in weeks and months. Most studies of successful treatment interventions show improvement in a majority of teens by twelve weeks of treatment, with the average length of the depressive episode being around eight months. The time it takes for recovery may vary from one adolescent to another. A number of factors may contribute to a longer recovery time, including more severe illness, ongoing stressors in the teenager's life, and the presence of comorbid psychiatric conditions, such as an eating disorder or an anxiety disorder.

Although depression usually responds well to treatment, unfortunately it is an illness with a tendency to reappear. It is estimated that somewhere between 30 and 70 percent of teenagers treated for depression will have a recurrence. With each episode of depression, the risk of having future episodes increases. Because many recurrences of depression follow closely on the heels of a previous episode, it is recommended that treatment for depression continue for at least six to nine months after an episode has ended. Teenagers who are at particularly high risk for having a relapse may need longer treatment.

Conclusion

During adolescence, depression is a common but serious problem. It is an illness that affects mood, sleep, energy, appetite, and ability to concentrate. The appearance of depression may be different in teenagers than in adults, with some symptoms such as irritability, anger, or low tolerance for frustration seeming more obvious than sadness. Left untreated, depression can have a dramatic impact on an adolescent's ability to function in almost all areas of life, and it places a teen at significant risk for attempting suicide. Treatment for adolescent depression often involves psychotherapy and, at times, medication. Intervention in other areas of a youth's life, such as family therapy and modifications to an educational program, are frequently an important part of treatment. Although depression usually responds well to treatment, it has a tendency to reappear. On a long-term basis, the teen requires close monitoring for warning signs of a reemerging depression.

References and Additional Reading

American Psychiatric Association. 2000. *Diagnostic and Statistical Manual of Mental Disorders,* 4th ed., text revision (DSM-IV-TR). Washington, DC: American Psychiatric Association.

Beresin, B., D. DeLuca, R. Falzone, M. Goldstein, L. Kutner, C. Olson, S. Schlozman, and D. Warner. 2006. "Diagnosing Adolescent Depression in Pediatric Practice." Video. Available at http://www.massgeneral.org/children/specialtiesandservices/adolescent_medicine/default.aspx.

Cheung, A. H., R. A. Zuckerbrot, P. S. Jensen, K. Ghalib, D. Laraque, R.E.K. Stein, and GLAD-PC Steering Group. 2007. "Guidelines for Adolescent Depression in Primary Care (GLAD-PC): II. Treatment and Ongoing Management." *Pediatrics* 120: e1313–e1326.

Cheung, A. H., C. S. Dewa, A. J. Levitt, and R. A. Zuckerbrot. 2008. "Pediatric Depressive Disorders: Management Priorities in Primary Care." *Current Opinion in Pediatrics* 20: 551–559.

Fergusson, D. M., L. J. Horwood, E. M. Ridder, and A. L. Beautrais. 2005. "Sexual Orientation and Mental Health in a Birth Cohort of Young Adults." *Psychological Medicine* 35: 971–981.

7 Bipolar Disorder

Bipolar disorder, formerly known as manic-depressive disorder, is estimated to affect more than five million adults in the United States, or 2.6 percent of the population in a given year. Until recently, it was believed to be relatively rare in children and adolescents. Over the past decade, however, the number of diagnoses of bipolar disorder made in younger patients has increased dramatically. There is some controversy surrounding this trend, and many people in both medicine and the media have argued that bipolar disorder is being overdiagnosed in teenagers. Others have countered that bipolar disorder is often overlooked and left untreated in teenagers because of difficulties in making the diagnosis. These questions remain an area of active research and debate within the field of psychiatry. Yet, it is clear that bipolar disorder can be a severe illness, which, if not properly diagnosed and treated, can have a devastating impact on teens and their families.

Symptoms and Warning Signs

One of the reasons for the increasing rate of bipolar disorder diagnoses in teenagers is a growing awareness among psychiatrists that the symptoms of this illness tend to manifest themselves differently in teenagers than they do in adults,

---

Sidebar 7.1 | Symptoms of Mania

- A period of abnormally elevated or irritable mood lasting at least one week, during which at least three of the following are present (or four if mood is irritable):
  - Inflated self-esteem or grandiosity
  - Decreased need for sleep
  - More talkative than usual
  - Flight of ideas or feeling that thoughts are racing
  - Distractibility
  - Increase in goal-directed activity or psychomotor agitation
- Excessive involvement in pleasurable activities with a high potential for painful consequences
- The mood disturbance is sufficiently severe to cause marked impairment in functioning or in relationships or to require hospitalization to prevent harm to self or others
- The symptoms are not the result of another psychiatric disturbance, effects from substance abuse, or a medical condition

Case Presentation

Bill was a sixteen-year-old boy whose parents took him for a psychiatric evaluation after becoming concerned by his increasingly erratic behavior. His parents reported that over the past several months, Bill had been flying off the handle with little or no provocation, becoming extremely angry and often yelling and screaming. These outbursts were happening with increasing frequency, such that they were now a nightly occurrence that his parents had come to dread. His parents had become frightened by his outbursts, as he appeared more aggressive and threatening. Over the past few weeks he punched two holes in the wall of his bedroom and broke his own laptop computer by throwing it against the wall in a fit of anger. In between his outbursts, Bill often appeared quite sad and depressed. On a few occasions his parents heard him make remarks such as "I have nothing to live for" and "My life is pointless. I wish I was dead."

Bill was also engaging in risky behaviors that worried his parents. When this behavior began, his parents thought that he was participating in "normal teenage rebellion," staying out past his curfew and getting a speeding ticket for driving fifty miles per hour in a twenty-five-mile-per-hour zone. However, even after he was grounded, Bill's behavior became increasingly dangerous. He started sneaking out of the house late at night, recently having been brought home by the police after being found wandering around a bus station late at night in a bad neighborhood. When his parents expressed concern about his safety, he told them, "Nobody would mess with me." His father lamented, "We have to watch him around the clock. We hear him all night walking around the house. . . . It's like he doesn't need to sleep anymore."

During the evaluation, Bill was talking extremely fast and shaking his legs, looking like he would rather be pacing around the room than sitting in a chair. Bill said that he had been feeling really down sometimes lately and that he had felt like his life was not worth living. He also acknowledged getting angered easily and being provoked especially by his parents and teachers. He reported feeling as if his thoughts were "going really, really fast," and he added, "I don't think other people can keep up with me." When asked about why his grades had dropped from a B to a D average, he said, "I'm too smart for school. That stuff is so boring. I don't see why I should have to sit through it."

The psychiatrist evaluating Bill thought that he might be suffering from bipolar disorder, with mixed features of both mania and depression. Because the psychiatrist was also concerned about Bill's safety, given his suicidal thoughts and recent dangerous behavior, he arranged to have Bill admitted to an adolescent psychiatric unit at the hospital. After a thorough evaluation at the hospital, Bill was diagnosed with bipolar disorder and started on a medication to stabilize his mood. After his discharge from the hospital, he began seeing a therapist on weekly basis. Through a combination of medication and therapy, Bill began doing much better. His mood improved, his anger outbursts became much less intense and frequent, his sleep patterns became more regular, and he appeared more in control of himself and his behavior.

particularly when they begin in early adolescence. As the condition's former name, manic-depressive disorder, implies, bipolar disorder typically involves episodes of depression like those that occur in major depressive disorder (described in chapter 6), as well as episodes of mania. Symptoms of a manic episode and the criteria that psychiatrists use to diagnose mania are listed in sidebar 7.1. In addition to these criteria, sidebar 7.2 lists the warning signs that parents should

Sidebar 7.2 | Warning Signs of Bipolar Disorder

- ► Extremely irritable mood.
- ► Severe outbursts of anger or aggression.
- ► Decreased need for sleep over a several-day period.
- ► Feelings of grandiosity, e.g., a sense of having special powers or abilities. These feelings may simply be exaggerated, such as believing that one can beat up the toughest kid in school, or may be bizarre, such as believing one can fly or read minds.
- ► Increased impulsivity, i.e., taking actions without considering the consequences.
- ► Periods of dramatically increased energy or activity, e.g., starting multiple, seemingly unrealistic projects at once.
- ► Agitation or inability to keep still.
- ► Risk-taking behavior such as driving fast or recklessly.
- ► Talking rapidly, loudly, and/or excessively.
- ► Feeling that one's thoughts are racing or having thoughts that seem disjointed.
- ► Hearing voices, having paranoid thoughts, or other psychotic symptoms. (These are not symptoms of bipolar disorder, but psychotic symptoms often accompany manic episodes in adolescents.)

look for if they are concerned that their teem may have bipolar disorder. Still, it is important to note that these symptoms are not specific to bipolar disorder but may occur in a variety of different psychiatric conditions. Thus, the presence of these warning symptoms does not suggest that a child has bipolar disorder, only that there is a problem that is in need of evaluation, and that bipolar disorder should be considered as a possibility.

The adult version of bipolar disorder typically has its onset in the late teens to early twenties, and those who have the disorder usually suffer from distinct episodes of depression and mania, with any one episode lasting for a period of several weeks to a few months. Recent research involving children and younger adolescents with bipolar disorder has shown that the pattern of symptoms that is typical in adults, with episodes of depression and mania that are clearly separated from each other, is much less common in younger patients. Rather, adolescents with bipolar disorder frequently have symptoms of both depression and mania occurring at the same time. Psychiatrists refer to this condition as a mixed mood state, as seen in the boy in the case presentation. Adolescents, particularly those in whom the disease presents in early adolescence, may also be more prone to rapid cycling, in which cycles of mania and depression occur over short periods of time, such as a few days or even several hours, rather than over the usual pattern of several weeks. Furthermore, adolescents with bipolar disorder may have a more chronic course, having symptoms over long periods of time without the periods of recovery between mood episodes that is often seen in adults with bipolar disorder.

Another important difference between bipolar disorder in adults and in adolescents involves the symptoms that make up a manic episode. Adults often feel a sense of emotional high or euphoria during a manic state, feeling "almost too good," as some patients describe it. This kind of elevated mood is much less common in adolescents with bipolar disorder. Rather, adolescents who are in a manic state tend to present with an angry, irritable mood. The degree of irritability involved in a manic episode goes far beyond the typical moodiness often seen in teenagers. During a manic episode, an adolescent may go into a rage over a seemingly minor event or comment, yelling, punching walls or throwing things, making threats, or even assaulting friends or family members.

Getting Help: What to Do If You Are Worried

If you are concerned that your child might have bipolar disorder, a thorough evaluation is the best first step toward getting the help your family needs. The evaluation should be performed by a clinician with experience in evaluating and treating adolescent bipolar disorder, which often means a referral to a child and adolescent psychiatrist. Although many pediatricians are comfortable diagnosing conditions such as ADHD or depression, the complexities involved in the diagnosis of bipolar disorder require the attention of a specialist in adolescent mental health. (See chapter 3 for advice on finding a psychiatrist for your teenager.)

As with most psychiatric disorders, there is no blood test or brain scan that can be used to diagnose bipolar disorder. Instead, the diagnosis of bipolar disorder is made by a clinician reviewing a thorough history of the symptoms that a child has been experiencing. Because adolescent bipolar disorder may resemble other psychiatric problems, it is a diagnostic challenge for even the most experienced clinicians. Thus, a psychiatrist often is not able to make a quick diagnosis. Generally only the most clear-cut cases can be diagnosed in a single visit. More often, the evaluation is extended over two or more visits during which the psychiatrist gathers information from the adolescent, the family, and other

---

Sidebar 7.3 | Differences between Adult and Pediatric/Adolescent Bipolar Disorder

► Mixed mood states (combined manic and depressive symptoms occurring together) are more common in pediatric bipolar disorder
► Elevated or euphoric mood is less common and extreme irritability more common in pediatric bipolar disorder
► Rapid cycling (shifting rapidly between manic and depressed states) is more common in pediatric bipolar disorder
► Mood disturbance in pediatric bipolar disorder may be more chronic and less episodic

important people in the adolescent's life, such as teachers, coaches, and pediatricians. Talking to people outside the family may be particularly helpful in learning how a teen behaves in settings outside the home, such as at school or during sports or other activities.

In many cases, the diagnosis of bipolar disorder remains unclear even after a thorough evaluation over several sessions. This can be frustrating for parents who are feeling desperate for a clear explanation of what is happening with their child. However, parents should be aware that this not unusual. Do not lose faith in your psychiatrist simply because he or she is unable to tell you with absolute certainty after only a few meetings whether your child has bipolar disorder. Most often, a psychiatrist needs to work with an adolescent over an extended period of time, observing symptoms and the response to treatment, before reaching a diagnosis. This is particularly the case early in the course of bipolar disorder, when symptoms are still evolving and may initially appear as depression.

In some cases of suspected bipolar disorder that are presenting a diagnostic challenge to a psychiatrist, neuropsychiatric testing may be helpful (see chapter 3 for a discussion of the role of neuropsychiatric testing in an evaluation). Although this testing alone cannot confirm or rule out a diagnosis of bipolar disorder, it may help in the process by identifying symptoms of a mood disorder that might otherwise be difficult to detect or by identifying other difficulties, such as attention problems or developmental delay, which could be mimicking symptoms of bipolar disorder.

The Parents' Role in Evaluating Bipolar Disorder

Given the challenges of diagnosing bipolar disorder in adolescents, what can a parent do to help in the process? Assisting the psychiatrist with a detailed history is most useful. It may help to allow some time before an evaluation to take notes about the problems you would like to discuss. In talking with the psychiatrist, try to avoid using jargon or terms that are vague or technical. For example, saying that your child is "explosive" or "grandiose" may be difficult for the psychiatrist to interpret, since these terms might mean different things to different people. In contrast, detailed and specific descriptions of your adolescent's behaviors that are concerning to you go a long way toward helping the psychiatrist make an accurate diagnosis. If some of the symptoms are episodic, such as outbursts of anger and aggression, it is helpful if you can provide information about how long these episodes last and how often they occur. Be sure to report any patterns in your child's symptoms that you might have noticed, such as your child's seeming more depressed in the winter months or anger outbursts that appear to happen only when discussing certain topics. Some psychiatrists will ask patients and parents to keep track of symptoms using mood charts, symptom logs, or journals. These tools may be helpful in identifying patterns of behavior. There are many versions of mood charts available online, through websites devoted to families affected by bipolar disorder (see appendix A for a listing of resources for families).

What If You Are Not Sure about the Diagnosis Your Doctor Has Made?

There is currently a great deal of controversy surrounding bipolar disorder in children and adolescents, which may place parents in a difficult position. In part, this controversy is related to the differences between the classic, adult version of bipolar disorder, for which the diagnostic criteria were developed, and the adolescent version of the disorder. The atypical nature of the symptoms in juvenile bipolar disorder, with more mixed episodes, rapid cycling, and irritability, both makes the diagnosis challenging and contributes further to the controversy. In addition, much of the research in this area has emerged only in the past decade, meaning that there are still many questions left to be answered, including the course that bipolar disorder takes from the diagnosis in adolescence through adulthood. The lack of consensus in the field of psychiatry regarding how common the illness is and how exactly it should be defined in younger patients means that there are differences between individual psychiatrists in the frequency that they make a diagnosis of bipolar disorder. Some child psychiatrists make the diagnosis very rarely and only in the clearest cases, and others are more inclined to make the diagnosis even though there is some degree of uncertainty. So what should a parent do?

If the possibility of bipolar disorder has been raised, and you are having doubts about your doctor's position, the best first step is to speak frankly to the doctor about your concerns. It is perfectly reasonable to ask the psychiatrist to explain in detail the reasons that he or she does or does not believe your child has bipolar disorder, including the symptoms that seem to fit with the diagnosis. It may be useful to ask your doctor about his or her own perspective on the controversy surrounding bipolar disorder and how he or she approaches the issue. Although you are in the office to help your child, not to debate a complex social and scientific issue, it is important to understand your doctor's perspective and potential biases. This is more than just a theoretical concern, as a psychiatrist who is biased against the diagnosis might be slow to recognize the condition, delaying the initiation of treatments that may help restore stability. Conversely, a psychiatrist who is biased in favor of diagnosing bipolar disorder might err on the side of making this diagnosis and starting treatments, including mood-stabilizing medications, that are unlikely to be effective and may cause harmful side effects if the symptoms are being caused by other problems.

After you have had an open discussion with the doctor, and if you still have doubts about the diagnosis, it is reasonable to seek a second opinion. If you do decide to seek a second opinion, it is generally best to mention to your primary doctor that you are doing so. Most psychiatrists are happy to receive input from another psychiatrist on a challenging case.

Other Problems to Consider

Differential Diagnosis: What Else Might Be Wrong?

A number of other psychiatric and medical problems as well as medications may present symptoms that resemble bipolar disorder, and these are listed in sidebar 7.4. Major depression (discussed in chapter 6) may be particularly difficult to distinguish from bipolar disorder in teens. This is in part because depressive symptoms are, by definition, part of the diagnosis of bipolar disorder. It is the presence of manic symptoms, such as racing thoughts and speech, agitated behavior, grandiose ideas, and a reduced need for sleep that allows a psychiatrist to make the diagnosis of bipolar disorder instead of depression. It is important to note that depression is also associated with sleep disruption, but in depression teenagers tend to have trouble sleeping despite feeling tired, whereas in mania they feel that they need little or no sleep, without slowing at all.

Depressed teenagers often show a great deal of irritability and anger to the outside world. Irritability and anger are also common manifestations of bipolar disorder, though the irritability associated with bipolar disorder tends to be more extreme. For example, a depressed teen might overreact to a minor request

---

Sidebar 7.4 | Conditions That May Be Mistaken for Bipolar Disorder

Mental Health Disorders
- ▶ Major depressive disorder
- ▶ Substance abuse
- ▶ Attention-deficit/hyperactivity disorder
- ▶ Behavior disorders:
  - ▶ Oppositional defiant disorder
  - ▶ Conduct disorder

Medications
- ▶ Corticosteroids
- ▶ Decongestants
- ▶ Anticonvulsants
- ▶ Tricyclic antidepressants

Medical Conditions
- ▶ Hyperthyroidism
- ▶ Seizure disorder
- ▶ Addison's disease
- ▶ Cushing's disease
- ▶ Vitamin B12 deficiency
- ▶ Systemic lupus erythematosus
- ▶ Huntington's disease
- ▶ HIV infection
- ▶ Herpes simplex encephalitis
- ▶ Brain tumor

(such as asking him to clean his room) with a few choice remarks and a slammed door. But a teen with bipolar disorder might have a dramatic outburst, shouting, becoming out of control, and making the family feel unsafe. These examples are oversimplified generalizations, of course, but they are meant to illustrate the fact that there is overlap in some of the symptoms of depression and bipolar disorder. Further, there may be differences in the particular quality of these symptoms that your psychiatrist may need to sort out in order to help distinguish between the two conditions.

Substance abuse is another common problem in adolescents that may cause symptoms that can be mistaken for bipolar disorder. Alcohol and marijuana may cause erratic behavior, impulsivity, and dramatic shifts in mood, activity, and energy level. Use of cocaine may mimic symptoms of mania, with feelings of euphoria, rapid thoughts and speech, increased activity, and grandiose ideas. Illicit use of stimulants, such as amphetamines, may have similar effects. Crystal methamphetamine, or crystal meth, is an illicit, potent, and highly addictive form of amphetamine that is a growing problem in many parts of the United States among adolescents and adults. Crystal meth intoxication leads to dramatic mood swings, erratic and sometimes violent behavior, and bursts of increased activity, followed by a dramatic crash during withdrawal that can resemble depression. Users of crystal meth may become paranoid, and repeated use can lead to psychotic symptoms that may persist long after use of the drug has stopped. If bipolar disorder is a suspected diagnosis, it is important to rule out substance abuse as the cause of your child's symptoms. This is not always straightforward, because substance abuse is often a comorbid problem in teens with bipolar disorder, as many will turn to substances in an effort to self-medicate the distress they are feeling.

Attention-deficit/hyperactivity disorder (ADHD), which is discussed in chapter 11, is another condition that may resemble some aspects of bipolar disorder. Symptoms of distractibility and hyperactivity are common to both conditions. Adolescents with ADHD may also show a low frustration tolerance and a tendency to get upset or even have a meltdown over small things, symptoms that may resemble the irritability of mania. However, in mania the outbursts tend to be much more extreme. Although ADHD can be an exasperating problem that may affect a teenager's mood, it is generally not associated with the severe disruption in mood that is seen in bipolar disorder. Moreover, symptoms of bipolar disorder are often episodic and fluctuating, whereas ADHD symptoms, though they may be more evident in some settings than in others, tend to remain fairly constant over time.

Behavioral disorders such as oppositional defiant disorder (ODD) and conduct disorder may also be mistaken for bipolar disorder and have several overlapping symptoms. These problems are discussed in detail in chapter 14. ODD is a disorder of childhood and adolescence that is defined by a pattern of negative, hostile, and defiant behavior over a sustained period of time. Similar to people with bipolar disorder, people with ODD may be argumentative, be easily annoyed, and have a short temper. Patients with conduct disorder also may demonstrate these characteristics, as well as a pattern of repeatedly breaking rules and showing disregard for the rights of others. Adolescents with conduct disorder may run away from home, deliberately destroy property, or commit crimes such as shoplifting or breaking into houses. On the surface, these behaviors can resemble the kind of risky, impulsive behaviors that are seen in bipolar disorder. When ODD or conduct disorder occurs alone, the adolescent does not demonstrate the dramatic disturbance of mood, with periods of depression, extreme irritability, or explosive outbursts, that are seen in bipolar disorder. This distinction may be difficult to make, even for a psychiatrist. Moreover, ODD and conduct disorder frequently occur with bipolar disorder as comorbid conditions, further clouding the diagnostic picture. This is one of the many challenges that make bipolar disorder a difficult condition to diagnose during adolescence, and it is one of the reasons why a thorough evaluation with a psychiatrist is necessary.

In rare cases, a medical condition may cause a severe disruption in mood resembling bipolar disorder. Some conditions may even cause mania. Hyperthyroidism, for example, may lead to excessive activity and an agitated state. Hormonal problems, including Cushing's disease and Addison's disease, may produce symptoms similar to bipolar disorder. Neurological disease that includes brain tumors and seizure disorders may cause, however rarely, changes in personality. The legitimate use of medications including corticosteroids, decongestants, anticonvulsants, and tricyclic antidepressants has been known to affect mood in this way in some patients. As with all psychiatric conditions, a thorough medical history is an essential part of an evaluation for suspected bipolar disorder. Consultation with a pediatrician or adolescent medicine specialist may also be necessary to rule out these or other medical conditions.

Comorbidities

There are several comorbid disorders that commonly occur together with bipolar disorder. As mentioned previously, substance abuse is fairly common in adolescents who also have bipolar disorder. Some of these comorbid disorders are also in the differential diagnosis of bipolar disorder, which can make the diagnosis that much more challenging. Identifying and treating a comorbid psychiatric condition may be an essential part of treatment for bipolar disorder. Unrecognized comorbid disorders may exacerbate mood symptoms in bipolar disorder and may be an obstacle in the path to stability.

Finally, bipolar disorder must be distinguished from the developmentally normal behaviors of adolescence. As part of healthy development, most teens show some degree of increased risk-taking behavior, a sense of invulnerability, and a tendency to act without always thinking through the long-term consequences. In a healthy teen, these tendencies may occasionally cause problems. When these behaviors are related to a normal developmental process, they are nowhere near the extremes that are seen in bipolar disorder. Behaviors that are part of a normal developmental process should not cause the degree of dysfunction and distress in nearly every area of a teen's life that is common in bipolar disorder. At times, this distinction may be hard for parents to make. If there is any question as to whether your child's problems are outside the range of normal development, it is reasonable to consult a professional.

Treatment

Treatment for bipolar disorder usually involves a combination of medications and psychotherapy. The primary goal of medication treatment is to reduce symptoms of mania and depression, helping to restore stability to the adolescent's life. When these symptoms are in remission, the goal shifts to maintaining stability and preventing future relapses.

Medications

Several different kinds of medications are commonly used in the treatment of adolescent bipolar disorder. While some people with bipolar disorder may require only a single medication to help them maintain a healthy mood and safely negotiate adolescence, it is not unusual for some people to require a combination of two or more medications to maintain their stability. A combination of medications may be used to treat different aspects of the illness, such as reducing manic symptoms with a medication such as lithium while treating depressive symptoms with a medication such as buproprion. Also, a combination of medications such as valproic acid and risperidone may be more effective than either one alone. The three general classes of medication that are commonly used to treat bipolar disorder are mood stabilizers (including the anticonvulsants), atypical antipsychotics, and antidepressants.

As the name implies, mood stabilizers are used to reduce symptoms of both mania and depression and to help maintain the adolescent's mood in a stable state between these dangerous extremes. Commonly used mood stabilizers include lithium (Lithobid, Eskalith, and others), valproic acid (Depakote), and several different anticonvulsant medications including carbemazepine (Tegretol), oxcarbazepine (Trileptal), and lamotrigine (Lamictal). These medications are discussed individually in more detail in chapter 5. It is important to note that in order to ensure safety, several of these medications, including lithium, valproic acid, and carbemazepine, require periodic monitoring of blood levels. But although these medications may be very effective in treating bipolar disorder, they carry some risk of adverse effects. Lithium, for example, may cause damage to the kidneys and thyroid gland in some patients. Valproic acid may cause liver damage; and lamotrigine has been associated with a rash that, in very rare cases, can progress to a life-threatening condition. Close monitoring by a psychiatrist, pediatrician, or adolescent medicine specialist that includes blood tests such as liver enzymes or thyroid levels is necessary to minimize the risk of these adverse effects or to identify them at the earliest stage.

A group of relatively new medications collectively called atypical antipsychotics has also been shown to be effective in stabilizing mood in adolescent bipolar disorder. Medications in this class include risperidone (Risperdal), aripiprazole (Abilify), quetiapine (Seroquel), and olanzapine (Zyprexa). Atypical antipsychotics may be particularly useful in helping to stabilize mood when mood episodes tend to be mixed with symptoms of mania and depression occurring together, as is often the case in adolescents. Blood levels of these medications do not need to be monitored. Because of their efficacy and the potential to use them safely without checking blood levels, many psychiatrists are now using atypical antipsychotics as a first-line treatment for mood symptoms in adolescent bipolar disorder. These medications may also be combined with mood stabilizers in cases that are difficult to treat and may work synergistically to reduce mood symptoms. However, treatment with atypical antipsychotics is not risk free, as there are potentially significant adverse effects including weight gain, sedation, and, with prolonged treatment, increased risk of diabetes mellitus and elevated cholesterol in the blood. (See chapter 5 for more detailed description of atypical antipsychotics and their potential side effects.)

Many medications used to treat bipolar disorder are better at reducing the highs of mania than they are at improving the lows of depression. Treating depression associated with bipolar disorder is essential. Teens with untreated depression may experience undue suffering and are at risk for suicide. Mood stabilizers and atypical antipsychotics by themselves may not be enough to address depressive episodes associated with bipolar disorder. For this reason, some teens require treatment with antidepressants as well. This may be a risky proposition because antidepressants have the potential to induce manic symptoms, agitation, or rapid cycling between manic and depressive episodes in people with bipolar disorder. These problems may arise with the use of any antidepressant in a person with bipolar disorder. Still, the risk of inducing mania or rapid cycling appears to be lower with buproprion (Wellbutrin) than with other antidepressants, such as the SSRIs including fluoxetine (Prozac) and sertraline (Zoloft). For this reason, buproprion is often used as the first-line medication treatment for depression in adolescents with bipolar disorder. SSRIs and other antidepressants may be used to treat adolescents with bipolar disorder, but they should be used with caution, starting slowly with low doses and close monitoring. It is generally safest to use antidepressants when the adolescent is already being treated with a medication such as an atypical antipsychotic or mood stabilizer that provides some protection against the potential for mania.

Psychotherapy

Because of the focus on medication use in treating bipolar disorder, many families and even some psychiatrists forget the important role that psychotherapy may play in achieving stability. Bipolar disorder causes a severe disruption in the lives of teenagers and has the potential to affect nearly every aspect of their lives, from sports to academics to relationships with friends and family. Psychotherapy may help teenagers minimize this disruption and make sense of their illness and the role it plays in their life. It encourages a healthy developmental track. A therapist may help teens learn about their illness and identify potential triggers for mood episodes or warning signs that symptoms are getting worse. Then they will have the tools to prevent emerging crises before they occur.

Prognosis and Risks

Bipolar disorder in adults tends to be a chronic, lifelong condition with periods of stability interrupted by episodic relapses. Though many patients suffering from bipolar disorder are able to manage their illness and lead healthy, successful lives, most often they require ongoing treatment. The long-term course of bipolar disorder in children and adolescents is less certain. It appears that when symptoms follow a more typical adult pattern, with distinct episodes of depression and mania, and when these symptoms begin late in adolescence, in the late teens or early twenties, the course tends to follow the more chronic pattern that is seen in adults. Less is known, however, about the course of bipolar disorder that is first diagnosed in younger teens or that presents with the atypical pattern of symptoms often seen in younger teens. This remains an area of ongoing research in the field. Some studies have suggested that many of the younger teens will not go on to develop the adult form of the disorder but that they are at increased risk for other serious forms of psychiatric illness later on, including substance abuse (see chapter 12) or personality disorders (see chapter 13).

What is fairly clear is the short-term risk associated with bipolar disorder. Adolescents with bipolar disorder are at very high risk for attempting suicide. Additionally, the symptoms of bipolar disorder may lead teens to engage in dangerous behaviors, such as unprotected and promiscuous sexual activity, driving recklessly, or performing physically dangerous feats. The risky behaviors associated with bipolar disorder can have potentially devastating consequences, ranging from criminal charges to serious injury or even death for teens and those around them. Bipolar disorder during adolescence can also have a profound and lasting psychological impact, contributing to social isolation, tumultuous family relationships, and low self-esteem during a critical period of psychological development and identity formation.

Adolescents who have been diagnosed with bipolar disorder and stabilized on a treatment regimen are at high risk for relapse in the months following their stabilization. This risk is high even with good treatment, but it skyrockets when teenagers are noncompliant with treatments, such as failing to take prescribed medications regularly. Monitoring for signs of relapse and assuring compliance as best as possible is particularly important, given the risks associated with bipolar disorder.

Conclusion

Bipolar disorder, once thought to be an illness more common in adulthood, is now diagnosed with increasing frequency in younger patients. Bipolar disorder involves a severe disruption in mood, with episodes of depression and episodes of mania. Symptoms of mania include abnormally elevated or extremely irritable mood, increased activity or agitation, grandiosity, rapid speech, racing thoughts, risky behaviors, impulsivity, and decreased need for sleep. In adolescents, bipolar disorder may be difficult to recognize, as the symptoms may follow different patterns than seen in adults, including symptoms of mania and depression often occurring together. The diagnosis of bipolar disorder may be complicated by that fact that a number of other psychiatric conditions can have similar or overlapping symptoms. It may be challenging to distinguish bipolar disorder from developmentally normal behaviors of adolescence, such as increased risk-taking behavior, a sense of invulnerability, and a tendency to act without always thinking through the long-term consequences.

Despite these challenges, it is important to recognize and treat bipolar disorder when it occurs in adolescence, as when it is left untreated, it can severely disrupt the life and healthy development of a teenager. Moreover, it carries significant risks, including suicide and the potentially devastating consequences of high-risk behaviors, including criminal charges, teen pregnancy, and automobile accidents. Treatment for bipolar disorder involves medications to treat symptoms of mania and depression as well as individual psychotherapy to help minimize the disruption the illness causes on a teenager's development. Family therapy and group therapy are often helpful as well.

References and Additional Reading

American Academy of Child and Adolescent Psychiatry. 2007. "Practice Parameter for the Assessment and Treatment of Children and Adolescents with Bipolar Disorder." *Journal of the American Academy of Child and Adolescent Psychiatry* 46: 107–125.
Belmaker, R. H. 2004. "Bipolar Disorder." *New England Journal of Medicine* 351: 476–486.

Freeman, A. J., E. A. Youngstrom, E. Michalak, R. Siegel, O. I. Meyers, and R. L. Findling. 2009. "Quality of Life in Pediatric Bipolar Disorder." *Pediatrics* 123: e446–e452.

Kessler, R. C., W. T. Chiu, O. Demler, and E. E. Walters. 2005. "Prevalence, Severity and Comorbidity of Twelve-Month DSM-IV Disorders in the National Comorbidity Survey Replication (NCS-R)." *Archives of General Psychiatry* 62: 617–627.

Anxiety Disorders

Feelings of worry are a usual part of everyone's life. Adolescence, with its rapid physical and emotional changes, increasing demands at school, and shifting social climate, may be a particularly anxiety-provoking time. During adolescence, some degree of anxiety is normal and may even serve a useful purpose. The teen who has been extremely stressed from attempting to write a twelve-page term paper in one night, after procrastinating for weeks, may remember that uneasy feeling with the next assignment and begin to think about changing his or her behavior. For many teenagers, however, anxiety is more than just an occasional, uncomfortable fact of life. At times, feelings of worry become so powerful that they cause daily suffering or interfere with healthy development, school, friendships, or family relationships. When this is the case, an anxiety disorder is the likely culprit.

Anxiety disorders are among the most prevalent psychiatric problems affecting adolescents. It has been estimated that as much as 20 percent of the population suffers from some form of anxiety disorder before reaching adulthood. Anxiety disorders are common in adolescent boys and girls, but on the whole they occur somewhat more frequently in girls. Despite their high rates of occurrence and because their symptoms may not be as outwardly apparent as the symptoms

---

Case Presentation

A specialist in adolescent medicine evaluated Max, a twelve-year-old boy who had problems with eating. Two months before the visit, Max reported that a piece of food became lodged in his throat, and he began to choke. Subsequently he became anxious whenever he would eat solid foods; as a result, he avoided solid foods of normal texture and insisted on eating only pureed foods. This led to social stigmatization at school. He had been previously evaluated by a gastroenterologist; the results of an upper endoscopic examination of his esophagus and stomach were normal.

The adolescent medicine specialist noted that Max was underweight and looked tired. He coughed and spit several times during the examination, complaining that he felt there was something in his throat. Otherwise, the examination was unremarkable, and the medical evaluation did not disclose a medical causation for the choking sensation. The boy was referred to a psychiatrist.

A psychiatric assessment revealed that Max had no body-image or weight concerns, essentially ruling out an eating disorder. Instead, he was diagnosed with an anxiety disorder, probably stemming from the memory of choking. In order to reintroduce solid foods, the psychiatrist treated him using a cognitive behavioral approach. Max did well in follow-up, with weight gain and an increasing intake of solid foods.

of other psychiatric disorders, anxiety disorders frequently go unrecognized or untreated.

Psychiatrists define several distinct disorders that fall under the general category of anxiety disorders. This chapter discusses five of the most common anxiety disorders: generalized anxiety disorder, specific phobia, social phobia, separation anxiety, and panic disorder. These disorders are grouped together in this chapter because they have a great deal in common with one another both in their symptoms and in the approach to their treatment. Two other frequent psychiatric conditions that are also classified as anxiety disorders, obsessive-compulsive disorder and posttraumatic stress disorder, are discussed separately in chapters 16 and 18, respectively.

Common Anxiety Disorders and Their Symptoms

Generalized Anxiety Disorder

Generalized anxiety disorder (GAD) is a condition in which symptoms of anxiety are not focused on one particular area but rather occur in a variety of situations and places. An adolescent with GAD will feel anxious most of the time, with worries that are difficult to control and out of proportion to the situation. In addition, the anxiety may be associated with the following symptoms: restlessness, feeling on edge, fatigue, difficulty with concentration, irritability, muscle tension, and sleep difficulties. Physical complaints, such as headaches or stomachaches, are also common, though they are not part of the criteria that psychiatrists use to diagnosis the disorder. In order to make a diagnosis of GAD, the symptoms must be present for at least six months.

A common cause of anxiety in adolescents with GAD is performance in school, sports, or other activities, such as playing a musical instrument. Although many teens have some degree of worry in these areas, teens with GAD experience anxiety that is out of proportion to the situation and that may be overwhelming and debilitating. Frequent worries about family are also common, with excessive concern about bad things happening to loved ones, such as a healthy parent suddenly dying. Catastrophic but unlikely events, such as a nuclear war or a natural disaster, may also be a preoccupation. Adolescents with GAD may require frequent reassurance that things are okay and that they and their families are safe. Left untreated, GAD may cause significant distress and problems in school, friendships, and family relationships. See sidebar 8.1 for signs of anxiety disorder.

Specific Phobia

As the name implies, the diagnosis of specific phobia is applied when a patient has a powerful fear of a particular object or situation, in contrast to the more

> ### Sidebar 8.1 | **Warning Signs of Anxiety Disorders in Adolescents**
>
> ► Feeling tense, worried, or on edge most of the time
> ► Frequent worry about bad things happening to themselves or family members
> ► Exaggerated fear of unlikely catastrophic events, e.g., earthquake or nuclear war
> ► Low self-esteem or frequently feeling unsure of oneself
> ► Excessive need for reassurance
> ► Clinginess or difficulty separating from parents
> ► Difficulties sleeping, including frequent requests to sleep in parents' bed or wanting to sleep with light or television on
> ► Frequent nightmares
> ► Frequent headaches, stomachaches, or other physical complaints
> ► Going to great lengths to avoid feared objects or situations, such as dogs, school, or public speaking
> ► Restlessness
> ► Difficulty concentrating
> ► Being easily fatigued
> ► Irritability

widespread worries of generalized anxiety disorder. Exposure to the feared object (such as wasps or snakes) or a situation (such as public speaking) brings about a powerful anxiety reaction and may even provoke a panic attack (see discussion of panic disorder later in this chapter). In order to diagnose specific phobia during adolescence, the symptoms must be present for at least six months. In a specific phobia, an adolescent may recognize that the fear is not rational but nonetheless feel powerless over it. He or she may go to great lengths to avoid fear. This avoidance behavior may cause temporary relief, but it ultimately serves to reinforce the fear, setting up a cycle in which the phobia may become more entrenched. Both the distress caused by a phobia and the associated avoidance behaviors may cause significant problems in a teen's life.

Social Phobia

Social phobia, also referred to as social anxiety disorder, is a form of anxiety disorder that is similar to specific phobia, but the fears are centered on social situations. Although it may occur in younger children and adults, it is often first recognized during adolescence. Affected teens show a pattern of severe anxiety in response to situations in which they feel that they may be scrutinized by others (such as giving a speech in class) or in which they must interact with unfamiliar people (such as at a party in which they do not know some of the attendees). In these situations, teens with social phobia may fear doing or saying something embarrassing. They may be especially sensitive to the reaction of other people, with a powerful fear of rejection and a tendency to assume people will respond negatively. The anxiety response that occurs in anticipation of a feared social situation, including flushing, sweating, or racing heartbeat, may make the situation even more challenging and unpleasant, leading to reinforcement of the fear. Avoidance is a common feature of the disorder. For example, teens with social phobia may develop a pattern of missing school, with feigned or anxiety-induced symptoms such as stomachache, on days when they are expected to give presentations in front of the class. As with specific phobia, the symptoms of social phobia must be present for at least six months before the diagnosis can be made in an adolescent patient.

Separation Anxiety Disorder

Separation anxiety disorder is a condition in which a child or adolescent experiences excessive anxiety related to being away from home or being separated from the primary attachment figure(s) (usually one or both of the parents). Separation anxiety disorder most commonly begins before puberty, but it may start in or persist into adolescence. An affected teen's fears may include worries that something bad will happen to his or her parent or that something will cause a prolonged separation from the parent (such as an overseas business trip). Teens with separation anxiety may avoid situations in which they are separated from their parents or their home, including going to school, overnight camp, or sleepovers at friends' houses. When separated from their parents, teens with separation anxiety may feel the need to check on their parents constantly, calling or wanting to know where they are at all times. They may even want to sleep in their parents' bed and have nightmares or difficulty sleeping related to their anxiety. Because of these symptoms, separation anxiety during adolescence may cause significant difficulties with school, peer relationships, and self-esteem.

Panic Disorder

Walter Cannon, a physiologist at Harvard, described the fight-or-flight response in 1915. This bodily response to stress can be lifesaving in times of danger, such as during an animal attack. Under stressful or dangerous conditions, bodily hormones are released, causing certain changes. For example, pupils dilate, allowing an individual to see more clearly, especially in the darkness. The heart pumps harder and faster, increasing blood circulation to muscles and the brain. Breathing speeds up, delivering more oxygen into the system. Blood vessels constrict to help diminish blood loss should there be an injury. And perspiration rapidly increases, allowing extra cooling of the body. The fight-or-flight response, though, is a primitive response to danger. In the contemporary world, life stressors are able to trigger this response all too often.

Although people use the term panic attack frequently in everyday speech, when psychiatrists use the term they have in mind a specific phenomenon with a clearly

---

Sidebar 8.2 | Symptoms of a Panic Attack

- Symptoms of feeling of one's heart racing or palpitations
- Sweating
- Trembling or shaking
- Shortness of breath or feeling smothered
- Feeling of choking
- Chest pain or discomfort
- Nausea or abdominal discomfort
- Dizziness or lightheadedness
- A feeling that things are not real or of being detached from one's body
- Fear of losing control of oneself or "going crazy"
- Fear of dying
- Numbness or tingling sensations in the body
- Chills or flushing

---

defined pattern of symptoms. According to the *Diagnostic and Statistical Manual of Mental Disorders* (DSM-IV-TR), a panic attack is defined as a discrete period of intense fear or discomfort that has a fairly sudden onset and is associated with at least four of the symptoms listed in sidebar 8.2.

Individual panic attacks may occur in response to a variety of situations, including in response to severe stress or as part of a variety of psychiatric conditions, including major depression, substance abuse, or generalized anxiety. However, panic disorder may be diagnosed when panic attacks are recurrent and result in frequent worry about having another attack or behaviors, such as avoiding particular places or situations in order to prevent panic attacks. Panic disorder is often accompanied by agoraphobia, which is characterized by an intense fear and avoidance of situations that may trigger a panic attack, particularly in crowds or public places.

Panic disorder is a common psychiatric condition in adults, with an estimated lifetime prevalence in the population of one in twenty. It often has its onset in late adolescence or early adulthood, and it is much less common in children and younger adolescents. Panic disorder may cause a great deal of distress and disruption in adolescents' lives. Fear of future attacks may lead to avoidance of school, sports, or social activities. In extreme cases, teens with panic disorder with agoraphobia may avoid leaving the house.

Getting Help: What to Do If You Are Worried

If you are concerned about the role of anxiety in your child's life, the first step is to talk to your teen about the problem. Anxious teenagers tend to avoid seeking help. They may fear the judgment of others if they were to talk about their worries and instead suffer quietly with the concern that there is "something wrong" with them. Some teens with anxiety may quietly worry so intensively and for so long that they assume their suffering is normal and that everyone else feels the same way. Thus, it is often parents' job to initiate the conversation about anxiety, and it is important for concerned parents to approach their child in an open, nonjudgmental way. Trying to understand your child's experience of anxiety is a key part of developing an effective solution. At times, what appears to be an anxiety disorder is, in fact, a response to a particular situation, such as a bully at school who has been targeting your child. It may be difficult for some teens to talk about these kinds of problems.

As with other issues, your teenager may not respond to your first attempt to talk about his or her anxiety. This may simply be a sign that the timing was not right. Let your child know that you are interested in how he or she is feeling and that you are willing to listen if he or she wants to talk in the future. Without pestering, after some time has passed, gently try to bring it up again.

If your child is willing to talk about anxiety, it is important to listen and ask questions, resisting the temptation to dismiss the worries too quickly. Being told "Don't worry so much" may be frustrating to a teen who would love to worry less but feels that the worry has become uncontrollable. Similarly, when a particular fear is described, an earthquake for example, simply stating "That's not going to happen" is unlikely to offer lasting relief and may make the teen less likely to talk about his or her fears in the future.

Adolescents with anxiety disorder may frequently seek reassurance from parents. So, it is not uncommon for them to call a parent at the grocery store to make sure that things are okay. Reassurance, though, offers only fleeting relief, enough to reinforce the reassurance-seeking behavior but not enough to reduce the anxiety in a sustained way. It may set up an escalating pattern in which reassurance is desperately sought with increasing frequency. It is often more helpful to listen, to try to understand the anxiety, and to work together with your child to come up with pragmatic ways of coping with the anxiety. Exercise, distraction with an enjoyable activity, and relaxation techniques including yoga, breathing exercises, or meditation are all useful coping skills.

Sometimes, parental guidance and support are not enough to help an adolescent cope with anxiety. When anxiety symptoms are causing a great deal of distress or are leading to significant problems at school, at home, or with friendships, it may be time to seek professional help.

Making the Diagnosis

As with many psychiatric disorders, the most important part of an evaluation for a possible anxiety disorder is a detailed interview with parents and the teen by a clinician with experience in diagnosing and treating anxiety disorders. Often, a teenager's pediatrician can help parents differentiate normal worries and behaviors of adolescence from a condition that requires further evaluation, and he or she can help refer parents to an appropriate mental health professional.

Although it is not unusual for a clinician to evaluate a teen over two or more sessions, an anxiety disorder may be diagnosed after a single visit. Because different forms of anxiety disorders can resemble one another, parents can help in

> **Sidebar 8.3 | Medical Conditions That May Present with Symptoms Similar to Anxiety**
>
> ▶ Brain dysfunction (encephalopathy) due to infection, toxins, or metabolic problems
> ▶ Brain tumor
> ▶ Cushing's disease (excess adrenal hormones)
> ▶ Hypocalcemia (low blood calcium)
> ▶ Hypoglycemia (low blood sugar)
> ▶ Hyperthyroidism (thyroid function too high)
> ▶ Hypothyroidism (thyroid function too low)
> ▶ Seizure disorder

the initial evaluation by giving specific, detailed information to the evaluating psychiatrist or therapist. Descriptions about particular worries ("He gets very worried that someone will break into the house when he's home alone") and particular symptoms ("She gets stomachaches almost every Monday morning before school, except during vacation") are very useful in guiding the diagnosis. In the days leading up to the evaluation, it may be helpful to pay particular attention to the symptoms and take some notes. Moreover, it is helpful for the adolescent's clinician to speak with other important people in your child's life, such as teachers or coaches. Since these sources can be contacted only with your permission (or your adolescent's permission, if he or she is eighteen or older), bring their contact information with you to the first appointment.

Before the first appointment, prepare your adolescent for the evaluation. Anxious teenagers will occasionally be reluctant to go to a strange place, meet someone new, and be asked a lot of questions. So the best approach is to let your child know your concerns. Explain why you want him or her to meet with a clinician. Do not wait until the last minute. That may undermine your teen's trust in you, and the visit with the clinician will be more challenging for everyone.

As with most psychiatric diagnoses, the diagnosis of an anxiety disorder is based on the description of symptoms. There is no laboratory test. Still, a medical history should be part of the evaluation process, and at times a medical workup, including blood tests, may be necessary to rule out medical conditions that might be causing an adolescent's symptoms. Sidebar 8.3 lists medical conditions that may be causing the adolescent's symptoms, and sidebar 8.4 lists medications and substances that could also cause these symptoms.

Testing

At times it may be difficult to diagnose an anxiety disorder. Adolescents may have trouble expressing themselves, and some may not even be aware that what they are feeling is anxiety. Instead, they may have physical symptoms such as stomachaches, headaches, or fatigue. When the diagnosis of an anxiety disorder is particularly difficult, psychological testing may be employed. Psychological testing is discussed in more detail in chapter 3.

When assessing anxiety, standardized symptom-rating scales are frequently employed. These are checklists of symptoms that are filled out by the patient and, on occasion, by parents or teachers. The responses may then be compared to the range of typical responses of children with and without anxiety disorders.

Although testing may be very helpful to clinicians in determining whether an anxiety disorder is present, the diagnosis is never based solely on the test results. The results must be interpreted and understood within the context of the adolescent's symptoms and the impact that they are having on his or her life.

Differential Diagnosis

A thorough evaluation for anxiety will also explore other possible psychiatric and medical conditions that may be mistaken for an anxiety disorder. One of the keys to successful treatment is ascertaining that the problem has been correctly diagnosed.

Mood disorders, including major depression and bipolar disorder, are conditions commonly confused with anxiety. Anxiety disorders and mood disorders frequently occur together. In addition, many of the symptoms of the two groups of disorders are similar or overlapping. Fatigue, feelings of restlessness, and disturbances in sleep and concentration are common to both mood and anxiety problems. Through a thorough exploration of the problem, a psychiatrist or other clinician may begin to distinguish anxiety problems from mood disorders. In part, this is achieved by reviewing the nature of the symptoms. For example, the fatigue that accompanies anxiety disorders is more of a tendency to wear down easily because of all the associated worrying, whereas the fatigue of depression is more of a general weariness and lack of motivation. The distinction between mood and anxiety disorders also involves recognizing symptoms unique to each condition, such as the persistent feelings of sadness in depression or the extreme explosiveness and erratic behavior that may be associated with mania in adolescents.

When anxiety symptoms occur in response to a specific stressor in an adolescent's life, the problem may be an adjustment disorder rather than an anxiety disorder. Adjustment disorder (discussed in chapter 14) is a condition in which mood and/or anxiety symptoms

> ### Sidebar 8.4 | Medications and Substances That May Present with Symptoms Similar to Anxiety
>
> ▶ Alcohol
> ▶ Amphetamines
> ▶ Barbiturates
> ▶ Benzodiazepines
> ▶ Caffeine
> ▶ Cocaine
> ▶ Hallucinogens
> ▶ Illicit and prescription inhalants
> ▶ Marijuana
> ▶ Methylphenidate
> ▶ Opioids
> ▶ Phencyclidine
> ▶ Tobacco

emerge in response to an identifiable stressor, but these symptoms do not reach the level of major depression or generalized anxiety. When the stressor is removed from the teen's life (which is not always possible, such as for teens who are reacting to their parents' divorce), the symptoms of an adjustment disorder resolve within a few months.

Substance abuse may induce anxiety symptoms. Marijuana, cocaine, and stimulants, such as amphetamines, may cause acute anxiety or even panic attacks. Excess caffeine intake also may cause anxiety symptoms. When substances that depress nervous system activity, including alcohol or benzodiazepines, are abused regularly, dependence on the substance may develop, leading to anxiety and related physical symptoms during withdrawal. Thus, a substance-use assessment is an important part of a thorough anxiety evaluation.

Some medical conditions can cause feelings of anxiety or symptoms resembling those of an anxiety disorder (see sidebar 8.3). One of the most common culprits of a medical cause of anxiety symptoms is hyperthyroidism (overactive thyroid), which is an excess of thyroid hormone in the blood. Hyperthyroidism may cause restlessness, nervous feelings, racing heartbeat, flushing, and palpitations. Other hormonal problems, including hypothyroidism (underactive thyroid), excessive adrenal hormones, and issues with blood sugar and calcium, can also cause symptoms similar to anxiety.

The side effects of several medications and substances have the potential to induce anxiety and related symptoms (see sidebar 8.4). Some asthma medications, including albuterol, frequently have this effect. In addition, several psychiatric medications may cause or exacerbate anxiety symptoms, including stimulants used to treat ADHD. Antidepressants, despite their effectiveness in treating many anxiety disorders, may worsen anxiety or cause severe restlessness in some cases.

Finally, an important possibility that must be considered in making the diagnosis of any one particular anxiety disorder is the diagnosis of another anxiety disorder. Most of the anxiety disorders share similar symptoms and features, and there is a high degree of comorbidity among them. This means that when one particular anxiety disorder is present, another related but distinct disorder may be lurking. This is true of the anxiety disorders discussed in this chapter as well as of two other common anxiety disorders discussed later in this book: obsessive-compulsive disorder and posttraumatic stress disorder.

There are other psychiatric conditions that often coexist with anxiety disorders. Identifying and treating a coexisting condition is an essential part of anxiety disorder treatment, because when these conditions are left untreated, they can impede the treatment of the anxiety disorder. As a result, a teenager who has both panic disorder and major depression might not see improvement in her panic symptoms until the depression is addressed. In addition to depression, other conditions that may coexist with anxiety disorders include substance abuse, learning and language disorders, and attention-deficit/hyperactivity disorder (ADHD).

Treatment

Treatment for adolescents with anxiety disorders is focused on reducing distress from anxiety symptoms, improving skills for managing anxiety, and helping teens maintain healthy development. The treatment approach is tailored to the particular teen, the specific disorder being treated, and the nature and severity of the symptoms. Generally, treatment consists of psychotherapy alone or in combination with medications.

Psychotherapy

Psychotherapy is often recommended as the first line of treatment for adolescents with anxiety disorders, and it may be very effective. By addressing some of the underlying psychological factors that generate anxiety disorders and giving teens the tools for addressing anxiety, psychotherapy can not only help deal with the problem in the short term but also reduce the recurrence of symptoms in the future. Several different psychotherapeutic approaches may be beneficial.

Cognitive Behavioral Therapy and Related Treatments. As discussed in more detail in chapter 4, cognitive behavioral therapy (CBT) is a type of psychotherapy that is based on the assumption that many psychiatric problems are rooted in unhealthy, distorted thoughts, or cognitions, as well as patterns of behavior that are related to these unhealthful cognitions. CBT aims to challenge distorted thoughts and alter patterns of unhealthful behavior that reinforce the thoughts. CBT can help a teenager identify and correct these patterns.

Because there is a great deal of evidence to support the efficacy of CBT, it is one of the preferred approaches to psychotherapy for adolescents with anxiety disorders. In treating anxiety, a CBT therapist may work with the patient to identify triggers for anxiety, including distorted thought patterns. The therapist will help the teen to modify patterns of behavior that reinforce anxious thoughts. Thus, in social phobia, a teenager may have a distorted view that everyone at the lunch table is paying attention to him, and he worries that he will say something inappropriate. These distorted ideas lead to avoidance: because of his fears, the teen may eat alone. This type of avoidance allows the distorted beliefs to continue. By identifying and challenging some of the inaccurate assumptions, a CBT therapist can help the adolescent confront his fears. The teen may start with small interactions, such as talking to someone in the hall before class, and build up confidence for bigger challenges, such as the lunch table. With time, anxiety diminishes, and social situations become easier for the teen.

CBT for anxiety disorders may incorporate the use of relaxation techniques, such as breathing exercises. These techniques can reduce symptoms and allow adolescents to gain a sense of control over their anxiety. Through practicing relaxation techniques, teens learn to slow down both heart rate and breathing, thereby modifying their body's physiological reaction to stress. This process may be further augmented by the use of biofeedback, a device that measures one or more of the body's responses to anxiety, such as heart rate, sweating, skin temperature, and muscle tension. Such feedback enables a teen to have better control over these responses.

Learning to master these physiological responses is useful in all kinds of anxiety, but it may be particularly important for panic disorder, when teens become overly aware of their body's physical reaction to stress, such as rapid breathing or a racing heartbeat. Teens misinterpret these signals and fear they have lost control. This causes greater stress, leading to even faster breathing and heart rate, and sets up a vicious cycle of mounting anxiety. Use of relaxation, with or without biofeedback, can break this cycle by teaching teens to identify their body's signals, modify the response, and regain a sense of control.

Another technique that is occasionally incorporated into CBT is exposure therapy. As the name implies, exposure therapy involves exposing the teen to the feared object or situation. This is typically accomplished in short steps called graded exposure, starting with mildly anxiety-provoking exposures and building up to the most feared situations. Relaxation techniques are used to help manage the associated anxiety. Exposure therapy is useful when specific triggers for anxiety are identified. It may be particularly effective in treating social phobia and specific phobias.

Psychodynamic Psychotherapy. As discussed in chapter 4, in psychodynamic psychotherapy the therapist works with the teen to explore the various mental forces, both conscious and unconscious, at work in generating psychiatric problems such as anxiety. This form of therapy tends to be less structured and more individualized than CBT. The therapist may encourage the teen to express the thoughts and feelings he or she has been experiencing. Through this process, a teen may understand unconscious conflicts that have been causing distress, learn better ways of managing feelings and, with time, experience a reduction in anxiety.

Adolescents with anxiety disorders may be effectively treated by psychodynamic psychotherapy. There is evidence to support its efficacy, though not as much evidence as there is to support the use of CBT. Psychodynamic psychotherapy is more challenging to study in a controlled, systematic way than CBT is. Nonetheless, it can reduce anxiety symptoms, allow for a better understanding of oneself, and promote healthy psychological development.

As with most forms of psychotherapy, a motivated adolescent and a good, trusting relationship with the therapist tend to lead to greater success in psychodynamic treatment. However, an anxious teenager who is initially wary of therapy can sometimes be guided into a greater willingness to engage in the process through a therapist who is patient and empathetic. Adolescents who have difficulty thinking and talking about themselves or who do not respond well to a lack of structure and clear goals may have more impediments to making progress with psychodynamic psychotherapy. Sometimes, these obstacles can be overcome with time and hard work, but for others a more structured treatment approach is preferable.

Group Psychotherapy. Group therapy is used in the treatment of a number of psychiatric conditions and can be particularly effective in treating anxiety disorders. By allowing adolescents who have anxiety in social situations to work together with other adolescents in a safe and supportive setting led by a therapist, group therapy can help improve their social skills and make them feel more confident in their social interactions. It can be a great comfort for teens to learn that other teens are facing similar challenges. As with other forms of therapy, the workings of group therapy may vary according to the guiding theoretical principle behind the treatment. Some groups employ skills and techniques from cognitive behavioral therapy, whereas others have a more psychodynamic approach. In the treatment of social phobia, group therapy may have an element of exposure therapy, as participants practice speaking in front of others. Some groups focus primarily on social skills training, helping teens to communicate more effectively. In finding a group, it is important for you to consider how your child may benefit from the group's particular therapeutic focus as well as the overall feel of the group and its leader.

The Family's Role

Taking an active role in a child's treatment for anxiety disorder appears to help parents manage their own concerns. The parents' role can take different forms, but often it involves meeting with their child's therapist on a regular basis to talk about the treatment and obtain guidance from the therapist on actions they can take at home to support their teen's progress. Through working with a therapist, parents can learn how to avoid reinforcing their teen's anxiety and related behaviors. They may receive guidance from the therapist on how to balance empathy for their child's suffering with exerting firmness in managing dysfunctional behavior. Parents may be called on to help their child practice skills that are being taught in individual therapy.

When the needs of the teen or the family are greater than the adolescent's own therapist can meet, the parents may be referred to a separate clinician for more intensive support and guidance. Patterns of interactions within a family sometimes play a role in fueling anxieties. Family therapy may be useful in identifying and treating these problems. Anxiety disorders tend to run in families, so it is not unusual for an anxious adolescent to have a parent or other member of the household who also struggles with anxiety. In this case, all who have anxiety should receive treatment. This reduces the overall stress level in the household and sets a good example for a teenager who may be ambivalent about treatment.

The School's Role

The school can play an important role in helping address a teenager's anxiety disorder, particularly when anxiety symptoms are having an impact on a teenager's academic functioning. In vulnerable adolescents, classrooms and crowded hallways may trigger anxiety symptoms, and frequent absenteeism is common with anxiety disorders. In these cases, it is important for parents and the outpatient treatment team to develop a collaborative relationship with the school to address the problem.

When a teen suffering from an anxiety disorder is avoiding school, schools may develop a program of gradually reintegrating the student back into the classroom. In these instances, the student may begin by attending school for a few hours each day and meeting individually with teachers and a counselor to ease the transition. Then, with support from the school and the outpatient treatment team, the demands and expectations may be slowly increased to a full schedule. Home tutoring or additional school-based academic support, such as use of a resource room for academic help, can assist students who have missed a good deal of school.

Placement in a smaller-sized classroom with access to academic and psychosocial support staff, such as school counselors and tutors, is a useful intervention that may be incorporated into a teen's educational plan. For teens who have many somatic symptoms (meaning that their anxiety frequently manifests itself as physical complaints such as headaches or stomachaches), it may be useful to work with the school nurse or health counselor to develop a plan for addressing these symptoms when they arise.

Medications

When psychotherapy alone is not sufficient to treat an anxiety disorder, medication should be considered. If the symptoms of anxiety are so severe that they are causing a great deal of impairment and interference with a teen's healthy development, medications are probably an essential part of treatment. For example, if a teenager rarely leaves the house and refuses to go to school because of severe anxiety, medications often help bring the disorder under control and set the teen back on track.

Selective Serotonin Reuptake Inhibitors (SSRIs). There are several different classes of medications that are used to treat anxiety disorders. Often, the first line of medications are selective serotonin reuptake inhibitors (SSRIs), such as fluoxetine (Prozac), discussed in chapter 5. Although SSRIs are classified as antidepressants, they are very effective in the treatment of anxiety disorders. They are relatively safe and well tolerated, with very low risk for abuse or dependence. However, SSRIs carry a risk for side effects. Common side effects include headache, dizziness, upset stomach, changes in appetite, dry mouth, and constipation. A rare but significant issue is that there is some evidence that the use of SSRIs may increase the risk of suicidal thoughts in some teenagers. This issue is discussed in more detail in chapters 5 and 6.

The side effects of medication vary from individual to individual. Some people feel a little drowsy while taking SSRIs, whereas others may feel an energy boost or sometimes a sense of restlessness. Although SSRIs normally help with anxiety, in some cases, after starting an SSRI anxiety may worsen. In rare cases, SSRIs can cause dramatic changes in mood or behavior, such as inducing a manic episode. It is thought that this occurs mostly in teens who have an underlying biological predisposition toward bipolar disorder, although it may be difficult to predict.

Another downside of SSRI treatment for anxiety disorders is that it usually takes some time for the medication to begin working. While some adolescents notice an effect sooner, most report that it takes two to four weeks before they feel a significant reduction in their symptoms. Sometimes, it may take up to six weeks for the medication to reach its full effect. Although, as mentioned, SSRIs are usually safe and well tolerated, the prescribing doctor should closely monitor the use of these medications in teenagers.

Benzodiazepines. When an SSRI alone is not effective or the symptoms are too severe to wait until the SSRI has an effect, other classes of medications may be used. The benzodiazepines are a class of anxiety medication that includes lorazepam (Ativan), clonazepam (Klonopin), diazepam (Valium), alprazolam (Xanax), and others. These medications are very effective in reducing anxiety and have the advantage of having an immediate effect, within minutes to hours. They can be used safely with SSRIs.

One of the primary differences between the various medications in this class is how quickly they act and how long they stay in the body. Medications that are fast acting and leave the body relatively quickly, such as lorazepam or alprazolam, are useful in situations when immediate relief of episodic symptoms is required. So a teen who experiences the early stages of a panic attack may stop the progress of the attack by taking a dose of a fast-acting benzodiazepine. Taking medications on an as-needed basis to stop a bout of symptoms is referred to as abortive treatment. Medications that are slower and stay in the body longer, such as clonazepam, are more effective in preventing symptoms from developing. This type of treatment is referred to as preventive treatment. Although these slower-acting medications may be given on an as-needed basis to keep symptoms at bay, they are often used on a regular schedule.

Benzodiazepines are powerful tools in managing anxiety, but they have several disadvantages that may limit their utility in adolescent patients. Most significantly, benzodiazepines are easily abused. When taken at moderate doses, they reduce anxiety, but at higher doses they can cause intoxication, with feelings of euphoria and reduced inhibition. In overdose, they depress the respiratory system and can be fatal; there is an even higher risk if these medications are taken with alcohol. As a result, in adolescents, benzodiazepines should be used with caution and under close supervision, particularly with teens who have a history of substance abuse or impulsivity. Parents may want to dispense the medications, and they should be aware of how many pills are remaining in the bottle.

Further, benzodiazepines can be habit forming. The body can become dependent on them, particularly when they are taken at high doses and on a regular basis. With long-term use, the body can develop a tolerance, requiring higher doses to achieve the same effect. On the other hand, discontinuing the medication suddenly or dramatically decreasing the dose can induce withdrawal symptoms that include confusion, increase in anxiety, elevation in heart rate and blood pressure, and a risk for seizures. In cases of extreme benzodiazepine dependence, withdrawal can be life threatening. Although some people are able to take benzodiazepines for a long time, tolerance and dependence tend to make these medications better at addressing anxiety in the short term.

Finally, benzodiazepines can have side effects that limit their use, with the most common side effect being sedation. This is a dose-related side effect, meaning that at higher doses there is greater sedation. Benzodiazepines may also interfere with concentration and learning, which is a significant concern for teenagers. Though less common, benzodiazepines may cause a paradoxical reaction in a small number of teenagers, especially in younger patients. When this reaction occurs, there is a dramatic change in behavior, with agitation, excessive talkativeness, silliness, or lack of self-control. In this case, the physician should be notified, and the teen should be kept safe. Avoid giving another dose of the medication until consulting the physician.

Other Medications. Several other medications may be used in the management of adolescent anxiety disorders. Buspirone (BuSpar) is a medication with a unique mechanism of action that affects serotonin receptors, and it has been shown to be effective in treating anxiety disorders in adults. While it may be useful in treating adolescents, buspirone does not appear to be as useful in reducing anxiety as other medications. It is often combined with an SSRI to boost the SSRI's antianxiety and antidepressant effects. Since it has minimal potential for abuse and dependence, buspirone has some advantages in treating anxiety disorders. Moreover, though side effects can occur, it is usually very well tolerated. Common side effects include nausea, headache, dizziness, sedation, and increased nervousness or restlessness.

Medications primarily recommended for other medical problems may be used to treat anxiety, particularly when trials of other medications have not been successful or have been limited by their abuse potential. Psychiatrists may use antihistamines, such as diphenhydramine (Benadryl) or hydroxyzine (Atarax, Vistaril), or even low doses of atypical antipsychotics, such as quetiapine (Seroquel). Although these medications may be valuable in some cases, before starting a medication that is outside the usual treatment regimen for anxiety, it is important to talk with your child's doctor to consider the risks and benefits.

Prognosis and Risks

Anxiety disorders in adolescents are sometimes quiet, with much of the suffering happening inside the mind of a troubled teenager. Still, it is important to recognize the signs of an anxiety disorder and get treatment as soon as possible. Without proper treatment, anxiety disorders can cause significant distress to your adolescent.

During adolescence, anxiety disorders can have a dramatic impact on school performance, setting up a child for a pattern of low self-esteem and underachievement that can carry into adulthood. Adolescence is also an important period for social development. Teens learn to negotiate friendships and romantic relationships and to have confidence in interactions with others. A disruption in this healthy development process caused by out-of-control anxiety can have a lifelong impact on a teen's social and occupational functioning.

Untreated anxiety disorders can also lead to a greater chance for other major problems. It is well known that the suffering and social isolation associated with untreated anxiety places a teenager at risk for depression. Furthermore, adolescents with anxiety disorders have been shown to have an increased risk for alcohol and other substance abuse. It is thought that this may in part be an effort by adolescents to self-medicate their anxiety symptoms.

Conclusion

Anxiety disorders are among the most common psychiatric disorders experienced by adolescents. But despite their frequency, the nature of their symptoms and the tendency of some teens to suffer in silence can cause anxiety disorders to go undiagnosed. Failure to obtain help interferes with healthy development and places teens at risk for many other problems, including low academic achievement, poor self-esteem, social problems, depression, and substance abuse.

Treatment for anxiety disorders may involve medications or psychotherapy, with each used either alone or in combination. Usually, psychotherapy is considered the first-line treatment, particularly in mild to moderate cases of anxiety. CBT is a popular approach with proven efficacy, though psychodynamic psychotherapy is also effective and commonly used. Group therapy may also be useful, especially in cases of social phobia or other cases in which social functioning in affected by anxiety symptoms.

When a teen with anxiety disorder is being evaluated, it is important to consider aspects of the adolescent's environment. Family therapy and parental guidance can help to identify and treat any patterns within the family that might contribute to the problem. Additionally, the school can collaborate with a teen's outpatient team to help address the symptoms occurring in school and to minimize the impact of anxiety on the teen's social and academic functioning.

References and Additional Reading

Bush T., L. Richardson, W. Katon, J. Russo, P. Lozano, E. McCauley, and M. Oliver. 2007. "Anxiety and Depressive Disorders Are Associated with Smoking in Adolescents with Asthma." *Journal of Adolescent Health* 40: 425–432.

Leger E., R. Ladouceur, M. Dugas, and M. Freeston. 2003. "Cognitive-Behavioral Treatment of Generalized Anxiety Disorder among Adolescents: A Case Series." *Journal of the American Academy of Child and Adolescent Psychiatry* 42: 327–330.

Safer, D. J. 2006. "Should Selective Serotonin Reuptake Inhibitors Be Prescribed for Children with Major Depressive and Anxiety Disorders?" *Pediatrics* 118: 1248–1251.

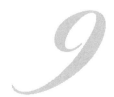

Psychotic Disorders

Psychosis is a condition in which the affected person has lost contact with reality. Psychosis may be the result of other psychiatric problems, such as substance abuse or a severe mood disorder, or it may present on its own, independent of any clear external causes. Although psychotic disorders are relatively uncommon during adolescence compared to other psychiatric problems such as depression and anxiety, primary psychotic disorders such as schizophrenia often begin to emerge during the adolescent years. Psychosis during adolescence is usually an extremely frightening and severely disrupting experience for teens and families alike. Without proper treatment it poses significant safety risks.

Case Presentation

John was a seventeen-year-old high school senior whose parents were concerned that he was behaving in a strange manner. Difficulties began late in his junior year, when his grades began slipping and his parents noticed he was spending increasing amounts of time in his room alone listening to music with headphones. John had always been fairly social, but he began spending less time with friends. The phone, which once seemed to ring incessantly, had gone silent. Over the summer, John's parents noticed that he began to neglect his hygiene, often going several days without bathing and wearing the same dirty clothes. At the start of his senior year, John's behavior grew more bizarre. He seemed to stare into space and sometimes uttered strange remarks. He refused to attend school. When his parents asked him why he did not want to go to school, he indicated that his teachers wanted to kill him. He said he knew "what was going on." When his mother asked what he meant, John said he knew there were cameras hidden in the house and that his parents had implanted a device in his brain to read his thoughts.

Because of these symptoms, John's parents brought him to a local emergency room, where he told the psychiatrist that he heard a voice saying bad things about him; the voice told him that he did not deserve to live. Concerned for his safety, the psychiatrist arranged to have John admitted to an adolescent inpatient psychiatric unit. There, a thorough evaluation ruled out medical problems, including drug abuse, that might be causing his symptoms. John was diagnosed with a primary psychotic disorder and treated with medications that helped clear his thoughts and, gradually, made him seem more like his former self.

After discharge from the hospital, John met regularly with a psychiatrist for medication monitoring and a therapist for counseling. John's parents enrolled him in a local support group, and he was able to catch up in his academics through tutoring and extra help and support from a school counselor. John graduated from high school on time and was doing well, without any psychotic symptoms. With input from his therapist, John and his parents decided together that it would be best if he attended a local college just in case his symptoms returned.

The Biology of Psychotic Disorders

The underlying biological causes of psychotic disorders are poorly understood. Though there is no clear pattern of inheritance and no single gene has been identified that causes any of the disorders, it appears that primary psychotic disorders such as schizophrenia and schizoaffective disorder tend to run in families and are likely to have a genetic component, probably involving several different genes that may increase one's risk. There is some evidence that environmental factors may also play a role in the development of primary psychotic disorders. For example, rates of schizophrenia appear to be higher in people born in winter and late spring, which has led some researchers to suggest that prenatal viral infections may play a role.

Because many of the drugs that treat psychosis block a chemical messenger in the brain called dopamine, theories about the biological causes of schizophrenia have focused on abnormal functioning of dopamine systems in certain parts of the brain. Research into the biological underpinnings of psychosis has expanded to explore the role of other brain pathways and chemicals, including serotonin. Also under investigation are abnormalities that occur during early brain development.

In secondary psychotic disorder, there is good evidence about the role of environmental factors. Thus, in a substance-induced psychotic disorder it is clear that the symptoms are related to the effects of the substance on the brain. It is also apparent that some people are more likely to develop a psychosis in response to a drug exposure. There is some thought that this increased likelihood is due to a genetic predisposition.

Symptoms and Warning Signs

The hallmark of psychosis is a severe distortion in the way that someone experiences the world. This distortion may involve a person's perceptions in the form of hallucinations, or it can affect a person's thoughts in the form of delusions or disorganized thinking.

Hallucinations are defined as perceptual experiences such as seeing or hearing things that are not real. Hallucinations may affect any of the senses, but auditory hallucinations, involving the perception of sounds that are not really there, are most common in psychotic disorders. Auditory hallucinations associated with psychosis often take the form of voices that are heard by the person. These voices may start out as subtle faint, indistinct mumbling or barely audible name calling. When they are more severe, the voices may be loud and intrusive. Often, they include negative comments about the person's behavior or commands telling the person to do something.

One might expect that a symptom as dramatic as hallucinations would be obvious to parents, but in fact they may be quite difficult to detect. Teens may hide their hallucinations, and it is not unusual for the voice that teens hear to order them not to tell other people. Sometimes, teens with psychotic disorders believe that if they tell others about the hallucinations, bad things will happen to them or their families.

It may be difficult for younger adolescents to distinguish auditory hallucinations from their own thought process, which may be perceived as an internal voice. A psychiatrist or appropriately trained clinician will know what questions to ask to make this distinction. In general, the voices associated with hallucinations are felt to be intrusive and uncontrollable, and they are experienced as happening in the outside world, as opposed to inside one's head.

A delusion is a false belief that persists despite overwhelming evidence that it is not part of the belief system of the particular culture or religion to which the individual belongs. Thus, a teenager may believe that aliens have implanted a device in his brain and are reading his thoughts or that the CIA is spying on him and has installed hidden cameras throughout the house. Delusions are held quite rigidly. The efforts of others to convince a person with psychosis that a particular bizarre idea is not true only serves as further evidence of the idea's truth.

Delusions are a distortion in the content of an adolescent's thoughts. Psychosis may also affect the process of an affected teen's thinking. The thoughts of someone affected by psychosis are described by psychiatrists as disorganized, meaning that they lack the normal, logical flow seen in most people's thought processes. The thought process in psychosis may be incoherent and difficult to follow, jumping around in unpredictable ways. Thinking in psychosis may also be dramatically slowed down, with the affected adolescent staring blankly and taking a long time to answer questions or freezing midthought for a period of time before resuming conversation.

Warning signs that your teen may be suffering from a psychotic disorder are listed in sidebar 9.1. It is important to note that many of these symptoms, such as social withdrawal or a decline in academic performance, are not specific to psychosis and may be the result of another psychiatric condition. The important

---

Sidebar 9.1 | Warning Signs of a Psychotic Disorder

- Dramatic decline in functioning in several areas
- Social withdrawal
- Hallucinations—seeing or hearing things that are not there
- Bizarre or erratic behavior
- Speech that is nonsensical, disjointed, or extremely difficult to follow
- Delusions—feelings of being watched by others who want to harm them
- Neglect of personal hygiene and complete lack of concern for one's appearance

point is that an adolescent who is demonstrating several of these symptoms should have a psychiatric evaluation as soon as possible.

Making the Diagnosis

Psychosis is not a specific diagnosis but rather a pattern of disordered thinking and perception that can be the result of many different underlying problems. These causes can be divided into two categories: psychosis that is the result of another psychiatric condition, such as bipolar disorder, and disorders in which psychosis manifests itself as the primary problem, with no identifiable underlying cause. In addition, several conditions can cause a disturbance in an adolescent's thinking that can resemble a psychotic state. When there is a disturbance in a teen's thinking, it is the psychiatrist's role to determine whether psychosis is present and, if so, to detect the most likely cause. See sidebar 9.2 for causes of psychosis.

Psychosis Due to Other Psychiatric Conditions

When psychotic symptoms begin during adolescence, substance abuse must always be considered as a possible cause. Drugs of abuse may produce an altered state of consciousness in the user that can mimic psychosis, with hallucinations, paranoia, and bizarre behavior. (See chapter 12 for a discussion of specific substances and their effects.) A teenager who abuses drugs over time may show other behavioral changes that resemble a psychotic disorder, including social withdrawal, apathy, poor hygiene, and a decline in school performance.

On rare occasions, the effects of a drug do not merely mimic psychosis. Rather, substances may actually induce a psychotic state that can persist for days or weeks after the substance is eliminated from the body. Referred to as a substance-induced psychotic disorder, this condition has been observed even with substances thought to be mild or benign, such as marijuana. It has also been seen with some prescription medications, such as corticosteroids. Substance-induced psychotic disorders appear to occur idiosyncratically and are probably related to a person's underlying predisposition. Other individuals treated with the same medication or the same batch of an illicit substance may not show any evidence of psychosis. Even when teens with psychosis are using drugs, often these substances are

> **Sidebar 9.2 | Possible Causes of Psychosis**
>
> ► Mood disorder (e.g., bipolar disorder, severe depression)
> ► Primary psychotic disorder
> > ► Brief psychotic episode
> > ► Schizophrenia
> > ► Schizoaffective disorder
> ► Substance-induced psychosis
> > ► Illicit substances
> > ► Prescription medications (e.g., steroids)

not the primary cause of the symptoms. Adolescents may turn to substances after psychotic symptoms have developed in an attempt to cope with a terrifying experience. It can be challenging to sort out which came first: substance abuse or a psychotic disorder.

Mood disorders such as bipolar disorder and major depressive disorder can also cause psychotic symptoms in adolescents, particularly when the mood symptoms are severe. When this happens, the psychotic symptoms may take on some of the features of the underlying mood disturbance. For example, a severely depressed teenager may begin to hear voices telling her that she is worthless (a symptom of depression) and that she should kill herself. When psychotic symptoms are due to an underlying mood disorder, they occur at the same time as other mood disorder symptoms. In some cases, a teen may develop a symptom such as feeling that people are talking about him and subsequently develop symptoms of depression. If psychotic symptoms begin before the mood disorder develops, or if they persist long after the mood symptoms have improved, then it is likely that the psychotic symptoms are not due to the mood disorder and that another psychiatric problem may be present.

Primary Psychotic Disorders

When psychotic symptoms occur as the primary problem, without any recognizable underlying cause such as substance abuse or a mood disorder, the condition is classified by psychiatrists as a primary psychotic disorder. Primary psychotic disorders are further characterized according to the duration and specific nature of the symptoms.

Schizophrenia. The best-known primary psychotic disorder is schizophrenia. People sometimes use the term *schizophrenic* to mean having a split personality. However, to a mental health professional, the term means something quite different. Schizophrenia is a chronic psychiatric disorder characterized by psychotic symptoms as well as impairments in cognition and social functioning. Schizophrenia rarely manifests itself before adolescence, but the incidence steadily increases throughout the teenage years to reach a peak age of onset in late adolescence through early adulthood. It is estimated that 1 percent of adults suffer from schizophrenia.

Psychiatrists classify symptoms of schizophrenia into two groups: positive and negative symptoms. Positive symptoms include delusions and hallucinations. Delusions in schizophrenia are often particularly bizarre and may involve the belief that others are controlling or reading the person's thoughts. Auditory hallucinations are the most common form of hallucinations in schizophrenia, usually taking the form of voices that may offer commentary on what the person is doing or instructions to tell the person what to do. Negative symptoms of schizophrenia, so called because they involve the absence of characteristics present in a healthy individual, include blunting of emotions, lack of interest in relationships, and the absence of motivation. Facial expressions in a teen suffering from schizophrenia may be flat, with little show of either positive or negative emotions. Alternately, sufferers may show inappropriate affect, meaning that their expressions are grossly abnormal for a situation, such as laughing hysterically when told something sad.

The behavior and speech of teens with schizophrenia may be disorganized, meaning that their words and actions do not make sense or fail to achieve a clear meaning or purpose. As a result, an affected teenager may frequently get off track when talking and be hard to follow; he may wander around a room, looking around and picking things up without a clear purpose. In some instances, the degree of disorganized behavior in schizophrenia can be so severe that sufferers become catatonic, remaining immobile or exhibiting no purposeful behavior or speech at all.

The symptoms of schizophrenia vary somewhat; psychiatrists refine the diagnosis into subtypes according to the constellation of symptoms demonstrated by the person. In the paranoid type, delusions are more prominent than symptoms of disorganization; in the disorganized type, disorganized speech and behavior are much more prominent than delusions and hallucinations.

In order to be diagnosed with schizophrenia, a person must have had a major disruption in functioning for a period of at least six months. Additionally, the person must demonstrate clear symptoms of illness, such as delusions, hallucinations, or disorganized speech or behavior, for at least one month (though an exception may be made if the symptoms subside before one month in response to treatment). A decline in a teenager's overall functioning usually precedes the onset of clear psychotic symptoms in schizophrenia. Months before hallucinations or delusions emerge, the teen will become increasingly withdrawn, with a deterioration of school or work performance and an increasing neglect for appearance and hygiene. This period of decline is referred to as a prodromal phase of the illness.

Before making the diagnosis of schizophrenia, a psychiatrist must determine that a teen's symptoms are not likely to be due to another cause, such as substance abuse or bipolar disorder. To worried parents eager to hear a diagnosis for their teen, the waiting time required to establish the diagnosis may appear too long. However, there is good reason to be cautious in diagnosing schizophrenia, as this diagnosis has major implications for adolescents and their family. Schizophrenia is a chronic, usually lifelong disorder that has the potential to inflict great suffering on its victims and their families. Further, it carries major risks, including an estimated 10 percent rate of suicide in a person's lifetime. The course and prognosis for people who are diagnosed with schizophrenia are discussed later in this chapter.

Other Primary Psychotic Disorders. Brief psychotic disorder and schizoaffective disorder are other primary psychotic disorders that should be considered in the diagnosis of an adolescent with psychotic symptoms. Brief psychotic disorder is relatively rare, and it involves the sudden onset of psychotic symptoms, often after severe stress in the person's life. With this disorder, the symptoms last less than a month before the person returns to his or her previous level of functioning. In contrast, schizoaffective disorder is a chronic disorder that often causes lifelong impairment. The symptoms of schizoaffective disorder are similar to those seen in schizophrenia, but the person also suffers from a major mood disturbance as well. This disorder is distinguishable from the psychosis that can occur with bipolar disorder or depression. A person with schizoaffective disorder may continue to have psychotic symptoms even when the mood symptoms are in remission.

Conditions Resembling Psychotic Disorders

Several different conditions can cause symptoms that may be mistaken for psychosis. Teenagers with pervasive developmental disorders, such as autism, may have several symptoms similar to those seen in psychosis disorders. For example, they may be socially withdrawn, be inwardly focused, or show little regard for their appearance and hygiene. Developmental disorders are often distinguishable from psychotic disorders because they are usually detected at a young age and because the symptoms remain fairly stable throughout childhood, whereas psychotic disorders most commonly have their onset during adolescence or young adulthood.

Medical conditions can also produce symptoms similar to psychosis, with severe disruptions in a person's thoughts and perceptions. Some of the most common of these conditions are listed in sidebar 9.3. Illnesses affecting the brain, such as seizures, infections, or brain tumors, are among the more common medical causes of apparent psychotic symptoms.

Teenagers who have undergone a major psychological trauma, such as witnessing a murder or surviving a near-fatal car crash, may display a pattern of symptoms that can be mistaken for psychosis. (Reactions to traumatic events

---

Sidebar 9.3 | Conditions That May Resemble Psychosis

- Medical conditions
  - Seizures
  - Brain tumor
  - Encephalitis (infection of the brain)
  - Rare metabolic disorders (e.g., Wilson's disease)
  - Rare genetic disorders (e.g., Huntington's disease)
- Developmental disorders (e.g., autism)
- Intoxication with a substance (e.g., PCP, LSD, cocaine)
- Psychological reaction to trauma (e.g., posttraumatic stress disorder, acute stress disorder)

are discussed in more detail in chapter 18.) These symptoms may include a feeling that nothing is real or a perception of being detached from one's own body and observing events from above. Teens who have suffered from a trauma may have vivid flashbacks similar to hallucinations in which they reexperience the traumatic event. They may have dramatic changes in their behavior, including becoming more withdrawn or frequently appearing spaced out and not paying attention to what is happening around them. Usually these symptoms do not represent a psychotic disorder, though a teen can have a psychotic break in response to a major stressor. Nonetheless, a teenager who is demonstrating these symptoms or other dramatic changes in behavior following a traumatic event should have an evaluation with a qualified mental health professional to determine what is happening and how best to respond.

Evaluation for Psychotic Disorders

An evaluation including a detailed review of the symptoms, a medical history, and any family information on psychiatric disorders is the first step in diagnosing a psychotic disorder. Essential components also include screening questions to assess for possible mood disorders or substance abuse. The psychiatrist should meet individually with the teen whenever possible to observe his or her behavior and thought process. Anxious parents should let their child speak for him- or herself during the evaluation. It is not unusual for parents to interrupt and answer if it seems to them that their child is not making sense, is evading the question, or is jumping around. But because your child's behaviors and responses are important for the psychiatrist to observe, the most helpful approach is to let your child answer for him- or herself. Wait for the psychiatrist to ask you directly before correcting inaccuracies or filling in the gaps in your child's response.

After taking a detailed history and based on this information, a psychiatrist will probably order tests to evaluate for possible causes of the adolescent's symptoms. More medical testing is done in teens with psychotic symptoms than with other psychiatric disorders. Usually a drug screen of blood, urine, or both is performed to determine whether there are any substances present in the teen's system that may be contributing to the symptoms. Blood tests may be ordered to rule out an infection such as syphilis or a metabolic abnormality such as copper poisoning. Tests of baseline liver and kidney functioning and of levels of cholesterol and fats in the blood and blood sugar may be ordered, as these may be monitored after medications are initiated. The initial evaluation may also include an electroencephalogram, or EEG, to measure brainwave activity and assess for possible seizures. A CT scan or MRI brain imaging is often performed to rule out a structural problem within the brain, such as a tumor, as a cause of the symptoms. Many psychiatrists believe that imaging is not necessary in most cases.

After a thorough review of the history and the results of medical and psychological tests, a psychiatrist should be able to determine the most likely diagnoses. Often, however, the exact diagnosis remains unclear in the early stages, and it is necessary to observe how the symptoms change over time. To make the diagnosis of schizophrenia, symptoms must be present for a period of six months. In the early stages, it may not be clear what course the illness will take. If a teen has a history of substance abuse, then he or she should be observed for some time after abstaining from substances.

Neuropsychological testing may be particularly helpful when the diagnosis remains unclear after a thorough psychiatric evaluation. It is not unusual for psychotic teens to be quite guarded about their symptoms, trying to hide them from parents and psychiatrists. Projective tests, such as the Rorschach inkblot test, require the examinee to respond to an ambiguous test item, offering his or her interpretation. The test item may be the start of a sentence that needs to be completed or, as in the Rorschach test, a pattern of smeared ink in which the examinee is asked to find a picture. Answering questions in this way provides a window into the mind of a person who may otherwise be guarded about his or her thoughts. People with psychotic disorders have been shown to have characteristic patterns of responses to projective tests that often seem strange and are quite distinct from the range of normal responses.

In addition to picking up subtle, hard-to-detect psychotic symptoms, neuropsychological testing can also help identify other problems that may be contributing to a teen's symptoms, including developmental disorders, cognitive impairments, and mood disorders.

Treatment

Psychosis is a sign of significant brain dysfunction. Restoring the brain to healthy functioning as quickly as possible is essential to maintaining the adolescent's safety. There is evidence that the psychotic state is damaging to the brain and that the longer it continues, the greater the likelihood future psychotic episodes will occur. Thus, quick and effective treatment that takes place as soon as possible is not only important for minimizing suffering for an affected adolescent and his or her family; timely treatment is also likely to reduce the risk of future episodes. It is also essential to treat any underlying problem such as substance use or depression to assure that the psychosis is ameliorated.

Medications

Medications are the mainstay of treatment for psychotic symptoms, and the primary medications used are called antipsychotics. These medications are discussed in more detail in chapter 5. Some of the older antipsychotics, called typical antipsychotics,, which include haloperidol (Haldol) and chlorpromazine

(Thorazine), can cause significant side effects, as previously stated. Neuroleptic malignant syndrome (NMS) is a rare complication of antipsychotic treatment in which patients develop a high fever, severe muscle rigidity, and confusion that can progress to coma or even death if not treated promptly. People may develop tardive dyskinesia may persist even when the antipsychotic medication has been discontinued.

As has been noted, a newer generation of antipsychotics, called atypical antipsychotics, has been used with increasing frequency in adolescents over the past decade. The atypical antipsychotics appear to be equally effective in treating psychosis but are much less likely to cause dystonia, NMS, and tardive dyskinesia. It is thought that atypical antipsychotics may be more effective than typical antipsychotics in treating the negative symptoms of schizophrenia, such as lack of motivation and emotional flattening.

Atypical antipsychotics do carry a risk of significant side effects, especially weight gain, which is of concern to many teenagers. It has been shown that up to half of patients treated with atypical antipsychotics will experience some degree of weight gain. The weight gain may be relatively small, on the order of a few pounds. Generally, it can be addressed by eating a healthier diet and finding time for more exercise. Some people do gain a significant amount of weight. When weight gain is substantial, parents should explore other management options with the psychiatrist or the teen's primary care physician. Diet, exercise, or a different medication may be indicated. In addition, referral to an obesity specialist or nutritionist may be indicated.

Electroconvulsive Therapy

Electroconvulsive therapy (ECT) involves the use of electricity to induce a seizure for therapeutic purposes and is described in chapter 6. The use of anesthesia to prevent the limbs from moving as they typically do in a generalized seizure have made this procedure much easier and safer for patients.

In adults, the use of ECT is effective for treatment of psychotic disorders such as schizophrenia. Use of ECT in adolescents has not been studied as extensively. Nevertheless, under some circumstances, ECT is used to treat adolescents. These circumstances may include an adolescent who is not compliant with medications or who is not responsive to multiple medication trials.

Psychotherapy

Psychotherapy alone is not very effective in directly addressing the primary symptoms of psychosis, such as hallucinations or delusions. For this reason, it is easily overlooked as a treatment for adolescents suffering from a psychotic disorder. But therapy can play a critical role in helping these teens, and it would be a mistake not to consider it as a part of the treatment plan for a psychotic disorder.

Sidebar 9.4 | Advantages of Psychotherapy for Adolescents with Psychosis

- ▶ Decreases social isolation and builds better social skills
- ▶ Helps teens manage stresses (for example in school) that have potential to worsen symptoms
- ▶ Improves teens' insight into their illness
- ▶ Encourages adolescents' participation in their treatment (e.g., better adherence to medication and appointments
- ▶ Assists adolescents in coping with their illness and understanding the role it has played in their lives
- ▶ Monitors for relapse of symptoms
- ▶ Surveys for and manages potential substance abuse

Psychosis wreaks havoc in teens and those around them. After the psychotic symptoms have been controlled, teens may find that they have fallen far behind in school and lost many friends. They may feel confused or frightened by what happened to them, and they may worry that the symptoms will return or that they will never be able to get their life back on track. This is where psychotherapy can be helpful. For adolescents with psychotic disorders, psychotherapy can have the advantages outlined in sidebar 9.4.

Psychodynamic psychotherapy, with the intense emotions it evokes and its exploration of intrapsychic conflicts, is generally not the best approach in managing psychosis, particularly in people who are actively psychotic. The disruption in thinking associated with psychosis makes it unlikely for psychotic people to be able to participate with any degree of success in psychodynamic psychotherapy. Moreover, the intense feelings it brings out may be stressful and overwhelming for psychotic people, potentially worsening their symptoms. A supportive approach is generally preferable. For teenagers with a psychotic disorder, supportive psychotherapy is usually focused on providing emotional support, improving coping skills, educating teens about the illness, and helping them problem solve the challenges they are facing. Some forms of cognitive behavioral therapy may also be helpful in treating psychosis, particularly in helping prevent relapse in teens who have been stabilized.

Help for Families

Psychosis is a major trauma for the entire family. Thus, it is important to be certain that everyone in the family is obtaining the help needed. Parents often find it useful to attend support groups to share their struggles with other families and hear about the challenges that others have faced. These groups may also be a good source of information about the resources in the area, such as a helpful after-school program or the name of a local child and adolescent psychiatrist.

Learning about your child's illness will enable you to be a better advocate for him or her and make informed decisions about treatment. In addition to books such as this one, websites provide useful information for parents looking to learn about their child's condition. As with all information on the Internet, it is important to consider the quality of the source. You probably already know that there is bad information mixed in with the good. The most trustworthy information can be found on the websites of government organizations or large medical groups. See appendix A for some recommended organizations.

If there are other children in the home, parents need to consider the impact of a sibling's psychotic disorder on them. Parents often find that caring for a child with a psychotic order is so stressful and demanding that the other children fall off the radar. Siblings of a teen with a psychotic disorder may be confused and frightened by what has occurred. They may fear that something similar will happen to them and wonder whether the family will ever get back to normal again. They may also feel that they are not receiving enough attention from their parents. You must talk to your other children about their experience and their worries. Explain what is happening, and tailor the discussion to fit the developmental level of each child. Your child's psychiatrist or therapist can help you develop the explanation you should offer.

Some families affected by a psychotic disorder find family therapy helpful. As with individual therapy, exploring highly charged, deep-seated conflicts is not the best approach in family therapy for psychosis. Once again, a supportive and educational role is most helpful. Working together with a therapist can help create a more supportive atmosphere at home to give your child the best possible chance of recovery.

Prognosis

For an adolescent with psychotic symptoms, the prognosis depends largely on the teen's particular diagnosis. In general, when psychotic symptoms are secondary to another underlying disorder, such as a mood disorder or substance abuse, the symptoms will recede, though not always right away, when the underlying condition is brought under control.

The prognosis for the primary psychotic disorders of schizophrenia and schizoaffective disorder is not as favorable as for psychosis that is secondary to other causes. These disorders usually follow a chronic, lifelong course. Though treatment with medications is effective in bringing psychotic symptoms into remission after an initial episode, there is a high rate of relapse for both disorders, with psychotic symptoms returning within a few years. A large study of people with schizophrenia and schizoaffective disorder showed that, following an initial psychotic episode, approximately 8 percent experienced a relapse within five years of stopping antipsychotic treatment. Relapse rates are lower when long-term antipsychotic treatment is continued. But because of the side effects of the medication, many people find this hard to do.

In addition to the risk of recurring psychotic symptoms, people with schizophrenia and schizoaffective disorder often experience a decline in their ability to live a semblance of a normal life. Their symptoms, which have the potential to severely limit their functioning in school, at work, and in relationships, are less responsive to treatment with medications than are other conditions.

People with schizophrenia and schizoaffective disorder have a shortened life expectancy compared to the general population. One of the major reasons for this is a significant risk of suicide. It is estimated that 5 to 15 percent of people with schizophrenia die by suicide. Suicide is of particular concern in adolescents with schizophrenia, who may be impulsive and may be overwhelmed when first faced with the diagnosis of a frightening, potentially lifelong illness. For this reason, assessment of suicidal thoughts and risk factors for suicide should be part of the evaluation and ongoing management for adolescents with psychotic disorders. Shortened life expectancy is also thought to be related to a number of other factors, including high rates of smoking, poor access to health care, and side effects, such as obesity and diabetes, associated with long-term medication treatment.

Despite the potential for serious, lifelong impairment in schizophrenia and schizoaffective disorder, there is a great deal of variability in the course of illness. And with treatment some people do quite well. It has been estimated that as many as 20 to 30 percent of people with schizophrenia are able to lead fairly normal lives, with only a mild degree of disruption or impairment. Another 20 to 30 percent of schizophrenic people have moderate impairment in their functioning, with ongoing symptoms and some limitations in their functioning. Finally, an estimated 40 to 60 percent of schizophrenic people will have significant, lifelong impairment from their illness, with major difficulties in their interpersonal relationships and limited ability to maintain employment and care for themselves.

Conclusion

Psychosis is a severe form of mental illness that often emerges during the adolescent years. The symptoms of psychosis involve a major disturbance in the affected teen's ability to perceive reality, usually in the form of delusions and hallucinations. Psychotic disorders can be divided into two categories, primary and secondary. The biology of psychotic disorders is poorly understood. Both genetic and environmental factors probably play a role.

Psychotic disorders cause major problems in nearly every aspect of an adolescent's life. Teens dealing with psychotic disorder have a severely impaired judgment and are at increased risk of suicide. Thus, it is essential for the safety of those affected to get appropriate treatment. Treatment for psychotic disorders usually involves a combination of medications to reduce the core symptoms of the disorder and psychotherapy and other forms of social support, such as social skills groups or a modified school program, to minimize the impact of the disorder on the teen's life.

The prognosis for a teenager diagnosed with a psychotic disorder may be difficult to predict and depends in part on the specific diagnosis. Some psychotic disorders, such as schizophrenia and schizoaffective disorder, are chronic disorders that have the potential to cause significant lifelong impairment. Yet even these disorders follow a variable course, with some people doing very well. Early identification and treatment of a psychotic disorder is the best way to improve the prognosis and quality of life for adolescents affected by them.

References and Additional Reading

Cancro R., and H. E. Lehman. 2000. "Schizophrenia: Clinical Features." In *Comprehensive Textbook of Psychiatry,* 7th ed., ed. B. J. Sadock and V. A. Sadock. Baltimore: Lippincott Williams & Wilkins.

Robinson D., M. G. Woerner, J. M. Alvir, R. Bilder, R. Goldman, S. Geisler, A. Koreen, B. Sheitman, M. Chakos, D. Mayerhoff, and J. A. Lieberman. 1999. "Predictors of Relapse Following Response from a First Episode of Schizophrenia or Schizoaffective Disorder." *Archives of General Psychiatry* 56: 241–247.

"Schizophrenia and Other Psychotic Disorders." 2000. In *Diagnostic and Statistical Manual of Mental Disorders,* 4th ed., text revision. Washington, DC: American Psychiatric Association.

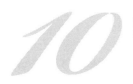

School-Related Problems

School is where adolescents spend many of their waking hours. As a cornerstone of adolescent development, school is more than a place to learn academics. When it goes well, school serves as a safe foundation from which teens can develop self-confidence, find adult role models, learn to negotiate social relationships, work through challenges, and practice the intellectual and interpersonal skills that they will need in adult life. School has the potential to serve as a laboratory of sorts for teens, where they can channel their developmental drive to experiment and take chances in healthy ways, such as trying out for a sports team, making friends in a new crowd, writing an editorial for the school paper, or asking out one's crush. Given school's critical role in adolescent development, when trouble arises at school, it has the potential to undermine teens' growing sense of individual identity and cause problems with self-confidence that can remain with them for years to come. Thus, it is important to identify and address these issues early on. In this chapter, we discuss some of the common psychiatric problems that arise in the school setting, including learning disorders, as well as the resources available within school systems to intervene when a psychiatric disorder threatens to interfere with an adolescent's success at school.

Case Presentation

Sam, a twelve-year-old boy, was seen in the adolescent medicine office early in the school year for recurrent back pain that started shortly after the beginning of the academic year. The back pain began early in the morning and seemed to improve after a few hours. He visited the school nurse often, missing several classes for each nurse visit. Sam was obese and had a history of attention-deficit disorder. Because of his back pain, he did not want to participate in athletics. His mother confided to his physician that her son was embarrassed by his weight and body shape.

Several months later, Sam was seen by the adolescent medicine specialist for a sore throat. Because of his frequent absences from school, the school administration required a note for him to return to class. In March, Sam's mother disclosed that he was failing two subjects and had average grades in the others. She requested a school evaluation.

Subsequently, school authorities completed an educational evaluation. Sam's educational program was modified, and the school, with the approval of his physician, required him to participate in physical education. It became apparent that the boy had a learning disorder and also was having school avoidance issues. He was referred to a specialist in adolescent weight problems as well as a therapist.

Overview of Schools and School Services

Public schools in the United States are charged with meeting the academic and developmental needs of their students. Federal law protects the rights of students to obtain an education suited to their needs. When parents interact with the public school system, they should be aware of these laws. The Rehabilitation Act of 1973 is a civil rights law that prohibits discrimination on the basis of disability in federally funded programs, including public schools. Section 504 of this act requires school districts to provide free appropriate public education (FAPE) to every qualified student regardless of disability. If adolescents have a physical or mental impairment that substantially limits their functioning in major life activities, including learning and behavior, they may qualify for services under Section 504 of the Rehabilitation Act. Impairments include psychiatric disorders, such as ADHD.

The Individuals with Disabilities Education Act (IDEA), first passed by Congress in 1990 and revised in 1997 and 2004, further defined the disabilities eligible for special services in public schools, expanded parents' rights to participate in the development of their child's educational plan, and outlined the process by which special education services are provided for students with disabilities. Under this law, each eligible student is provided an individualized education plan (IEP) that is specifically designed to meet his or her educational needs. The categories of disability outlined by IDEA include autism (which includes other autistic-spectrum disorders), hearing or visual impairment, mental retardation, orthopedic impairment, serious emotional disturbance (which includes severe mood disorders such as depression and bipolar disorder), specific learning disabilities, speech or language impairment, traumatic brain injury, visual impairment including blindness, and other health impairment (under which services for ADHD are categorized). Despite the guidelines for the provision of services outlined by federal law, there may be significant variation in how the eligibility criteria are interpreted and the kinds of services that are available across different states and school districts.

Getting Help for Your Child's School Problems

When it appears that your child may be having difficulty in school, the first step is to open lines of communication with the school. Prior to the initiation of a formal evaluation, families can request a prereferral meeting, in which they get together with their child's teachers, guidance counselors, a principal or vice principal, and anyone else at the school who has had significant interaction with their teen. Such a meeting helps to establish a collaborative relationship with the school and can give parents a sense of the behaviors that the school is observing. Many concerns can be addressed by problem solving together with the school without initiating the sometimes time-consuming process of formal educational evaluation. Often, the school has dealt with similar difficulties in the past, and it may already have ideas about changes that can be implemented. However, if major problems persist after a prereferral meeting, it is often necessary to request an educational evaluation. The federal laws provide an outline for the procedures that schools must follow in performing an educational evaluation and determining the need for services. It is best to submit this request in writing, in the form of a letter addressed to the school principal or special education director. The letter should be short and to the point. Include the following: the date of the request, your child's name and date of birth, a brief description of the difficulties that are leading you to make the request, and your ultimate goal. Generally, parents hope to determine if their child has a disability that should be addressed by special educational services or other school-based interventions. To ensure that the letter is read, some parents choose to send it by certified mail. After sending a letter, parents may want to follow up with a phone call to the school.

Within ten school days of receiving a request, public schools are obligated to initiate the evaluation process. Depending in part on the nature of the teen's difficulties, the available resources in the school district, and the school's assessment of what is necessary in a particular case, the specific components of the evaluation may vary. Parents may request that the school assess for particular concerns, such as a learning disorder. Components that may be included in the evaluation are listed in sidebar 10.1. Depending on the complexity of the problem, the testing that is performed, and the school's efficiency, the educational evaluation process may require months to complete. At the conclusion of the evaluation, the school provides parents with a written report summarizing the findings.

No later than forty-five school days from the initial request, the school is required to hold a team meeting, which includes parents, to discuss the assessment and develop a plan for addressing the educational needs of the student, including eligibility for special educational services. Parents may also invite others to the meeting who they feel may be helpful, including supportive family members, educational advocates (discussed later in this chapter), or their child's psychiatrist

---

Sidebar 10.1 | Components of a School Evaluation

► Classroom observations by the child's teacher and/or outside observers such as other teachers or consulting mental health professionals

► Achievement testing, which is a measure of academic accomplishment, that shows whether a student is performing at grade level in a particular subject

► Neuropsychological testing, which provides information about a student's cognitive and emotional functioning (discussed in more detail in chapter 3)

► Input from outside professionals such as a therapist or psychiatrist who is working with your child

or therapist. Sometimes, mental health clinicians may participate via telephone conference.

At the team meeting, members of the school staff will determine whether the student has a disability that makes him or her eligible for services, and if so, they will recommend the appropriate services. There is a broad range of interventions that the school might offer. When a student appears to require relatively minor accommodations, such as preferential seating or more time to take tests, the school may recommend a 504 plan. Under a 504 plan, which takes its name from Section 504 of the Rehabilitation Act, a student participates in the same curriculum as other students. Accommodations are made to allow the student to make progress in this curriculum despite his or her disability.

When a student's disability is more impairing and the student is unable to make progress in a general curriculum even with accommodations, the student may be deemed eligible for an individualized education plan (IEP). The criteria for qualifying for an IEP are stricter than for a 504 plan, and an IEP generally involves a greater degree of intervention. Under an IEP, the curriculum itself is modified to fit the needs of the student. Modifications may include specialized instruction with professionals, such as occupational therapists or speech therapists. Instruction for some or all classes is held in a separate setting, such as a special education classroom with a smaller class size, and there is probably more support. Students on an IEP receive progress reports, usually on a quarterly basis. The IEP is reviewed by the school every year, and the evaluation process, including testing when appropriate, is repeated every three years. This enables the school to reassess the student's needs and update the IEP. However, if parents feel that their child is not making progress or that a change in their child's condition requires modification to the IEP, they may request a meeting of the evaluation team at any time.

At times, a student's disability is so significant that a regular, mainstream public school is unable to meet his or her needs. When this occurs, a student may be placed in a separate therapeutic school setting under an IEP. There are a number of conditions that may require this level of intervention, but some examples include an autistic student with significant developmental delay and self-injurious behavior that requires intensive behavioral intervention or an adolescent with a severe, treatment-resistant eating disorder that requires extremely close monitoring to keep the teen safe.

Therapeutic schools vary widely according to their areas of expertise, their philosophy and approach to problems, the services they offer, and the level of supervision and intervention they provide. There are therapeutic day schools with a schedule similar to that of a mainstream school, and there are therapeutic residential schools, in which students live at the school. Some therapeutic schools provide psychiatric care, including medication evaluation and management by a child and adolescent psychiatrist.

If you believe that your child requires this level of intervention, it may be useful to work with an educational advocate who is familiar with the schools in your area. The advocate can help find an appropriate match for your child's needs and help guide you through the often complicated process of arranging an appropriate placement. Before settling on a particular school, explore the options that are available. Visit schools, and while there, talk with staff and students. Thoroughly review the schools' literature or websites. Generally, it is best to involve your teen in the process.

Most educators are interested in improving the lives of children and adolescents, and schools want to meet the needs of all their students and to provide them with the best possible education. Still, public schools often work within tight budgetary constraints. Thus, the needs of an individual student who requires costly specialized services may be at odds with the needs of a school system with myriad demands on the budget. At times, it may seem to parents that the school is not offering the services that their child requires. When this occurs, parents have rights defined by federal law to allow them to have a voice in the process and to help protect the needs of their child.

However, if you do not agree with the school's initial proposal for your child's educational plan, try to avoid assuming a hostile, confrontational attitude. By maintaining a positive, collaborative relationship with the school, parents may be able to develop a more satisfactory arrangement. It may be useful to arrange a separate meeting with the special education director to discuss your concerns, as this may be less intimidating than the IEP meeting and may allow for better discussion.

Finding a good educational advocate may take research. Your child's psychiatrist, therapist, or pediatrician may be able to recommend an educational advocate. Other parents and school officials may also be able to provide you with names of advocates. A valuable resource is the Council of Parent Attorneys and Advocates, a national nonprofit special education advocacy organization that provides a database of advocates and educational attorneys organized by state. Visit its website at www.copaa.org. Many areas have local advocacy groups that may also locate advocates and provide other useful information. In Massachusetts, for example, the Federation for Children with Special Needs (www.fcsn.org) has a listing of advocates and runs educational programs for parents of children with disabilities. Similar organizations in your area can be found by searching the Internet or talking with your child's mental health providers.

In general, if parents do not agree with the recommended education plan, they can request an independent educational assessment by an evaluator outside the school system. Under some circumstances, this assessment may be funded by the school. Parents can also contact their state's department of education to discuss options for appealing the school's decision. At times, parents may wish to hire an attorney with expertise in education law to explore legal avenues for obtaining more services for their child. This is often a measure of last resort. The legal process can be time consuming and expensive, but in some instances it can be very effective.

Learning Disorders

Learning disorders are a group of conditions in which the affected individual's performance in one particular area of cognitive and academic functioning, such as reading, written expression, or mathematics, is substantially below that which would be expected for the individual's overall age, intelligence, and educational level. Learning disorders are one of the most common causes for school-related difficulties, and when they are not recognized and addressed, they can cause significant emotional distress for a teenager.

Symptoms and Warning Signs

Learning disorders are more common in boys than in girls, with the exception of mathematics disorder, in which the gender distribution is about equal. Learning disorders are generally recognized prior to adolescence, when it becomes clear that a child is having a great deal of difficulty in one particular area. However, learning disorders vary in the degree of severity, and in milder cases they may go unrecognized until the demands of school increase during the middle school and high school years. In addition, the symptoms of a particular learning disorder vary among adolescents. For example, some children with mathematics disorder have a great deal of difficulty with learning concrete math facts, such as memorizing multiplication tables, whereas others have more trouble with abstract concepts, such as using formulas or conceptualizing sets of objects. It is likely that each of the major learning disorders including reading, mathematics, and written expression actually represent a heterogeneous mix of different underlying processing problems.

Reading disorder, which is by far the most common of the learning disorders, often first becomes apparent when young children have difficulty learning the letters of the alphabet and the sounds they make. As these children progress through school, they may have trouble sounding out words. They read slowly and show poor reading comprehension. If the disorder is not identified in early childhood, by middle school it can lead to problems in multiple areas.

Mathematics disorder may present with a range of symptoms. Early in school, children may have trouble learning to count and may confuse the meaning of arithmetic symbols, such as the plus and minus signs. Outside school, children may have difficulty keeping score in games, learning to tell time, or making change. Some children have trouble determining left from right or being able to think spatially when reading a map.

As with the other learning disorders, a disorder of written expression may manifest itself in a range of symptoms. In general, children are slow to write and make many errors. Difficulties may range from the more concrete, basic aspects

> **Case Presentation**
>
> Joe, a sixteen-year-old boy, was evaluated in adolescent medicine to determine if there were physical causes for his illegible handwriting. The illegibility had led to academic problems in examinations in which Joe had to write essay answers, as his teachers could not read his writing. There was family and personal angst over his academic performance. The results of a complete physical and neurological examination were normal.
>
> The handwriting issues had not been addressed previously by the adolescent or his family. His school made an accommodation so he could use a computer for examinations. His academic average improved, and he eventually enrolled in a top engineering school.

of writing such as letter formation, spelling, punctuation, and legible handwriting to more general problems in finding words and organizing thoughts. Children with this disorder may refuse to hand in assignments, or they may submit unfinished work.

If learning disorders are not identified in early childhood, their indirect effects may manifest themselves during adolescence. Teens with unrecognized learning disorders may become frustrated with their schoolwork and develop poor self-esteem. In order to protect their fragile sense of self, they may devalue certain subjects, or school in general, calling it "stupid" or "a waste of time." They may appear lazy and unmotivated, which may be a front designed to conceal their underlying difficulties. Most teens would rather be perceived as an unmotivated student, which may be interpreted as a cool insouciance, rather than being labeled "stupid." To disguise or compensate for their difficulty, some teens with learning disorders will act out. They may be disruptive in class or take on the identity of a class clown.

Learning disorders may trigger significant anxiety. If teens are asked to read in class or sit through a seemingly endless math class, they may develop a sense of dread. Often, teens will try to avoid the subject areas that give them trouble. They may remain quiet and try to hide in the back of the room, or they may avoid a certain class by frequently arriving late or visiting the nurse's office with various complaints. Others may skip school. Teens with disorders of written expression may fail to turn in assignments. Teachers may feel that they spent little time or attention on assignment, when in fact the student agonized for many hours to produce a short, disorganized essay.

Making the Diagnosis

Standardized testing of both cognitive functioning (i.e., IQ tests) and achievement is an essential part of a learning disorder evaluation. This testing may be conducted by a school psychologist as part of an educational assessment or by an outside neuropsychologist. If your child's scores on achievement tests are below his or her intelligence level and level of education, there is a very good chance that you are dealing with a learning disorder.

Despite the importance of formal testing in diagnosing learning disorders, the diagnosis cannot be made on test results alone. Rather, to ensure an accurate diagnosis, adolescents with suspected learning disorders should be evaluated by a psychologist or psychiatrist. The clinician can help integrate the information gathered from testing with information from other sources, including classroom performance and history provided by the teen and parents. In addition, a psychiatrist or psychologist can screen for other conditions or problems that may be occurring with the learning disorder, such as ADHD, or as a result of the learning disorder, such as depression and anxiety.

Depending on the nature of the problem and the history that the clinician gathers, some children and adolescents with suspected learning disorder may be referred for additional sensory or neurological testing. For example, before reading disorder is diagnosed, it is important to rule out a visual problem as a cause of the reading difficulty. Inadequate motor control can contribute to writing problems, and impaired hearing can cause a variety of academic difficulties that may resemble a learning disorder.

Comorbidities

Teenagers with one learning disorder are at high risk for having another learning or communication disorder. In fact, most children with either mathematics disorder or disorder of written expression also have reading disorder. Furthermore, ADHD is very common in adolescents with learning disorders, which may well compound academic difficulties.

Treatment

Treatment of learning disorders is focused on educational intervention. The goals of intervention include a combination of remediation (i.e., trying to fix the underlying problem to the greatest extent possible) and accommodation (i.e., helping the student learn to work around the problem in order to minimize its impact). Students with significant learning disorders usually require an individualized education plan to help them address the problem. The IEP should be tailored to fit the student's needs, but interventions may include specialized instruction in the area of difficulty, individual tutoring, and added time on tests and quizzes. Students may be allowed to use tools, such as a laptop computer for teens with writing disorders or a calculator for those with mathematics disorder.

The identification and treatment of other coexisting problems is also an important part of managing a learning disorder. Psychotherapy, such as cognitive behavioral therapy, may be helpful for some teens in boosting self-esteem or bolstering problem-solving skills. Although medication does not play a role in addressing the learning disorder itself, it may be indicated for treating comorbid conditions such as ADHD.

Prognosis

Learning disorders are generally thought to be lifelong conditions. Nonetheless, with early identification and appropriate interventions, sufferers may gain a degree of competence in the area of disordered learning and minimize the impact that the disorder has on their lives. The outcome may vary depending in part on the degree of severity and on the interventions provided during childhood and adolescence. Many adults with learning disorders migrate toward fields that place minimal demands on their area of difficulty. Without appropriate intervention, adolescents with learning disorders are at high risk of academic underachievement, premature dropout, behavioral problems such as conduct disorder, and limitations in occupational functioning later in life.

School Refusal

Poor school attendance is a common problem that can be a huge strain on parents, schools, and, though it may not be apparent, the student him- or herself. School avoidance or school refusals are not a diagnosis in their own right, but they are generally symptoms of some other underlying process. Thus, the first step in helping a teen who is having major attendance concerns in school is a thorough assessment of the problem. Typically, psychiatric evaluation is indicated in this case.

Comorbidities

A psychiatrist or other mental health professional can identify potential psychiatric problems that may be contributing to the adolescent's behavior. Common psychiatric problems underlying poor school attendance include mood disorders, anxiety, and behavioral disorders such as oppositional defiant disorder or conduct disorder (discussed in chapter 14). Difficulties with peers, including bullying, frequently play a role as well. To help the clinician identify the nature of the problem, you should have discussions with teachers, school counselors, or other staff. Often, an educational assessment through the school is an important step toward understanding the cause of the problem. It should mobilize the school to address the issues. Testing through a school-based assessment can help identify potential learning disorders that may be playing a role in an adolescent's school refusal.

Treatment

Treatment of school refusal obviously depends on the nature of the underlying problems that are contributing to the behavior. For example, a teenager whose school refusal is rooted in a severe anxiety disorder may need appropriate therapy and medication. In addition, there should be a plan to increase the teen's exposure to the school environment. Supports need to be available at the school to help the student in times of stress and to build on techniques learned in therapy for managing anxiety. In contrast, students with conduct disorder may need increased direct supervision, greater communication between parents and the school, involvement of truancy officers or other community resources, and consistent enforcement of consequences for continued school refusal or other behavioral problems. Regardless of the nature of the underlying problem, management of school refusal almost always involves a collaborative approach among mental health providers, the school, parents, and the adolescent.

Conclusion

School is one of the fundamentals of adolescent life. Problems in school that arise during adolescence have the potential to cause significant distress and, if not addressed, can have negative effects that can last a lifetime. Struggles in school can lead to poor self-esteem, underachievement in one's career, and difficulties with relationships later in life. Thus, identifying problems early and obtaining appropriate help and services is essential to your child's well-being. Often, addressing mental health problems that are affecting an adolescent's school performance is a joint effort among the school, the family, and the teen's mental health providers.

In the public school system, federal laws protect the rights of students with disabilities, including mental illness, to receive services that meet their educational needs. Usually, the most successful approach is for parents to establish a positive, collaborative relationship with the school, with good communication in both directions. However, parents must balance this approach with the need to know their rights and advocate for their children when necessary.

References and Additional Reading

Beitchman, J. H., and A. R. Young. 1997. "Learning Disorder with a Special Emphasis on Reading Disorders: A Review of the Past 10 Years." *Journal of the American Academy of Child and Adolescent Psychiatry* 36: 1020–1032.

Stein, M. T., and B. Lounsbury. 2004. "A Child with a Learning Disability: Navigating School-Based Services." *Pediatrics* 114: 1432–1436.

Svetaz, M. V., M. Ireland, and R. Blum. 2000. "Adolescents with Learning Disabilities: Risk and Protective Factors Associated with Emotional Well-Being: Findings from the National Longitudinal Study of Adolescent Heath." *Journal of Adolescent Health* 27: 340–348.

11 Attention-Deficit/ Hyperactivity Disorder

Attention-deficit/hyperactivity disorder (ADHD) is a chronic condition that affects children, adolescents, and adults. ADHD affects 5 to 8 percent of children and adolescents, and it is believed to be the most common mental disorder diagnosed in childhood. Approximately 65 percent of children with ADHD continue into adolescence with symptoms related to their illness. The spectrum of ADHD varies from childhood to adolescence, making ADHD more difficult to diagnose in adolescents because observable hyperactivity, seen more commonly in preadolescents and young children, is less likely to be noted in teens. Moreover, children are unlikely to have academic failure problems.

It seems that no psychiatric diagnosis affecting adolescents receives as much media attention as ADHD, including controversy about whether it is a real disorder or merely a byproduct of our sped-up lifestyle or some other aspect of modern American culture. Over the past two decades, evidence emerging from research supports the position that ADHD is a very real disorder with consistently identifiable symptoms, biological underpinnings, and significant impairments and risks. Imaging studies have demonstrated consistent differences in the brain structure and activity patterns in individuals with ADHD compared to those without the disorder. These findings include a decrease in size in regions of the brain, such as the prefrontal cortex, that play a role in modulating attention. Medical professionals believe that genetics play an important role in ADHD, since it tends to run in families. In sets of twins, when one twin suffers from ADHD, there is a 90 percent chance that the other one will as well. ADHD is not preventable.

Academic issues may herald a diagnosis of ADHD in the adolescent years, and starting middle school or high school may precipitate an academic crisis in teens who have not yet been diagnosed with ADHD. Adolescents who had previously been able to function in school find that they are unable to keep up with the extra cognitive demands. In addition, teens are expected to organize and do their work with less adult supervision. Since adolescents with ADHD are usually less able to focus and set goals for their academic work, and they seem emotionally immature compared to their peers, they experience a decline in the quality of their schoolwork and in their grades.

Moreover, there is a higher risk that teens with ADHD will initiate tobacco and substance use compared to their peers who do not have ADHD. These risky

Case Presentation

Ben, a fourteen-year-old boy in the eighth grade, was brought to a psychiatrist for evaluation because of school difficulties. Ben's parents reported that he was a bright and precocious child but that ever since he was a young boy he had been forgetful, had trouble following directions, and was never "a good listener." Described as a very active child during elementary school, he was chastised by his teacher for talking excessively and getting out of his chair during class. Many of these problems seemed to resolve after he entered middle school in the sixth grade, but by seventh grade, his grades dropped from a mostly A average to a B and C average. His struggles with English and math were particularly difficult. In his first semester of eighth grade, he was receiving mostly Cs, and he failed his prealgebra class. His report card indicated that many teachers felt that he was not "working up to his potential." Ben said he found school "boring" and "didn't care" how he did. His father said he feared that Ben was becoming "lazy and unmotivated."

After reviewing a thorough history with Ben and his parents, the psychiatrist spoke with Ben's teachers, who reported that Ben made careless mistakes on tests. Incomplete or late homework assignments contributed to his declining grades. He seemed to have many problems with long-term projects. His English teacher noted that despite Ben's being bright and insightful in class, his writing assignments were disorganized and seemed "thrown together" at the last minute. Ben's math teacher gave a somewhat different story, stating that he was concerned Ben was "really struggling" and did not seem to understand the basic math concepts.

In a second meeting, the psychiatrist asked Ben's parents to complete a standardized ADHD symptom checklist. He also sent copies to the school for Ben's teachers to complete. He recommended that Ben's parents make a written request for an individualized educational assessment from the school. When Ben talked with his parents in private, he discussed feeling frustrated with school and said he felt as if "it's just not worth the effort." As an example, he said he worked many hours on his last English paper, but he really had trouble "getting going with it." When he received the low grade, he was disappointed and felt he had wasted a lot of time.

After Ben's psychiatrist reviewed all the information he gathered from Ben, Ben's parents, and the school, he diagnosed Ben with ADHD and prescribed a stimulant medication. Ben immediately reported feeling better able to focus. Almost immediately, with the exception of math, Ben's schoolwork improved.

Through the individualized educational assessment, Ben participated in testing with the school psychologist. The tests showed that he had high intelligence but problems with executive functioning, which refers to higher-level abilities that control or regulate other lower-level abilities such as memory, attention, and motor skills. Goal-directed behavior, planning, and decision making, as well as other functions, may be affected by executive functioning problems. Achievement testing indicated a level of performance in math that was below what would be expected for Ben's intelligence. The psychiatrist and school psychologist agreed that Ben probably had a learning disorder in mathematics.

Ben was started on a 504 plan, and modifications were made to his academic work. For example, Ben's teachers helped him break long-term projects into smaller, more manageable tasks. They allowed him extra time on tests and created a homework log to help him keep track of assignments. Ben was also assigned a tutor in math and met weekly with his math teacher to review the material. By the end of the school year, Ben's grades were back up to As, and, more importantly, his spirits were decidedly improved. Ben's father was pleased that Ben seemed to be putting in more of an effort. Ben said, "Before it felt like no matter how hard I tried, things weren't right, and it would get me really upset. Now it feels like everything is coming together for me."

behaviors can have a profound affect on the adolescent's academic performance as well as on his or her adjustment outside school.

See appendix A for further resources on ADHD, such as the National Institute of Mental Health.

Symptoms and Warning Signs

ADHD is known to affect more boys. The rates of diagnosis are much higher in boys, probably due to earlier diagnosis in childhood. Because boys are more likely to act out or have behavioral problems with ADHD, they come to the attention of teachers earlier than do girls, who tend not to have ADHD-related behavioral issues. Girls with ADHD often have academic problems that become apparent in middle school. The disorder is categorized into subtypes according to the group of symptoms that is most prominent: primarily inattentive subtype (formerly called attention-deficit disorder, or ADD), primarily hyperactive subtype, and combined type, in which problems with both hyperactivity and inattention are present. The symptoms of ADHD inattention subtype are noted in sidebar 11.1, and the symptoms of ADHD involving a problem with hyperactivity are listed in sidebar 11.2.

Symptoms of ADHD begin in early childhood, and the disorder is often diagnosed before adolescence. However, at times it goes unrecognized until the teenage years, particularly in those teens with the primarily inattentive type. Bright, resourceful children may be able to compensate for their problems for some time, but in the middle school and high school years, demands on an adolescent's at-

---

Sidebar 11.1 | Symptoms of ADHD Inattention Subtype

- ► Difficulty maintaining attention during schoolwork or other activities
- ► Being distracted easily
- ► Careless mistakes or lack of attention to detail in schoolwork
- ► Appearance of not listening, even when being addressed directly
- ► Difficulty following directions
- ► Frequently failing to finish school assignments, household chores, or other duties
- ► Difficulties with organization
- ► Complaints of feeling bored
- ► Avoidance or dislike of tasks that require sustained attention
- ► Forgetfulness, e.g., not remembering to turn in completed homework assignments or to bring home the books needed to complete an assignment
- ► Tendency to lose things

> **Sidebar 11.2 | Symptoms of ADHD Hyperactivity Subtype**
>
> ► Excessive activity and/or talking
> ► Frequently fidgeting or getting out of one's seat when required to sit still (as in a classroom)
> ► Often feeling restless
> ► Having trouble quietly engaging in activities on one's own
> ► Difficulty waiting for one's turn in the classroom, in sports, or in other activities
> ► Impulsively blurting out answers or making other comments in class
> ► Interrupting the conversations of other people

tention and organizational skills increase dramatically. Teens with ADHD find longer-term projects and more open-ended assignments more problematic.

Making the Diagnosis

ADHD is a clinical diagnosis that is based on the presence of characteristic symptoms. The diagnosis may be made by a child and adolescent psychiatrist, another mental health professional, or a pediatrician. To make a diagnosis, it is important for the evaluating clinician to have an accurate picture of the child's behavior in a variety of settings, including at home and at school. The clinician may wish to speak with the child's teachers, coaches, or other important people in his or her life. Clinicians often use symptom checklists or standardized scales, such as the Conners Rating Scale, in an effort to obtain an objective measure of the degree of symptoms present in school and at home. To determine if the therapy is effective, these scales may be used during treatment.

Though research studies have identified potential genes and brain abnormalities that may play a role in ADHD, at present there are no laboratory tests or brain imaging studies that are used to diagnose ADHD. Some practitioners claim to be able to diagnose ADHD using seemingly scientific methods such as findings on an electroencephalogram (EEG) or levels of certain chemicals in the blood. In general, these claims are misleading at best and often downright dishonest. There is no good scientific evidence to support such claims. The diagnosis of ADHD is always a clinical one, made according to the presence of symptoms and the degree of difficulty they are causing. At times, the diagnosis of ADHD may be unclear. Thus, a learning disorder or another psychiatric condition may make it difficult to determine whether a teen's symptoms are related to ADHD. In these situations, neuropsychological testing can be helpful. It is important to note that a diagnosis of ADHD does not imply deficit in intelligence. It is possible to have a very high IQ and still have ADHD.

Other Problems to Consider

Differential Diagnosis: What Else Might Be Wrong?

An adolescent's attention and activity level involve complex, coordinated brain functions. A number of disruptions in the brain's healthy functioning can cause problems in these areas that may resemble the symptoms of ADHD. It is important to consider other possible causes for a teen's difficulties before settling on a diagnosis of ADHD.

Mood disorders, including depression and bipolar disorder, frequently cause major problems with attention. The symptoms of these conditions, including restlessness, impulsivity, and problems with concentration, have some overlap with the symptoms of ADHD. As a result, a mood disorder should be considered in a teen suspected of having ADHD, particularly if the symptoms seem to have begun in the adolescent years. Similar to adolescents with depression, those with ADHD may seem irritable or easily frustrated, and they may appear to lack motivation. However, if they are demonstrating persistent periods of depressed mood, dramatic mood swings, aggressive or erratic behavior, or suicidal thoughts, there is probably a problem with mood instead of or in addition to ADHD.

Learning disorders may resemble ADHD. Teens suffering from them may become restless and bored in class and have difficulty completing assignments. Yet in learning disorders the problems should appear exclusively in the particular area of difficulty, and the student should be able to sustain attention in other subjects. Thus, a student with a specific learning disorder in math should not have great deal of difficulty in history or English classes. In contrast, students with ADHD are likely to have global troubles not only in all or most of their classes but also in other areas of their life. In cases in which a learning disorder is suspected, neuropsychological testing can help confirm the diagnosis. Testing generally shows performance in a particular area that is below what would otherwise be expected given a teen's grade level and overall intelligence.

Teens who have patterns of frequent oppositional behavior, as seen in oppositional defiant disorder (ODD) and conduct disorder (discussed in chapter 14), may also have behavior patterns that resemble ADHD. They may refuse to complete homework assignments or engage in disruptive behavior. To confuse matters further, ADHD commonly occurs together with behavioral disorders such as ODD. But teens who have ODD or conduct disorder without comorbid ADHD should have the ability to sustain their attention and regulate their behavior when they are sufficiently motivated. This may be difficult to differentiate, and it may require a thorough evaluation by an experienced clinician to make an accurate diagnosis.

Comorbidities

Adolescents with ADHD are at increased risk for having other psychiatric conditions. In particular, rates of substance abuse are higher in teens diagnosed with ADHD. In part, this may be due to increased impulsivity as well as an attempt by teens to self-medicate. The risk of substance abuse in adolescents with ADHD appears to be reduced when they receive proper treatment. Adolescents with ADHD are also at increased risk of developing mood disorders, possibly due to the low self-esteem that can result from ADHD. The relationship between ADHD and bipolar disorder is less clear. The two conditions share several overlapping symptoms, leading researchers to suggest that some children and teenagers initially diagnosed with ADHD may in fact be showing early manifestations of bipolar disorder, which becomes clear later as the illness progresses. Between half and three-quarters of teens with ADHD may meet criteria for oppositional defiant disorder (see chapter 14).

Treatment

Treatment for adolescents with ADHD generally involves some combination of medication, educational accommodations, and behaviorally focused therapy. There is no single treatment plan that works for every child. Rather, the best treatment plan is one the takes into account the teen's individual needs. The severity of the ADHD symptoms, the presence of comorbid problems such as depression or a learning disorder, the availability of supports, the adolescent's areas of strength, and the family's views on medication and other treatments are factors that play a role in deciding on an appropriate treatment plan. Collaboration with the school and your child's mental health provider is essential in developing an effective approach to treatment.

Medications

Medications are a very effective treatment for ADHD. They can dramatically improve teens' focus and reduce their impulsivity and hyperactivity, helping them feel more in control in school and beyond. Still, the decision to start medication is never an easy one. In addition to the potential for side effects, medications can stir up strong feelings in teens who are in the process of finding their identity. In addition to weighing the benefits of medication versus its risks, it is important that you explore your child's feelings about taking medication and include them in the decision process as much as possible.

Stimulants are the first line of medications used to treat ADHD. These medications include methylphenidate (Ritalin) and amphetamine salts (Adderall). The stimulants increase levels of the brain chemicals dopamine and norepinephrine in the connections, or synapses, between brain cells. The activity of these chemicals in specific brain regions appears to play a major role in the modulation of attention and impulse control. Unlike many psychiatric medications that take effect gradually, stimulants can have an immediate impact on the symptoms of ADHD, leading to improvement even after the first dose.

The body metabolizes stimulants fairly quickly. As a result, they wear off after a few hours. In order to provide symptom control throughout the day, the medication must be taken several times each day. Or it may be administered in a controlled-release formulation that allows for less-frequent, more-convenient dosing while providing optimal levels of medication in the teen's system. Amphetamine salts are available in a controlled-release form such as Adderall XR. Controlled-release forms of methylphenidate include Ritalin LA, Concerta, and Metadate CD. There is also a controlled-release methylphenidate topical patch called Daytrana.

Unfortunately, these medications have side effects, such as headaches, stomachaches, decreased appetite, and difficulty sleeping. Sleep problems can be addressed by switching to a different time-release formulation or changing the timing of the doses. Sometimes, teenagers can become more irritable or moody when taking stimulants. Often, this occurs as the medication is wearing off late in the day, and this too can be addressed by changing to a different medication formulation.

There has been some concern that stimulants may slow the rate of skeletal growth, but this is controversial. Some studies indicate that stimulants do not significantly affect growth, and others suggest small differences in a minority of people. Nonetheless, while adolescents are taking stimulants, they should have their height and weight monitored by their pediatrician.

Stimulants may also cause increases in blood pressure and heart rate. These increases are negligible and do not have any significant medical implications in an otherwise healthy teenager. However, blood pressure and pulse should also be monitored by the prescribing doctor during treatment.

As noted in chapter 5, the most serious concern about stimulant medications is also the most controversial. Cases of sudden death due to cardiovascular problems such as arrhythmias have been reported in a small number of adolescents who were taking stimulants. Although these unfortunate events are extremely rare and also occur in adolescents who are not on medications, they have raised the question of whether stimulants increase the risk of potentially fatal heart problems. The extreme infrequency of these events makes this a difficult area to study. Findings from studies that have attempted to answer this question have been mixed, with some suggesting that there is no increase in risk for teens on stimulants. However, a recent large study suggested that stimulants may be associated with a slight increase in risk of unexplained sudden death, though these events continue to be extremely rare.

In general, it is advised that stimulant medications be used with caution in those adolescents whose medical history suggests that they may have cardiac disease, which may include a history of congenital heart disease, irregular heart beat, fainting, and sudden death in children or young adults. If the teen has such cardiac history, then a medical consultation with his or her pediatrician should be done. However, the American Academy of Pediatrics issued a policy statement in August 2008 suggesting that is not necessary to routinely obtain an electrocardiogram screening on children before beginning medication for ADHD treatment.

Adolescents may abuse stimulants. Inappropriate use of stimulants, including taking excessive doses or snorting or smoking them, can cause a high, with feelings of euphoria and a surge of energy. Also, some adolescents may abuse stimulant medications in order to decrease their appetite and lose weight. This may be an issue in teens who have an eating disorder as well as ADHD. Thus, weight should be monitored for teens on stimulant medications. Stimulant abuse can lead to severe problems, including physiological and psychological dependence on the medication, extreme mood swings or irritability, and even paranoia and psychosis (see chapter 12 for further discussion of stimulant abuse). For this reason, parents and physicians should give careful consideration to the risk of abuse before giving stimulants to teens who have a history of problems with substances. Still, a history of substance abuse does not mean that stimulants should never be used. Close parental supervision of medication administration and storage or use of stimulants formulations with chemical properties that make them more difficult to abuse may allow for the safe use of stimulants in teens.

A commonly used nonstimulant medication for ADHD treatment is atomoxetine (Strattera). This medication has a unique mechanism of action, blocking the reuptake of the neurotransmitter norepinephrine after it is released by brain cells. Blocking reuptake of norepinephrine increases its transmission between cells and indirectly increases levels of dopamine in certain parts of the brain. Atomoxetine has been shown to be effective in treating both the inattentive and hyperactive symptoms of ADHD. Unlike stimulants, atomoxetine may take some time to reach its full therapeutic effect. With daily use, there may be continued gradual improvement in symptoms over a period of four to eight weeks.

Most teens tolerate atomoxetine. Yet, it does have potential for side effects, some of which are similar to those seen with stimulants. Common side effects include decreased appetite, upset stomach, dry mouth, constipation, fatigue, and difficulty sleeping. As with stimulants, atomoxetine has the potential to cause small increases in heart rate and blood pressure; therefore, it is advised that these be monitored when the medication is started.

Some teens taking atomoxetine may experience effects on mood, including irritability or anxiety. Rarely, they may have onset of manic episodes following initiation of treatment with atomoxetine. This is thought to occur primarily in teens who have an underlying biological predisposition to bipolar disorder (see chapter 7 for a description of manic symptoms). Probably related to atomoxetine's potential to affect mood in a small number of people, some studies have indicated that its use can cause a small but significant increase in the risk of suicidal thoughts in adolescents (see appendix A for reference). Because of this concern, the Food and Drug Administration (FDA) has added atomoxetine to a list of several medications, including SSRIs, that may increase the risk of suicidal tendencies. This is a controversial issue that is still being studied, and it is discussed in more detail in the discussion of antidepressant treatment in chapter 6.

Although the risk of suicidal thoughts appears to be small (well under 1 percent in existing studies), adolescents on this medication should be closely monitored by the physician and parents, particularly in the early stages of treatment. When the medication is started, frequent visits with the doctor may be required. In addition, parents should look for changes in their child's mood or behavior. When changes do occur, the physician should be notified.

Even though stimulants and atomoxetine are the primary medications used to treat ADHD, when the more established treatments do not work or cannot be used, several other medications may be employed as a second line. Buproprion (Wellbutrin) is an antidepressant that affects transmission of the neurotransmitters dopamine and norepinephrine, which have been shown to play a role in ADHD. While it has not been approved by the FDA as a treatment for ADHD, several studies have suggested that it may have some efficacy in reducing ADHD symptoms. Common side effects include headache, stomach upset, decreased appetite, anxiety, and insomnia. Buproprion may also lower the seizure threshold and should be used with caution in teens who are at risk for having seizures.

Clonidine is a medication that is primarily used to treat high blood pressure. It also has effects on the central nervous system and has been shown in several studies to be effective in the treatment of ADHD. Clonidine is useful in treating tic disorders, including Tourette syndrome, and thus may be a good choice of medication when an adolescent is suffering from tics as well as ADHD. It appears that clonidine may have greater efficacy in reducing the hyperactive symptoms of ADHD and less efficacy in addressing the inattentive symptoms. Side effects include sedation, which may be significant in some people, decreased blood pressure, dizziness or lightheadedness, dry mouth, and depressed mood. Clonidine may also increase risk of a cardiac arrhythmia in teens who have an underlying heart condition.

Modafinil (Provigil) is a relatively new medication with a poorly understood mechanism of action. Its effects include increased alertness and wakefulness, similar to stimulants. Currently, it is approved only in the treatment of certain kinds of sleep problems involving excessive daytime sleepiness, such as narcolepsy and shift-work sleep disorder. However, some preliminary studies have suggested that it may be useful in the treatment of ADHD. At present, there are few data supporting its safety and efficacy in adolescents. With further research, it may prove to be another ADHD treatment option.

Therapy

Psychotherapy can be a powerful tool in ADHD treatment. Therapy can play a role either as an adjunct to medication or as an alternative approach for parents and adolescents who prefer not to use medication. Behavioral therapy, focused on changing behavioral patterns and learning concrete skills, is generally the most helpful therapy approach in addressing ADHD symptoms. Unstructured and open-ended approaches, such as psychodynamic psychotherapy, are less likely to be helpful and may be frustrating for some adolescents with ADHD.

Through therapy, adolescents can learn strategies for managing their symptoms. Education is also an important aspect of therapy, as teens have a better recognition of the symptoms of ADHD and the ways that it can affect them. Through this strategy, they can work to minimize the impact that ADHD has on their lives.

Parents can also benefit from education about ADHD. Clearly, it is challenging to live with a teen affected with ADHD. Parents may confuse symptoms of ADHD, such as forgetting to do a chore, with selfishness or a lack of responsibility. Help with homework may lead to frustration on both sides and may result in arguments. By working with their teen's therapist, parents can learn how to tell what problems may be ADHD symptoms, what is "normal teenage stuff," and what signs may indicate a larger problem. A therapist can help teach parents strategies for working with their adolescent at home and how best to advocate for their adolescent at school.

Coaches, Advocates, and Other Supports

To improve organizational skills, some teens with ADHD may benefit from working with a tutor or an ADHD coach. Coaches are often professionals with some background in education who have experience working with adolescents who have ADHD. Your teen's psychiatrist, therapist, or school may be able to provide you with suggestions.

Educational advocates can help parents work with the school system to develop an appropriate plan to meet a child's academic needs. They often become involved when parents feel that the school is not offering a plan that adequately meets their child's needs. In this case, advocates can educate parents about their rights and help them to negotiate the educational system into developing an appropriate plan. Advocates may be able to offer insight into the kinds of modifications and accommodations helpful for your teen's situation.

Parent support groups and advocacy organizations are also useful resources for many families. Your teen's mental health provider should be familiar with the resources in your area and may be able to direct you to a local group. A national organization called Children and Adults with Attention Deficit/Hyperactivity Disorder (CHADD) has branches throughout the country that offer support groups, educational sessions, and parent training classes. Details about local chapters and other useful information can be found on the organization's website, www.chadd.org. See appendix A for other helpful resources related to ADHD.

Educational Modifications

Working with the school can be an important aspect of managing ADHD. Public schools are required to meet the educational needs of their students without discriminating on the basis of a disability, including psychiatric disorders such as ADHD. By offering a modified academic program tailored to fit a child's needs, schools can help students with ADHD continue to thrive and progress academically. Different teens will require different degrees of intervention in the school according to their individual needs. Students with ADHD symptoms that are well controlled by medications or other treatments and who do not have a great deal of difficulty in other areas may do well with only minor adjustments to their school program. Students with more severe problems, such as difficult-to-manage ADHD along with other comorbid psychiatric problems, may require a greater degree of intervention, such as an individualized education plan (IEP).

Because ADHD is a common problem, many schools have experience in developing modified education plans to meet the needs of students with ADHD. After evaluating your child's needs, school psychologists and counselors may offer suggestions about specific modifications. In this process, it is important to obtain the input of the people who have the most direct, hands-on experience with your child, including teachers and classroom aides. Your child's psychiatrist or therapist is also likely to have valuable input about what interventions would be useful. It is reasonable to invite your child's mental health providers to attend school meetings to offer their insight and suggestions. If they are unable to attend, they may still communicate with the school via telephone conference or by providing a letter with written recommendations.

Although your adolescent's plan should be customized to meet his or her individual needs, modifications that can be helpful for students with ADHD include those listed in sidebar 11.3.

Alternative Treatments

Understandably, parents are often reluctant to put their children on medication for ADHD, and many explore alternative treatments and natural remedies. Although some of these treatments have shown promise, in general, alternative medicine approaches to ADHD treatment have not been well studied. None has

> ### Sidebar 11.3 | School Modifications for Adolescents with ADHD
>
> ▶ Seat the student in a location with the fewest distractions, such as away from the door and near the front of the classroom.
> ▶ Help the student use organizational tools, such as colored folders, to keep track of papers for different subjects and a calendar to keep track of assignments and tests.
> ▶ Break down large, longer-term projects into smaller steps with intermediate deadlines. For example, a term paper may be broken down into steps such as deciding on a topic, finding relevant background resources, writing an outline, completing a first draft, and then writing revisions until the finished assignment is submitted on time.
> ▶ Provide duplicate sets of text books or other class materials for home and school. This avoids the potential to forget materials that are essential to completing assignments.
> ▶ Allow extra time on tests or other assignments.
> ▶ Grant access to a study skills class or "resource room" where the student can get closer attention and help with organization.
> ▶ Develop frequent communications between parents and teachers. Try a daily e-mail or progress report.

the same degree of proven efficacy as the more established treatments. Nevertheless, if a particular approach does not pose any significant health risk to your child, incorporating alternative medicine into your treatment plan for ADHD may be helpful.

Some treatments may have advantages beyond reduction of ADHD symptoms. For example, yoga, exercise, and meditation can reduce stress and improve a teen's overall health. Still, it is important to note that these approaches have not shown great results in reducing ADHD symptoms. When you are considering alternative treatments, avoid those in which the safety is not well established. Focus on treatments that are known to have some efficacy.

For many years, there have been theories about links between diet and ADHD, with particular focus on high sugar intake. This idea is based on the observation from many parents that their children seemed more hyper after eating or drinking a lot of refined sugar from sweetened cereals, junk food, or soda. There is no evidence that diet, including food additives, causes or complicates ADHD.

However, there may be environmental toxins that do have a role in childhood ADHD. Several different groups of researchers have noted the role of lead poisoning in hyperactivity, distractibility, and restlessness in children. Moreover, prenatal exposure to alcohol may give rise to behavioral problems in children. Children who are diagnosed with fetal alcohol syndrome often are hyperactive, disruptive, and impulsive. And finally, a few studies have noted a link between maternal smoking during pregnancy and ADHD symptoms in the child. Obviously, to avoid toxin-induced ADHD, pregnant women should avoid alcohol and tobacco, and children should live in lead-free homes.

Herbs and Supplements. There are a number of products advertised on the Internet and elsewhere promising "natural" treatment of ADHD through herbs or formulations of vitamins or supplements. Most supplements used for the treatment of ADHD have been poorly studied, and none has shown the degree of efficacy that is seen with established ADHD treatments. In addition, "natural" does not mean safe. Many of the world's most potent poisons are naturally occurring, and the FDA does not hold vitamins or herbal supplements to the same standards for proving safety as it does prescription medications. Even vitamins, when given in large doses, can be harmful.

Omega-3 fatty acids, a "natural" remedy, holds promise for the treatment for ADHD. Omega-3 is a polyunsaturated fatty acid required by the body and available in certain fish, nuts, and flaxseed. These compounds have been the source of great attention in recent years, as they have been touted to have a number of health benefits. There is some evidence that supplementation with omega 3 fatty acids, which can be taken in capsules derived from fish oil or flaxseed oil, may reduce ADHD symptoms in some children. Obviously, more research needs to be done in this area. Currently, omega-3 fatty acid supplements are not viewed as a first-line treatment for ADHD, but they may be reasonable as an adjunct to other treatments.

When taken in recommended amounts, omega-3 fatty acids are fairly safe, but they may have side effects in high doses, such as bleeding and stomach upset. Children with seafood allergies should avoid taking supplements derived from fish oil. In general, it is best to consult with your child's pediatrician or psychiatrist before starting omega-3 fatty acids or any other supplement.

Prognosis and Risks

With proper treatment, adolescents with ADHD can thrive and reach their full potential. Untreated ADHD during adolescence can have a major impact that can extend beyond the teenage years. Academic struggles related to ADHD may lead teens to become frustrated with academic work and feel badly about themselves during a time that is critical to the formation of self-image, potentially setting them up for a lifelong pattern of poor self-esteem. For some adolescents, ADHD causes major social problems as well. Hyperactivity and impulsivity may result in behaviors that annoy their peers and make it more difficult to fit in. Some teens compensate by becoming the class clown or the antiauthoritarian rebel.

In addition to concerns about self-esteem and social development, researchers have identified more concrete risks associated with untreated ADHD. For example, teenagers with untreated ADHD have higher rates of automobile accidents and lower occupational and academic achievement in later life, including higher rates of school dropout and lower salaries in adulthood. An even bigger concern is a significantly increased risk of substance abuse and tobacco use in teenagers with untreated ADHD. This risk is probably due to a combination of factors, but it may be a form of self-medication for some teens, as well as an indirect effect of low self-esteem.

Course

The course of ADHD through adolescence and into adulthood is an area of active research. It was once believed that ADHD almost always resolved by early adulthood. In recent years there has been a growing appreciation that symptoms can persist well beyond adolescence. Though the precise numbers vary widely across different studies depending on the methodology that is used, in general it appears that the majority of adolescents will outgrow their symptoms by the time they reach adulthood. Still, a significant minority will have persistence of symptoms, which may range from a few mild areas of difficulty to full-blown ADHD that continues to cause significant difficulties into adulthood.

Conclusion

ADHD is the most commonly diagnosed mental condition in children and adolescents. Most cases of ADHD have a genetic basis, although prenatal exposure to alcohol or tobacco and postnatal exposure to lead may also precipitate this illness. Teens with ADHD are more likely to have substance abuse problems, oppositional defiant disorder, and learning problems. There are a number of medications that are helpful in reducing ADHD symptoms, and generally these medications are safe to use in adolescents. With proper treatment, teens with ADHD often reach their full potential.

References and Additional Reading

Brown, R. T., R. W. Amler, W. S. Freeman, J. M. Perrin, M. T. Stein, H. M. Feldman, K. Pierce, and M. L. Wjolraich. 2005. "Treatment of Attention-Deficit-Hyperactivity Disorder: Overview of the Evidence." *Pediatrics* 115: e749–e757.

Gould, M. S., B. T. Walsh, J. L. Munfakh, M. Kleinman, N. Duan, M. Olfson, L. Greenhill, and T. Cooper. 2009. "Sudden Death and Use of Stimulant Medications in Youths." *American Journal of Psychiatry* 166: 992–1001.

Polanczyk, G., and L. A. Rohde. 2007. "Epidemiology of Attention-Deficit/Hyperactivity Disorder across the Lifespan." *Current Opinion in Psychiatry* 20: 386–392.

Rappley, M. D. 2005. "Attention Deficit–Hyperactivity Disorder." *New England Journal of Medicine* 352: 165–173.

12 Substance Abuse

Adolescence is a time for experimentation. New interests, friends, and self-expression are all part of the process. Therefore, it is not surprising that adolescence is a time when problems with substance abuse first emerge. Because teens often fail to consider the long-term consequences of their actions and have a tendency to see themselves as being impervious to harm, they are particularly vulnerable.

Although most teens may experiment with alcohol, tobacco, or marijuana without developing a problem, a significant minority will progress to patterns of problem usage. If this occurs, an adolescent has the best chance of overcoming a substance abuse problem by obtaining appropriate help as soon as possible. In this chapter, we discuss which adolescents are at highest risk for abusing substances, warning signs that your teen may have a problem with substance abuse, and approaches to treating this problem.

Even though it is perceived that adolescent drug use has been climbing in the United States, in fact, overall substance use among teens has decreased to some extent, with usage of alcohol, marijuana, and cocaine on the decline. However, trends in drug use are ever changing. While the use of some drugs may be declining, there is concern that use of others may be on the rise. For example, salvia divinorum is a powerful hallucinatory agent unknown to many parents and health professionals that is still legal in most of the United States. Thanks in part to easy availability over the Internet, its use appears to be on the rise. There is concern that abuse of prescription drugs, including pain killers and stimulant medications, is on the rise as well.

Influenced by the torrent of information sharing and communication that takes place over the Internet, teen drug use has changed dramatically. Photos and videos of intoxicated teens are posted on the Internet on sites such as YouTube, Facebook, and MySpace. There are also social networking sites that provide a forum for teens to discuss drug use and other risky behaviors. Sites provide information with varying degrees of accuracy about substances and ways to get high. Some sites promote drug use and have message boards for teens to share their knowledge and compare experiences. For example, the website Erowid (www.erowid.org) is a massive compendium of information and postings about psychoactive substances, some accurate and some less so, with an overall pro-drug, pro-experimentation bias. Other sites, including government sites such as the National Institute on Drug Abuse (www.nida.nih.gov) warn of the dangers from drug use and provide useful information for kids and parents. It is obvious

---

Case Presentation

Paul, a sixteen-year-old boy, was brought to the hospital emergency room because of frostbite and low body temperature. He had been found lying in the snow with ice around his bare right foot about seven hours after leaving a party with other teens. His blood alcohol level, taken at the hospital, was almost 0.12 (more than legally drunk). He had no recollection of the events that had taken place during the preceding seven hours.

The teen had a history of experimenting with alcohol and marijuana in the past. Because of the extensive and deep frostbite, he had a significant amount of tissue injury and required hospitalization in the intensive care unit. A toe amputation was needed because of gangrene. The adolescent was referred to a therapist during the hospitalization.

---

that we are living in an era when teens are surrounded by much information, and parents must remain educated and vigilant in order to protect their children.

Risk Factors

There are a number of factors that have been identified that may increase an adolescent's risk of developing a substance abuse problem. These factors can be divided into three categories: individual factors, family factors, and community factors.

Since males are more likely to abuse substances than are females, individual risk factors include being male. Teens with psychiatric illness are at significantly increased risk of abusing substances, particularly when the psychiatric disorder goes untreated. Conduct disorder, attention-deficit/hyperactivity disorder, learning disorders, mood disorders, and post-traumatic stress disorder appear to place teens at particularly high risk of substance abuse. Psychiatric illness may increase risk in several different ways. Teens may try to self-medicate their symptoms, they may have impaired judgment or increased impulsivity and risk-taking behavior, or the illness may contribute to their low self-esteem. Low self-esteem itself appears to be an important risk factor for substance abuse even in the absence of a psychiatric disorder. Similarly, academic underachievement, poor social skills, and limited coping skills have been associated with high rates of teen substance abuse.

Family factors play a significant part in teens' risk for substance abuse. There is strong evidence that genetic factors play a part in determining an individual's predisposition to addiction. Thus, even when an adolescent is not directly exposed to parental substance use, a strong family history of substance abuse may place that adolescent at risk. However, the example set by parents is even more powerful than genetic influence, as teens who are exposed to substance abuse in the home are at very high risk of developing substance abuse problems. Parents' actions in modeling responsible behavior for their children are much more powerful than the verbal messages they communicate. Loose supervision and chaotic home environments also raise the risk for adolescent substance abuse problems. In addition, the quality of teens' relationship with their parents influences their likelihood for substance abuse. Teens who report that they view their parents as supportive and as people they can talk to if they have a problem have lower rates of substance abuse than teens who lack this degree of trust.

Community is also an important factor in determining adolescents' risk for substance abuse. It is not surprising that teens living in areas with high rates of substance abuse are at increased risk for abusing substances. Availability of substances is one key factor, but attitudes about substance abuse in the community, including at school, may be just as important. Communities that convey a message of tolerating substance abuse, for example, by turning a blind eye to drinking at school events, may increase risk for the adolescents in that community.

Prevention and Protective Factors

Parents can help lower their children's risk of developing a substance abuse problem. First, set a good example with your own behavior, and maintain a positive and communicative relationship with your child. Teens who feel they can turn to a parent when they have a serious problem and who argue infrequently with their parents also have lower rates of substance use. Provide good supervision by knowing where and whom your teenager is with at all times. As is so often the case in parenting teenagers, when it comes to substance use it is essential to find the right balance between providing clear and consistent limits and avoiding an overly harsh or judgmental approach that might shut down lines of communication. Finally, parents can help minimize their children's risk of substance abuse by acknowledging and addressing problems in the family, including conflict, relationship issues, or a possible mental health issue, before these problems cause further damage.

Schools and communities can also play an important role in prevention. Teens who participate in sports and other organized activities have lower rates of substance abuse. Similarly, involvement of concerned adults such as coaches, teachers, and school counselors can be a positive influence on teens' lives in many ways. Schools can provide education about the potential dangers associated with substance use and convey a message that they do not condone the use of drugs or alcohol, such as through zero-tolerance policies and anti-drug programs. And finally, schools can help lower rates of substance abuse by providing academic help and social and emotional support to students who are struggling.

> **Sidebar 12.1** | **Warning Signs for Adolescents Abusing Substances**
>
> ► Dramatic changes in mood or behavior, including irritability, angry outbursts, or erratic behavior
> ► Decline in school performance or attendance
> ► Dropping out of activities such as sports teams or school groups
> ► Loss of motivation
> ► Distancing oneself from friends and developing a new peer group, especially with peers who have delinquent behavior or little interest in school
> ► Sudden changes in appearance, including adopting more eccentric styles or paying less attention to hygiene
> ► Violating curfew, sneaking out of the house, or other delinquent behavior
> ► Stealing money from parents or asking for money more often
> ► Becoming increasingly secretive about whereabouts and activities and avoiding parents when returning home after being out
> ► Frequently appearing or complaining of feeling tired

Symptoms and Warning Signs

Teens with substance abuse problems are likely to give warning signs that parents and other adults can detect, as seen in sidebar 12.1. It is important to note that these signs do not necessarily indicate a substance abuse problem. When not accompanied by other warning signs or with signs of a decline in overall functioning, a change in interests, clothing styles, or groups of friends may be part of normal adolescent experimentation. Many of these warning signs may also signify other psychiatric disorders, such as depression. Nonetheless, if several of these signs are present, it is important to look into the situation.

Making the Diagnosis

What to Do If You Suspect a Substance Abuse Problem

If you are concerned that your child is using drugs or alcohol, it is important to discuss these concerns with your child. It may be difficult for teens to be completely honest about their use of substances. Many will try to minimize or normalize their behavior. Nonetheless, it is important to give your child the message that you are aware of a possible problem and you are concerned. Doing so will also help keep your teen from feeling blindsided if you later confront him or her about the need to get help. Approaching the issue from a concerned, nonjudgmental standpoint rather than from an angry, punitive point of view is more likely to be productive.

After this discussion, if you are still unsure whether your child may have a substance abuse problem, then talk with other people in your child's life. Contact parents of your child's friends, teachers, school counselors, and coaches to see if they have noticed a potential problem. Siblings may be aware of a problem, but they may be afraid to get their brother or sister in trouble. Letting them know that your goal is not to be punitive but rather to get help for a problem may make them more likely to tell you what they know.

Teens who may be abusing substances need to be monitored closely. This means knowing with whom your child is socializing and where they plan to go. Checking in when your child comes home after being out with friends can help parents pick up signs of substance use.

If you suspect your child is using substances and is not being honest with you, it may be necessary to search their room for evidence of substance use. This may feel like spying on your child, but it may be necessary in order to protect him or her. You could also ask your child's physician to run a urine drug screen; however, it is best to tell your child about the screen beforehand.

Getting an Evaluation for Substance Abuse

An evaluation for substance abuse may be performed by a child psychiatrist, a social worker, a psychologist, or another mental health professional with experience in this area. The evaluation begins with a detailed history from the parents and the teen. This history should be comprehensive, exploring not only the teen's use of substances but also exploring his or her overall mental and physical well-being. A thorough substance abuse evaluation should screen for other psychiatric problems, such as depression or ADHD. The teen's past medical and psychiatric history is also an essential component of the evaluation. Additionally, the clinician may explore family issues, as these often play a role in adolescent substance abuse.

Laboratory tests, including a urine drug screen, are a common part of the evaluation. A teenager may refuse to take such a test, but refusal itself can be revealing, as it is rare for teens to refuse a drug screen unless they have something to hide. Possible associated medical problems can be assessed. For example, to screen for alcohol-related liver damage, levels of liver enzymes may be checked in teens who are heavy drinkers.

Sidebar 12.2 | Signals of Serious Substance Abuse

► Substance use is causing problems in the teen's activities, such as school, home life, sports, or work
► The adolescent is repeatedly using substances in dangerous situations, e.g., drinking and driving
► The teen is involved in violence as a result of substance use
► The adolescent is arrested for reasons related to substance abuse

---

Sidebar 12.3 | Symptoms of Substance Dependence

▶ Developing a tolerance to the substance, in which increasing amounts of the substance are needed to produce the same effect

▶ Having withdrawal symptoms when use of the substance is stopped

▶ Frequently taking more of the substance than planned

▶ Repeated, unsuccessful attempts to cut down or stop using the substance

▶ Spending a great deal of time using the substance, trying to obtain it, or recovering from its use

▶ Giving up important activities (e.g., dropping out of school, quitting a sports team) for reasons related to substance use

▶ Continuing to use a substance despite knowing that it is causing major physical or psychological problems (e.g., depression)

How does a mental health professional distinguish between normal adolescent experimentation and a more serious problem with substances? The line is not always clear. In general, use of a substance can be considered abuse when it is repeatedly causing problems in a teen's life. Sidebar 12.2 lists signals that indicate that an adolescent's substance use may have moved beyond experimentation and into the realm of abuse.

Repeated use of drugs or alcohol may lead to *substance dependence,* a term used by mental health professionals to refer to a condition in which an individual loses control of the substance use, persistently using the substance despite clear signs that it is causing harm. Symptoms of substance dependence are noted in sidebar 12.3.

When tolerance and withdrawal are present, the individual is said to have *physical dependence,* which means that the body has adjusted to the regular presence of the substance and that abruptly stopping its use can be physically uncomfortable and even dangerous. (Specific withdrawal symptoms related to particular substances are discussed later in this chapter.) The degree to which physical dependence occurs varies according to the particular substance. For example, physical dependence to opiates may develop fairly rapidly. By contrast, physical dependence to marijuana is less common, and there is some controversy as to whether it occurs at all. It is important to note that a substance dependence disorder may occur with predominantly psychological and behavioral symptoms.

What If Your Child Refuses to Go for an Evaluation?

Difficulty acknowledging the problem is a common feature in substance abuse, and many adolescents will resist going for an evaluation and treatment. In fact, often the early stages of treatment are focused on helping teens recognize the ways in which their substance use has become harmful. Thus, parents' initial goal in obtaining help is to have their teen appear for treatment.

One approach is to engage your adolescent in treatment by framing it according his or her concerns and priorities instead of your own. For example, despite your point of view, a teen might not feel that his daily use of marijuana is a problem, and he may even see it as something that helps him cope with stress. However, he may acknowledge difficulties with anxiety and problems managing stress at school. By encouraging him to get help for those problems, he may be willing to begin meeting with a therapist who can, after establishing a trusting relationship, begin to explore the role that marijuana plays in the teen's life.

Often, parents must use a carrot-and-stick approach to getting their child into substance abuse treatment. By threatening strict consequences, such as grounding or taking away access to the car, for refusing to go and by offering additional privileges (without compromising close supervision) for going, parents may be able to pressure teens to get the help they need.

If a substance abuse problem is severe and the adolescent has reused to obtain help, it may be necessary to enlist the resources of the juvenile justice system. If an adolescent has been arrested, parents can request that a judge order substance abuse treatment and mandatory drug testing as terms of probation, even if the crime was not directly related to substance use. Many states have arrangements through which parents can request services for their child, such as the assignment of a probation officer and court-mandated treatment, even if the teen has not been arrested. Fear of legal consequences, including incarceration, is a powerful incentive. Many parents are reluctant to invoke these services, for fear of getting their teen into legal trouble. Still, when an addiction becomes severe and it is not being addressed, problems with law are usually not far behind. It may be preferable to enlist legal help voluntarily before a problem becomes too entrenched than to sit idly by and let an adolescent risk his or her life and the lives of others.

Other Problems to Consider

A number of other psychiatric problems may have symptoms similar to the warning signs of substance abuse. Depression may cause teenagers to seem more irritable with little motivation and energy and may cause a decline in school performance (see chapter 6). Bipolar disorder may cause these same symptoms during a depressive episode and may also cause impulsive, erratic, or explosive behavior during a manic or mixed episode (see chapter 7). Psychotic disorders, such as schizophrenia, may resemble some of the symptoms of substance abuse, in that teens with psychosis may say or do strange things, stop taking care of themselves, isolate themselves from others, and seem secretive or guarded with parents (see chapter 9).

Substance abuse is closely intertwined with other forms of psychiatric illness. Other psychiatric illnesses can increase an adolescent's risk of developing a substance abuse problem, and substance abuse can also cause other psychiatric disorders by altering brain chemistry. Frequent use of many substances, including alcohol, marijuana, and cocaine, may cause mood disorders in susceptible individuals. Psychiatrists diagnose this condition as a *substance-induced mood disorder*. The features of such a disorder may be identical to those seen in depression or bipolar disorder except that they appear to have been triggered by heavy substance use. Similarly, several substances, including cocaine, marijuana, and hallucinogens such LSD, may cause what is referred to as a *substance-induced psychotic disorder*, sometimes even after a single use. In this condition, psychotic symptoms such as delusions, disordered thinking, and hallucinations may persist for weeks after the substance is out of the teen's system.

Treatment

As with other forms of psychiatric treatment, treatment for substance abuse disorders can take a variety of different forms according to the needs of the individual. The cornerstones of substance abuse treatment for adolescents are individual therapy, treatment for any comorbid psychiatric issues, group therapy (including support groups), and family therapy.

Individual Treatment

Individual therapy focuses on helping adolescents build insight into the role that substances play in their life and teaching skills for establishing and maintaining abstinence. Since many teens entering treatment do not initially recognize their substance use as a problem, in the beginning, treatment may be focused on helping adolescents understood the ways in which substances have been harmful to them or those around them and become open to change. As adolescents' insight and motivation for change improves, the therapist can teach them skills to help them abstain from drug use and avoid relapse. Skills involve recognizing and avoiding triggers for use, managing urges to use, and learning ways of dealing with stress and difficult emotions without turning to substances.

Several different theoretical approaches may be used in individual therapy for substance abuse. Cognitive behavioral therapy, or CBT (discussed in chapter 4), is a frequent, skills-based approach with proven efficacy. Another technique that is commonly used in the treatment is motivational interviewing, which involves an empathetic, nondirective approach to help guide teens toward appreciating the need for change and finding the motivation to make changes in their substance use.

In addition to addressing the substance abuse problem, it is important for clinicians working with adolescents to recognize and treat any comorbid psychiatric issues. Failure to do so can place a teen at high risk for relapse. For example, an adolescent with an anxiety disorder may turn to alcohol and marijuana as a way of trying to deal with her symptoms. Even if the substance abuse is brought into remission, anxiety will remain an ongoing trigger for relapse until the disorder is treated.

While medications may be used to treat coexisting psychiatric disorders, often they do not have a direct role in the treatment of substance abuse disorders in adolescents. However, there are medications that have been used as part of the treatment for adults with alcohol abuse. Acamprosate (Campral) and naltrexone (Revia) appear to work by reducing one's craving for alcohol. Naltrexone may also treat opiate abuse by blocking the receptors in the brain to which opiates bind in order to produce their effects. Another medication, disulfiram (Antabuse), helps promote abstinence by causing an unpleasant reaction, including anxiety, flushing, headache, nausea, and vomiting, when an individual taking the medication drinks alcohol. These medications may be considered for adolescents with severe, treatment-resistant substance disorders. Since these medications can have potentially dangerous side effects, they should be used under the close monitoring of a psychiatrist who is experienced in their use.

Group Therapy

Group therapy is often an important component of treatment for adolescents with substance abuse disorders. Groups help teens recognize that there are other kids who are struggling with similar issues, and allow them to get support and advice from their peers. Adolescents are particularly attuned to the opinions of their peers, so they may be able to hear a message from a fellow group member that would be ignored if given by a therapist or parent.

Involvement in twelve-step programs, including Alcoholics Anonymous (www.aa.org) and Narcotics Anonymous (www.na.org) can be another important part of substance abuse treatment. Although such programs were designed for adults, studies have shown that they may be effective for adolescents. Adolescents are welcome at AA and NA meetings, and many areas have specific "young people" groups. These programs may be more effective if a teen attends meetings regularly and identifies a sponsor/mentor who has been in recovery for a long period of time. Other programs such as Al-Anon and Alateen (www.alanon.alateen.org) are two branches of an organization that offers support to family members of people with alcoholism or narcotic abuse. They may be a useful resource for parents and siblings of a teen with substance abuse problems.

Family Treatment

Effective treatment of an adolescent with a substance abuse disorder often means involvement of the entire family. Parents may need guidance from a teen's therapist or other involved clinicians on how to manage their child's issues with substance abuse. Family therapy can be helpful when there are issues at home that are contributing to the adolescent's substance problem and can help improve communication and strengthen relationships within the family. Individual psychiatric treatment for a parent may be warranted if that parent is suffering from a mental health or substance problem. It is very difficult for adolescents to address their own problems with substances if there is someone at home who is continuing to abuse drugs or alcohol.

Inpatient Substance Abuse Treatment

Many adolescents with substance abuse disorders need more intensive treatment than they can receive as outpatients. Inpatient programs provide intensive treatment in a safe, structured, and highly supervised environment; these programs may be located on a locked psychiatric unit or in an unlocked residential facility. Good candidates for an inpatient program include those teens who have developed physiological dependence to a substance. In this case, the adolescent needs to be monitored for withdrawal symptoms and potentially dangerous medical consequences of withdrawal that could occur with such substances as alcohol and benzodiazepines. It should be noted that in therapeutic doses, benzodiazepines may be helpful for adolescents who are withdrawing from alcohol abuse. Adolescents with a severe substance abuse problem, poor insight into their problem, and little motivation to change may also need inpatient treatment. For these teens, inpatient treatment can establish a period of enforced abstinence, laying the groundwork for recognition of their problem and initiating motivation for change. In addition, in order to maintain their safety and stability inpatient treatment may be necessary for adolescents who have a severe comorbid psychiatric illness that also requires intensive psychiatric treatment. Thus, a teen with bipolar disorder and alcohol abuse who is suicidal may need to be treated on a locked psychiatric unit until her symptoms begin to improve.

Other Programs

Inpatient substance abuse treatment is usually short term, typically lasting a few weeks, though the duration can vary according to the program and the needs of the adolescent. Once the teen has been stabilized and begins to improve, he or she may be stepped down to a day treatment program or to outpatient treatment. Occasionally, adolescents with substance problems that have been particularly difficult to treat may be referred from a psychiatric unit or short-term residential unit (sometimes called "acute residential treatment," or ART) to a long-term residential program, where treatment may continue over a period of months.

Some adolescents with substance abuse disorders benefit from wilderness programs. These programs offer treatment for adolescents with substance abuse and behavioral problems in a remote setting. Furthermore, these programs usually provide intensive individual and group therapy interspersed with outdoor activities such as hiking and camping, which may help some teens become more self-reliant and self-confident. Some programs take a very harsh disciplinary stance and may not be the best fit for certain adolescents. Before sending your child to such a wilderness program, it is advisable to research it thoroughly and to obtain input from clinicians who know your child well. Wilderness programs can be quite expensive and are generally not covered by insurance.

Common Drugs of Abuse and Their Effects

Alcohol

Because alcohol is relatively easy to obtain and its use is more socially sanctioned in our society than other substances are, it is the most commonly used substance during adolescence. According to 2007 survey data from the federal Substance Abuse and Mental Health Service Administration (SAMHSA), approximately 16 percent of adolescents between the ages of twelve and twenty have used alcohol in the past month (www.oas.samhsa.gov). Since alcohol use is so common among adolescents, there is a tendency for adults to normalize it. Yet frequent experimentation with alcohol appears to lead to a greater prevalence of problem use. According to SAMHSA, over 4 percent of youth in the twelve-to-twenty age range appear to meet the criteria for a diagnosis of alcohol abuse or dependence.

It is risky for adolescents to consume alcohol. The adolescent brain is different from that of a mature adult, and there is some evidence to suggest that at-risk adolescents may progress more rapidly than adults from occasional use of alcohol to problem use. Studies have shown that more than half of adult alcoholics began to abuse alcohol during adolescence.

Occasional use poses other threats as well. Automobile accidents are the leading cause of death for fifteen- to twenty-year-olds in the United States, and alcohol plays a role in a significant portion of these accidents. According to the 2007 Youth Risk Behavior Survey conducted by the U.S. Centers for Disease Control, over 29 percent of ninth- to twelfth-graders rode in a car with a driver who had been drinking alcohol in the past thirty days, and over 10 percent had driven while drinking. Even for those teens who avoid drinking and driving, drinking may lead to other risky behaviors, such as unprotected sex.

The effects of alcohol are well known. After one or two drinks, alcohol can produce a pleasant, relaxed feeling. As the level of alcohol goes up, there is greater impairment of attention and reaction time and a decrease in inhibition. Alcohol can induce a feeling of euphoria, but it can also bring about sudden shifts in mood, including anger outbursts or feelings of intense sadness. At higher levels, alcohol depresses activity of the central nervous system, leading to drowsiness, confusion, impaired balance and coordination, slurred speech, and ultimately unconsciousness. At high levels, alcohol is toxic to the brain and liver, with potential for permanent damage even with a single binge. At very high levels, alcohol intoxication can be fatal.

Regular alcohol consumption can lead to tolerance, meaning that it requires consumption of increasing amounts in order to produce the same effect. Alcohol overuse can produce physiological dependence, in which withdrawal can occur with physical symptoms. These symptoms may include significant increases in blood pressure, heart rate, and temperature. Alcohol withdrawal may also cause delirium tremens, a potentially dangerous condition involving hallucinations and confusion. Severe cases of alcohol withdrawal can lead to seizures and death. Thus, when teens who are very heavy drinkers with physiological dependence stop drinking, they may require medical monitoring and treatment in an inpatient medical or psychiatric setting. Medications, including benzodiazepines, can prevent serious symptoms from withdrawal.

Heavy alcohol use can have a number of undesirable physical and psychological effects, including cirrhosis (or scarring) of the liver, pancreatitis, gastritis (inflammation of the stomach), stomach or intestinal ulcers, heart problems, and anemia. Psychologically, alcohol can induce mood disorders, most commonly depression, or worsen the symptoms of an existing psychiatric illness. Alcohol can also interfere with function and metabolism of psychiatric medications, rendering them less effective. Over time, toxicity from alcohol can cause problems with memory and cognition that may be irreversible. Needless to say, adolescents who drink heavily are at risk for unprotected sex and physical/emotional trauma.

Marijuana

Marijuana is the illicit drug most often used by adolescents. Despite the common belief that use of marijuana and other illegal drugs is increasing in the United States, it appears that marijuana use has actually declined somewhat in recent years. Data from the National Survey on Drug Use and Health, conducted by SAMHSA, indicate that the percentage of adolescents ages twelve to seventeen who had used marijuana in the past month declined from 8.2 percent in 2002 to 6.8 percent in 2005 and has remained fairly steady at this level since then (www.oas.samhsa.gov). Nonetheless, marijuana continues to be a problem for many teens.

Parents should be aware that the marijuana that is used today is not the same drug that some of them may have used years ago. Changes in cultivation practices over the past twenty years have produced more potent strains of marijuana with higher concentrations of THC, the primary psychoactive chemical in marijuana. The U.S. Department of Justice, in cooperation with the University of Mississippi, has reported data from an analysis of the marijuana seized in drug raids showing that the average concentration of THC more than tripled between 1986 and 2006. Marijuana also may be laced with other substances, including cocaine, heroin, PCP, or even embalming fluid.

There are countless slang terms for marijuana and related paraphernalia. The following are some of the more common names for the drug itself: pot, weed, bud, herb, ganja, reefer, chronic (this sometimes refers to marijuana laced with cocaine), dope, grass, indo, skunk, and sensimilla. A marijuana cigarette may be referred to as a "joint," "spliff," or "doobie."

Marijuana is usually smoked. It can be rolled in cigarette paper to make a joint, put into a hollowed-out cigar (called a "blunt"), or smoked from a hand pipe or water pipe (called a "bong"). When marijuana is smoked, its effects are felt within minutes and generally last a few hours. Marijuana can also be ingested, such as by baking it in brownies. When the drug is ingested, the onset of its effect is delayed but lasts longer, usually over a period of several hours, depending on the amount ingested.

The acute effects of marijuana may vary from teen to teen and be influenced by the user's expectations. A typical high involves an initial feeling of euphoria, which may be followed by a feeling of relaxation and calm. Common effects include giddiness, drowsiness, lightheadedness, heightened sensitivity to lights and sounds, increased appetite, and altered perceptions of space and time. Marijuana causes impaired concentration and problems with short-term memory and motor coordination, which is likely to interfere with schoolwork and make driving dangerous. At times, marijuana may induce a feeling of intense anxiety or paranoia or a panic attack.

The long-term effects of marijuana may vary and are the subject of some debate. Some frequent users can develop amotivational syndrome, which, as the name suggests, is characterized by lack of motivation and energy. Frequent marijuana use has been associated with a number of psychiatric problems, including depression, anxiety, psychotic disorders, and delinquent behavior. However, there is some controversy as to whether these disorders are caused by marijuana use or whether people with these disorders are more likely to use marijuana. Heavy marijuana use can lead to lasting memory impairment, and smoking marijuana can cause significant damage to the lungs and airways.

While marijuana is not as addictive as some other substances, it is possible to develop dependence. With frequent use, teens may develop psychological dependence, in which they have little control over their marijuana use. There is some debate about whether marijuana causes physical dependence, with tolerance and withdrawal symptoms, but it appears that some heavy users may develop a physical dependence. Withdrawal symptoms include irritability, depression, anxiety, headaches, intense cravings for the drug, insomnia, restlessness, and decreased appetite. These symptoms may continue for over a week after the last use of marijuana.

Cocaine

Cocaine is a dangerous and highly addictive drug. Although cocaine use among adolescents has decreased slightly over the past several years from a peak in late 1990s, according to a 2007 survey conducted by the Centers for Disease Control and Prevention, 7 percent of adolescents between the ages of twelve and seventeen have tried cocaine (www.cdc.gov).

Usually cocaine is sold either as a white powder or in the highly addictive derivative form called crack cocaine. Crack cocaine consists of crystalline pellets of varying sizes and shapes that are generally off-white to yellowish in color and smoked from a specialized pipe that is typically crafted out of a narrow tube of glass. The powder form of cocaine is normally snorted into the nose, but it may be rubbed into the gums or ingested. Cocaine may also be injected beneath the skin ("skin popping") or into a vein. The extremely dangerous and often lethal combination of heroin and cocaine injected together is referred to as a "speedball." The effects of cocaine are felt within minutes of use, with smoked or injected cocaine taking effect more rapidly than cocaine that is snorted. The effects can last from a few minutes to several hours, depending on the amount taken and the method of consumption. The drug is a powerful stimulant to the central nervous system, resulting in a high that is usually experienced as a feeling of euphoria accompanied by a surge in energy, activity, and talkativeness. Users may develop a temporary grandiose sense of themselves or feel invincible. These positive feelings may be accompanied by acute anxiety or paranoia. A person high on cocaine may behave erratically or have explosive fits of rage. When the effects of cocaine wear off, the user often experiences a crash, with depressed mood and extreme fatigue.

Physical side effects of cocaine use include increases in heart rate and blood pressure and dilation of the pupils. When snorted or rubbed on the gums, it acts as a local anesthetic, causing numbness and decreasing blood flow. Cocaine is also a potent appetite suppressant.

In overdose, cocaine can be lethal, as it can lead to a cardiac arrhythmia or cause a myocardial infarction (heart attack), even in a young, healthy person. Cocaine can also cause seizures or stroke. Because dealers commonly cut the drug with other materials to increase their profits, cocaine use is particularly risky. This variable potency can make it difficult for even an experienced user to gauge the amount of drug that will be sufficient to produce a high without getting into lethal territory.

Chronic cocaine use can cause changes in brain chemistry that strongly predisposes a teen to depression. The constriction of blood vessels caused by cocaine can lead to stomach ulcers or kidney damage. Snorting cocaine can cause erosion of nasal tissue, including perforation of the septum between the two nostrils. Smoking crack cocaine can be highly toxic to the lungs.

Perhaps the biggest concern about repeated cocaine use is the highly addictive nature of the substance, with the potential for the drug to take over an adolescent's life and place him or her at high risk of overdose. When an adolescent develops cocaine dependence, there is an unpleasant withdrawal syndrome that occurs when the drug is stopped. These symptoms include powerful cravings for the drug, depression, fatigue, excessive sleep, inability to experience pleasure, increased appetite, poor concentration, achiness, chills, and runny nose.

Opiates

Opiates are a group of chemically related substances that includes the street drug heroin, as well as a number of prescription pain killers including morphine, codeine, and methadone. These drugs are highly addictive, and their use among teenagers appears to be on the rise, due in part to the growing illicit sale of prescription medication such as Oxycontin (often called "OCs"), and Percocet (or "Percs").

Depending on the particular opiate, they may be snorted, smoked, or injected, usually directly into a vein but sometimes beneath the skin ("skin popping"). Prescription opiates that come in pill form are frequently ingested or pulverized and snorted.

Opiate use produces a high characterized by feelings of euphoria, relaxation, and well-being, usually accompanied by drowsiness and often by itchiness, flushing, and dry mouth. Physiologically, opiates are depressants to the central nervous system that relieve pain at lower doses and produce unconsciousness or confusion at higher doses. Overdose on opiates is potentially lethal, usually by suppression of a person's drive to breathe.

Because opiates are highly addictive, users quickly develop tolerance to these drugs, requiring increasing amounts to get high. When opiates are stopped, those teens who have developed physiologic dependence experience a very unpleasant withdrawal syndrome. Symptoms of opiate withdrawal include anxiety, restlessness, insomnia, sweating, chills, nausea, vomiting, diarrhea, and leg and stomach cramps.

Moreover, opiate use carries other risks. Many users of these drugs progress to intravenous (IV) use, often heroin, as injecting the drug provides a more rapid and intense high than other means. Intravenous injection carries many risks, including possible transmission of HIV and hepatitis B infection through shared needles, abscesses of the skin, emboli (small blood clots or particles of foreign material in the blood stream that can block blood supply to vital organs), and cardiac infection (endocarditis). Adolescents who use opiates may be predisposed to depression and other psychiatric problems.

Hallucinogens

Hallucinogens are a group of drugs that alter a person's senses and perception of reality. Commonly used hallucinogens include LSD ("acid"), PCP ("angel dust" or "embalming fluid"), and psilocybin mushrooms (which may be called "'shrooms" or "magic mushrooms"). An herb called salvia divinorum is growing in popularity among adolescents. Currently, it may be purchased legally, and it is readily available on the Internet. Ketamine ("Special K") and MDMA ("ecstacy"), which may also be considered hallucinogens, are discussed later in this chapter, in the section on club drugs.

The effects of hallucinogens vary widely. The expectations and mindset of the user may heavily influence the effects of an individual drug. LSD, short for lysergic acid diethylamide, is usually taken by placing in the mouth a small piece of blotting paper (or a "tab") soaked in the substance. LSD produces a "trip" that is often characterized by altered perception of space and time and vivid perceptual distortions, including seeing colors, geometric patterns, and objects shifting in their appearance. Additionally, LSD can also cause changes in the user's perception of self, which some users view as a spiritual experience. LSD's effects can be unpredictable, and some adolescents become paranoid, anxious, or delusional on the drug. These effects can lead to unpredictable and potentially dangerous behavior.

LSD may cause dilated pupils, fever, increased heart rate and blood pressure, insomnia, tremors, decreased appetite, and dry mouth. The drug is not thought to produce tolerance or withdrawal symptoms, although psychological dependence is possible in frequent users.

Effects of LSD typically last for six to twelve hours, but it has the potential to cause chronic psychological effects even after a single dose. Some users experience flashbacks, in which the effects of the drug are reexperienced long after it has left the body, sometimes in an intrusive and potentially impairing way. In some users, LSD appears to carry risk of inducing a chronic psychotic state.

Psilocybin is a naturally occurring psychoactive substance that can produce distortions in a person's perception of reality similar to the effects of LSD. The drug is taken by ingesting dried mushrooms of various species that contain the substance. After ingestion, psilocybin's effects last several hours, including perceptual distortions or hallucinations, such as experiencing colors or sounds more intensely or seeing "after-trails" of moving objects. Time perception distortions are also common. On occasion, users can have a bad trip, in which they experience intense fear or anxiety. Psilocybin can induce psychotic symptoms in susceptible individuals and can cause flashbacks similar to those seen with LSD. High doses of the drug may cause nausea, vomiting, unsteady gait, pupillary dilation, and drowsiness. Although overdose on the drug is not believed to be fatal, there is a danger that users may mistake a poisonous mushroom for a psilocybin mushroom and suffer dire medical consequences.

PCP, short for phencyclidine, also has unpredictable effects. At times it produces a detached, trancelike state, and at other times it can induce extreme agitation, paranoia, confusion, or feelings of invincibility. Hallucinations are possible at higher doses. A person high on PCP may demonstrate bizarre, unpredictable, and potentially violent behavior, and many teens have seriously injured themselves or those around them under the influence of this drug. PCP may cause rapid and shallow breathing, flushed skin, sweating, fluctuations in heart rate and blood pressure, numbness of the extremities, rapid flickering eye movements, muscle spasms, and lack of coordination. At higher doses, PCP can cause seizures, coma, and even death. PCP is addictive, and chronic use can lead to dependence, with withdrawal symptoms including powerful cravings for the drug, memory and cognitive problems, and depression. These symptoms may persist for many months after the drug is stopped.

Salvia divinorum is a psychoactive plant in the mint family that has been growing in availability and popularity among American teenagers over the past decade. The drug is usually referred to as "salvia" by teens, but it may also be called "magic mint," "sally d," or "diviner's sage." At present, there are no federal laws against the possession or use of salvia divinorum, though its legal status may change at the state level. It is available over the Internet.

A teen may consume Salvia divinorum by chewing or smoking the leaves or by drinking a liquid extract made from the plant. The drug's effects are short-lived, beginning minutes after use and lasting for about thirty minutes. Saliva divinorum is reported to produce psychedelic effects, with altered perceptions of space and time and auditory and visual hallucinations. It may cause a trancelike state and uncontrolled laughter. Some users may experience depressed mood or anxiety. While intoxicated, the adolescent's judgment and functioning are markedly impaired, and he or she may be prone to engage in risky behavior. There are concerns that the drug may worsen mood problems in vulnerable individuals. There have been some highly publicized cases of adolescents who were frequent users of salvia divinorum who committed suicide. It is difficult to determine what role the drug may have played in these tragic deaths.

Benzodiazepines

Benzodiazepines (or "benzos") are prescription medications used to treat seizures, insomnia, and anxiety (see chapter 5 for a discussion of their clinical use). Drugs in this class include includes lorazepam (Ativan), clonazepam (Klonopin), diazepam (Valium), and alprazolam (Xanax). When abused, the pills may be ingested or ground and snorted.

The effects of benzodiazepines are similar to those of alcohol, as they produce feelings of relaxation, disinhibition, and well-being. They may cause drowsiness, slurred speech, lack of motor coordination, and delayed reaction time.

Abuse of benzodiazepines is risky: physiological dependence is very common, and withdrawal from these drugs is not only uncomfortable but also dangerous and potentially fatal. Withdrawal symptoms include severe anxiety, restlessness, mood changes, rapid heart rate, and elevated blood pressure. More severe withdrawal symptoms include confusion, hallucinations, agitation, and seizures.

By suppressing a person's respiratory drive and brain activity to the point of inducing coma, benzodiazepines carry a risk of lethal overdose. The risk from overdose on benzodiazepines is increased when they are mixed with other substances, particularly with other nervous system depressants including alcohol or opiates.

Stimulants

Stimulants are a group of related drugs that work in a similar fashion to increase activity in certain parts of the brain. They may be referred to as "speed" or "uppers." The stimulants include the prescription medications methylphenidate (Ritalin, Metadate, Concerta, and others, sometimes referred to as "ritz" by adolescents) and amphetamine (Adderall, Dexedrine), which, when used appropriately, can be very effective in the treatment of ADHD and other disorders. When these medications are absorbed gradually into the bloodstream at moderate levels, they increase alertness and, in patients with ADHD, improve attention and reduce symptoms of impulsivity and hyperactivity. On the other hand, when the level of stimulant in the blood is very high or increases very rapidly, which can be achieved by grinding up and snorting pills, they can produce a high that leads some teens to abuse these medications.

The high is characterized by a feeling of euphoria accompanied by alertness, increased energy and activity, decreased need for sleep, and talkativeness. At higher levels, stimulants may bring about aggressive behavior, agitation, paranoia, delusional thinking, hallucinations, and a sense of grandiosity. Stimulants increase heart rate and blood pressure and cause dilated pupils. They also decrease appetite, a common side effect of ADHD medications, and for this reason they are sometimes abused by teens with eating disorders or those who are self-conscious about their weight. In overdose, they are potentially fatal and may cause seizures, cardiac arrhythmias, or coma.

While appropriate use of prescription stimulants under the supervision of a physician rarely leads to dependence, abuse of these medications with frequent consumption in high doses can produce dependence. Stimulant withdrawal symptoms include fatigue, excessive sleep, depression, and strong drug cravings.

Methamphetamine is an illicit drug that is related to the other stimulants, but it deserves special mention. It is dramatically more potent, deadly, and addictive than its prescription medication cousins. Also called "crystal meth," "speed" (which may also refer to other stimulants), "tweak," "crank," "ice," "crystal," or "glass," methamphetamine is among the most devastating substances of abuse, and its use is on the rise in the United States.

This substance is synthesized, or "cooked," in illegal laboratories and sold on the street in whitish crystal chunks. It is most commonly smoked in glass pipes, similar to crack cocaine, but may also be snorted, ingested, or dissolved in liquid and injected into a vein. Methamphetamine's effects are similar to those of the other stimulants, but it is much more potent and produces a more intense high and is more likely to induce paranoid thoughts and erratic, impulsive, and often violent behavior. Users may be more sexually promiscuous while under the influence of the drug. High doses of methamphetamine appear to be directly toxic to the brain and may cause lasting brain damage. Overdose and need for emergency medical care are more likely with methamphetamine than with other stimulants.

Methamphetamine is notorious for being extremely addictive, with users frequently falling into a precipitous downward spiral in which the drug takes over their lives. Addicts may develop a number of psychiatric problems, including paranoia or psychotic symptoms that may persist long after the drug is stopped. Chronic users frequently suffer significant weight loss and malnutrition due to appetite suppression and poor self-care. Burns on the hands and face are common among those who smoke the drug. Users' teeth often erode and fall out, sometimes within a short period of time. This is referred to as "meth mouth."

The addiction resulting from methamphetamine abuse can be difficult to treat. The outlook for a teen's recovery is better if the treatment is intense and extended over time.

Club Drugs

Club drugs are a diverse group of substances that are commonly used in clubs, bars, and parties. Drugs in this category include MDMA, GHB, rohypnol, and ketamine. In the 1980s and 1990s, when these drugs became part of the rave scene, their use grew rapidly. (A rave is a large, late-night underground party held in an illegal location such as an abandoned warehouse.) Though the rave scene has been on the wane in recent years, use of these drugs is still quite common.

MDMA is an illicit substance produced in illegal laboratories that is most commonly referred to as "ecstacy" (or "XTC"), "E," or "X." This drug may come in different colors and often bears an imprint on the surface, such as a dollar sign or other popular icon, to distinguish a particular brand. In these pills, MDMA is often mixed with other substances such as cocaine, methamphetamine, ketamine, or caffeine. Indeed, one of the dangers of club drugs, as with many drugs of abuse, is that the user cannot be certain about what he or she is taking.

The effects from MDMA use are usually felt within an hour of consuming the drug and last for several hours thereafter, including a feeling of euphoria, a sense of calm and well-being, and an increase in intensity of perceptual experiences. Many users wear fluorescent, glow-in-the-dark clothes and accessories or carry glow sticks at parties to enhance the perceptual effects of MDMA. Users frequently report feeling an increase in feelings of empathy and a desire to connect with others. MDMA also acts as a stimulant, increasing energy and sweating, raising heart rate and blood pressure, dilating pupils, and decreasing appetite. Users frequently grind their jaws and may suck on lollipops or pacifiers to counteract this effect.

MDMA use can have a number of harmful consequences effects including hyperthermia, in which the body's temperature becomes dangerously elevated, liver and kidney damage, cardiac arrhythmias, and an imbalance of electrolytes in the blood. MDMA use can be fatal, and it can also create physical dependence, with withdrawal symptoms including depression, fatigue, and difficulty with concentration.

Ketamine was originally manufactured as an anesthetic agent and is still commonly used for veterinary purposes, but it has limited clinical use in humans because of the drug's powerful psychoactive effects. Ketamine is referred to as "Special K" or "Vitamin K." It may be sold as a liquid, powder, or pill, and it used through a variety of means including injection into a vein, ingestion, or snorting. It is frequently taken via a nasal inhaler, called a "bumper." A dose of the drug taken in this fashion is called a "bump." Ketamine is sometimes mixed with other substances, such as marijuana, and smoked.

The effects from ketamine occur quickly after use and typically last thirty minutes to an hour. The effects include a trancelike disconnected feeling, visual hallucinations, and decreased sensitivity to pain. Users refer to an intense experience on ketamine in which there is a deep sense of detachment from reality or an out-of-body experience as "the K-hole" or "K-land." Ketamine can also cause significant confusion and memory loss.

Physical effects of ketamine include increased heart rate and blood pressure, impaired movement, unsteady gait, and dilation of the pupils. At high doses, ketamine may cause rigidity and spasm of muscles, impaired vision, nausea, vomiting, seizures, and suppression of the respiratory drive. Psychosis after ketamine use has been reported. Deaths from ketamine overdose are rare but may occur and are more likely when ketamine is mixed with other drugs. The detached state induced by ketamine places users at significant risk, as they may be unable to respond normally to their environment or protect themselves.

The long-term effects of ketamine include flashbacks, possible brain toxicity with cognitive impairment, and damage to the bladder with associated urinary symptoms. Ketamine is known to produce psychological dependence, and it appears that ketamine can produce physical dependence in some heavy users, though this is somewhat controversial. Withdrawal symptoms include stomach cramps, muscle twitching, restlessness, nightmares, and strong urges to use the drug.

Similar to ketamine, the drug GHB was initially developed as an anesthetic agent. In the 1980s, the drug was reborn when it was sold as a nutritional supplement to help build muscle and reduce fat. When the harmful effects of GHB and the drug's potential for abuse became increasingly clear, the nonprescription sale of GHB was banned by the FDA in 1990.

GHB is also referred to as "liquid ecstacy," "liquid X," or "soap" (for its soapy taste). It is sold as a powder or dissolved into a liquid, which may be sold in a water bottle or eye dropper and consumed by mixing it with a beverage. The drug effects are felt ten to twenty minutes after ingestion. They reach a peak after about an hour but may persist for several hours. GHB's effects include a feeling of euphoria, decreased inhibition, and increased pleasure from sensory experiences such as movement or music. At higher doses, it may produce muscle relaxation, amnesia, dizziness, confusion, drowsiness, and loss of balance. Physical effects include excessive salivation, lowering of heart rate and blood pressure, and suppression of the respiratory drive. GHB overdose can be fatal and is a serious risk because of the variability in the concentration of drug doses sold on the street. Overdose symptoms include headache, vomiting, hallucinations, seizures, loss of consciousness, coma, and respiratory arrest.

Because GHB appears to increase muscle mass and decrease body fat by increasing levels of human growth hormone, it is sometimes abused by bodybuilders. GHB has also been used as a date-rape drug. The colorless, odorless liquid form of the drug can be slipped into a drink to mask its flavor, leaving the victim in an impaired, vulnerable state while under its influence.

GHB is very addictive, and users may quickly develop a tolerance to the drug. Withdrawal symptoms in those who are physically dependent on GHB include anxiety, tremor, insomnia, confusion, and even psychosis.

Rohypnol is a fast-acting benzodiazepine that is not used clinically in the United States. It is usually taken in the form of pills, which are smuggled into the United States. Rohypnol pills are frequently referred to as "roofies." The effects of Rohypnol are similar to those of other benzodiazepines, but it is extremely potent compared to prescription benzodiazepines. It is included here because it is commonly used on the club scene, and it may be mixed with other club drugs such as MDMA. Similar to other benzodiazepines, Rohypnol can be fatal in overdose and can lead to physical dependence with significant, potentially dangerous withdrawal symptoms. Rohypnol is sometimes used as a date-rape drug.

Inhalants

The term *inhalants* refers to a broad variety of chemical products that are inhaled to produce a high. Inhalants include a number of items that can be found around the house, including glue, rubber cement, paint thinner, nail polish remover, spray paint, aerosolized hairspray or deodorant, correction fluid, lighter fluid, gasoline, and nitrous oxide gas from whipped cream containers (called "whippets"). Use of these inhalants to get high is sometimes called "huffing." On the rise among adolescents is a new form of inhalant abuse called "dusting," which refers to the abuse of computer cleaners containing compressed gas.

Inhalants may be used in a variety of ways. Teens may breathe directly from a container of a liquid or put it into a plastic bag to concentrate the fumes. Alternatively, the substance may be applied to a rag that is placed in the mouth. Aerosolized products may be sprayed directly into the mouth or nose. Some inhalants, such as nitrous oxide, may be breathed in through a balloon containing the substance.

Because a variety of substances may be abused in this way, the effects vary depending on the particular substance that is used. In general, however, the intoxicating effects are felt by the user almost immediately and last only a short period of time, sometimes for only a few seconds. These effects include a feeling of euphoria, giddiness, hallucinations, and dizziness. Users may have slurred speech and poor balance similar to alcohol intoxication. The high from some inhalants may be followed by a crash with depressed mood, fatigue, and headache, which may prompt some teens to use the substance again.

The availability of inhalants makes their abuse quite common, particularly among younger adolescents. Nonetheless, the effects of inhalant use can be devastating. Even one-time experimentation can be deadly, as high concentrations of inhalants in the blood can cause sudden death due to cardiac arrest or a cardiac arrhythmia. Inhalant use can cause brain and nerve damage, leading to significant neurological problems including hearing loss and impairments in cognition and memory. With repeated use of many inhalants, damage to the kidneys and liver is also common. Use of some inhalants can cause severe, potentially irreversible damage to the bone marrow, which produces new blood cells. Adolescents who use plastic tents to inhale these substances can die from suffocation.

It is nearly impossible for parents to block their children's access to inhalants, as many of them can be legally purchased by minors. Instead, parents should educate their children about the dangers of inhalant use and look for signs that their child may be using these drugs. These signs include dramatic changes in mood and behavior and a decline in the teen's academic performance. More specific signs of inhalant abuse include sores or a rash around the nose and mouth, a chemical smell on the teen's breath or clothes, paint or other suspicious stains on clothes, and seeing a hidden sock or rag soaked in chemicals.

Steroids

Anabolic steroids are a group of drugs that are chemically related to the hormone testosterone. They promote muscle growth. Some anabolic steroids are available by prescription and are used for medical purposes. Those that are used illicitly may be diverted from legitimate medical use, smuggled from other countries, or synthesized in illicit laboratories.

Steroids are not used for their psychoactive effects but rather are used to help change the adolescent's appearance or gain a competitive edge in sports. Steroids are most frequently injected into a vein or muscle, but some forms come as pills or gels that are rubbed onto the skin. Users must take them repeatedly in order to get a benefit, and bodybuilders often develop complex regimens of dosing and weightlifting designed to maximize their effect.

In addition to increasing muscle mass, steroids have effects throughout the body. They lower the voice and promote growth of facial and body hair. They may cause hair loss on the scalp and acne on the face and torso. In males, steroids may cause impotence, lowered sperm count, testicular shrinkage, and the development of breast tissue (due to conversion of steroids into estrogens by the body). In females, steroids disrupt the menstrual cycle, promote a masculine appearance, and cause clitoral enlargement. More serious side effects of steroid use include increased cholesterol, blood-clotting abnormalities, and liver damage. Steroids may trigger cardiovascular problems including elevated blood pressure, heart failure and risk of heart attack, sudden cardiac death, and stroke. In adolescents, steroids can cause premature maturation of the bones and subsequent stunting of growth. Steroids also carry risk associated with illicit needle use, including skin infection or abscess and HIV or hepatitis infection from shared needles.

Steroids also produce a number of adverse psychological effects. These include increased aggression and fits of anger, colloquially called "roid rage." Users may experience profound changes in mood, including mood swings, depression, or mania. In rare cases, psychosis related to steroid use may occur. After chronic use, withdrawal symptoms from steroids may occur, including depression, fatigue, restlessness, insomnia, and decreased appetite.

Conclusion

Substance problems are among the most common psychiatric issues during adolescence. Although some degree of experimentation is common among adolescents, a small but significant minority of teens will develop serious problems with substances that may result in significant impairment in their lives and place them at risk for a number of negative outcomes, including psychiatric issues, overdose, and accidents.

Several risk factors have been identified related to adolescent substance abuse. These include individual factors, such as low self-esteem, poor school performance, and comorbid psychiatric illness; family factors, such as a high degree of conflict, poor teen supervision, and substance abuse in a parent; and community factors, such as high rates of substance use and easy availability of substances. Parents can help reduce their teens' risk of substance use by setting a positive example with their own behavior, talking to their children about the dangers of substance use, and providing close supervision.

When substance problems do emerge, it is important for parents to recognize the warning signs and seek help from a professional as soon as possible. Depending on the needs of the teen, treatment may take many forms, including outpatient, residential, and inpatient programs, The most effective treatment often involves multiple approaches, including individual therapy, support groups, family treatment, educational or vocational programs, and treatment of comorbid psychiatric issues.

References and Additional Reading

American Academy of Pediatrics, Committee on Substance Abuse. 1996. "Testing for Drugs of Abuse in Children and Adolescents." *Pediatrics* 98: 305–307.

———. 2000. "Indications for Management and Referral of Patients Involved in Substance Abuse." *Pediatrics* 106: 143–148.

———. 2005. "Use of Performance-Enhancing Substances." *Pediatrics* 115: 1103–1106.

Johnston, L. D., P. M. O'Malley, J. G. Bachman, and J. E. Schulenber. 2008. "Monitoring the Future National Survey Results on Drug Use, 1975–2007: Volume I, Secondary School Students." NIH Publication No. 08-6418A. Bethesda, MD: National Institute on Drug Abuse.

Sheridan, R. L., M. A. Goldstein, F. J. Stoddard, and T. G. Walker. 2009. "A 16-Year-Old Boy with Hypothermia and Frostbite." *New England Journal of Medicine* 361: 2654–2662.

Toumbourou, J. W., T. Stockwell, C. Neighbors, G. A. Marlatt, J. Sturge, and J. Rehm. 2007. "Interventions to Reduce Harm Associated with Adolescent Substance Use." *Lancet* 369: 1391–1401.

13 Personality Disorders

Personality disorders are a distinct group of psychiatric disorders that involve persistent patterns of inflexible, unhealthy ways of interacting with others and distorted responses to life events. These patterns of behavior are markedly different from the normal range of behavior in a culture and may cause the teen a significant degree of distress or lead to an impairment in healthy functioning.

Because most psychiatric disorders seem, to varying degrees, foreign to the true nature of the affected adolescent, personality disorders are somewhat different from other psychiatric illnesses, The illness leads to changes in the teen's thoughts or behaviors, and these changes resolve after treatment. For example, when a teen is depressed, she may perceive matters in a darker, more pessimistic way than normal. She may spend less time with friends, miss school, sleep excessively, and eat less. These thoughts and behaviors represent a noticeable change from her usual self. After the depressive episode resolves, the teen returns to her "old self." In contrast, personality disorders are likely to be a stable part of an adolescent's identity. As the name implies, they represent a problem with a teen's personality, including one's view of oneself and others, one's approach to relationships and social interactions, and one's reactions to stress. These maladaptive personality traits can change with time and treatment, but this change takes time and effort.

Because the personality of an adolescent is still a work in progress, personality disorders are relatively common in adults, but they are diagnosed much less frequently in adolescents. Some of the traits that characterize personality disorders, such as impulsivity, instability in relationships, or an excessively egocentric focus, are a normal part of adolescent psychological development. These traits, as well as others that may be more problematic, are likely to evolve during adolescence. In adolescence, caution should be exercised in labeling these patterns as a disorder before they are truly fixed.

Nonetheless, personality disorders tend to emerge first during late adolescence and early adulthood. Furthermore, psychotherapy aimed at addressing unhealthy patterns of behavior may be more effective during adolescence, before these patterns become too ingrained in the teen's personality. Parents may be able to recognize the early stages of potentially unhealthy behavior patterns and seek advice from a mental health professional. However, a diagnosis should be made only after careful consideration and a thorough evaluation by an experienced clinician.

Case Presentation

Rebecca was a nineteen-year-old who was referred for psychotherapy after discharge from an inpatient psychiatric facility where she had been hospitalized for an overdose of over-the-counter medications. During the evaluation, Rebecca explained that she had taken the overdose after her boyfriend ended their relationship. She spent considerable time in the initial meeting with the therapist expressing vehement anger toward her ex-boyfriend. In addition, she also described feeling "hollow inside" most of the time, and she reported that she often cut herself superficially on her arms in an effort to relieve these feelings or when she felt emotionally overwhelmed.

She began seeing the therapist weekly and discussed a history of stormy relationships throughout her high school years with friends and boyfriends. Rebecca developed an intense attachment to the therapist early in the treatment, telling him in the third session, "I feel like you understand me like no one else has before." Yet when the therapist told Jessica that he was planning to go away for two weeks, she expressed a great deal of anger toward him, stating, "How can you abandon me like this when I'm just starting to feel better? I don't think you care about me—you just want my money!"

In the weeks leading up to the therapist's vacation, Rebecca settled down and seemed more calm, although somewhat more distant. When the therapist returned from vacation, he was surprised to learn that Rebecca had been hospitalized. She had carved the words "hate" and "die" into her arms with a razor blade and overdosed on medications. After discharge, Rebecca refused to return to see the therapist, telling him angrily that she thought he was "pathetic" and obviously did not know what he was doing. The therapist, who suspected a diagnosis of borderline personality disorder, convinced Rebecca to see a colleague who specialized in dialectical behavioral therapy (DBT). She also began attending a weekly DBT skills group for women with similar difficulties.

Rebecca gradually improved over the next several years. She learned more effective ways to manage her intense mood swings, unhealthy impulses, and anger. She began cutting less often and eventually stopped altogether. Rebecca's symptoms worsened periodically, and she overdosed after she lost her job because of an argument with her boss. Still, as timed passed, these periods became fewer and farther between.

Symptoms and Warning Signs

Personality disorder symptoms involve longstanding problematic patterns in a teen's thoughts, feelings, relationships, or impulse control that are far outside the normal behavior seen within the culture. For the diagnosis to be made, it must be determined that the symptoms are not exclusively due to some other psychiatric illness (such as depression), a medical condition (such as brain injury), or substance abuse. Furthermore, the symptoms must occur in a broad range of situations, not just in particular circumstances. Personality disorders are categorized into three distinct groups, or "clusters," named Cluster A, Cluster B, and Cluster C. Disorders within each cluster share some similar features.

In Cluster A disorders, behaviors are odd and eccentric. These disorders include paranoid personality disorder, schizoid personality disorder, and schizotypal personality disorder. The symptoms of the Cluster A disorders are summarized in table 13.1. Adolescents with these disorders tend to be isolative, forming few relationships and preferring to keep to themselves. Their strange behavior and unusual, often bizarre beliefs help solidify their "outsider" status. Although people with other personality disorders frequently have problems with interpersonal relationships, what distinguishes those with Cluster A personality disorders is that they have little interest in forming relationships, and as a result they are usually not distressed by their isolation. They may migrate toward occupations that involve little interaction with others.

Cluster B personality disorders are associated with some of the most difficult and troubling symptoms of any psychiatric illness. This group is described as the "dramatic, emotional, or erratic" cluster of personality disorders. These disorders can cause significant difficulty in an adolescent's life and can present a major challenge to family members and mental health providers as well. The Cluster B personality disorders are antisocial personality disorder (also discussed in chapter 14 on behavior disorders), borderline personality disorder, histrionic personality disorder, and narcissistic personality disorder. (See table 13.2.) Cluster B disorders are more likely than those in the other clusters to come to clinical attention because, whereas people with Cluster A disorders may keep quietly to themselves, people with Cluster B disorders have symptoms that are dramatic and problematic both for themselves and those around them.

Cluster C personality disorders are summarized in table 13.3. They include avoidant personality disorder, dependent personality disorder, and obsessive-compulsive personality disorder (not to be confused with obsessive-compulsive disorder, which is discussed in chapter 16). Collectively, these disorders are known as the anxious and fearful disorders, as all of them are associated with a high degree of anxiety.

Borderline personality disorder deserves further discussion, as it is the most common personality disorder to be diagnosed during adolescence, and it is the disorder that can cause significant dysfunction and distress. This personality disorder occurs more commonly in females and in those who have suffered abuse or neglect during childhood. Those who suffer from this disorder show a great deal of instability in their emotions, their behavior, and their relationships. One of the core features of the disorder is an intense fear of abandonment by others, and people with borderline personality disorder may go to great lengths to avoid feeling abandoned. They often complain of feeling empty inside and lack a stable sense of their own identity. They may develop intense attachments to others in a desperate effort to relieve this sense of emptiness. People with this disorder tend to have a black-and-white view of others, seeing them in either an exaggeratingly positive fashion or in a distorted, negative view. Psychiatrists refer to this tendency as "splitting." Teens with borderline personality disorder may devalue a person in their life that they once idealized, suddenly holding a harsh, negative view of that person. This often occurs when the teen feels abandoned and may represent an unconscious attempt to ward off this feeling.

Table 13.1	**Cluster A Personality Disorders: Odd and Eccentric Behavior**	
Personality Disorder	**Symptoms**	**Differential Diagnosis** (conditions with similiar symptoms that may be confused with the disorder)
Paranoid	Pathological distrust and suspiciousness of others, including ▶ Unfounded suspicion that others may want to harm or deceive one ▶ Preoccupation with doubts about loyalty of friends ▶ Not confiding in others because of fear that the information may be used against one ▶ Reading hidden negative meaning into benign statements ▶ Persistently bearing grudges ▶ Tendency to interpret events or statements as an attack on one's character and being quick to react angrily ▶ Recurrent suspicions about the fidelity of a spouse or romantic partner	Psychosis, including paranoid schizophrenia Delusional disorder, a disorder in which someone holds rigidly to a delusional belief Drug abuse, including of substances such as cocaine, stimulants, and marijuana, that can cause paranoid thoughts
Schizoid	Lack of interest in relationships and limited range of emotional expression, including symptoms such as ▶ Not desiring or seeking out close relationships, including romantic relationships ▶ Preferring solitary activities ▶ Taking pleasure in few activities ▶ Lack of close friends ▶ Indifference to others' reactions ▶ Emotional coldness or limited range of expression	Schizophrenia and related psychotic disorders, which can lead to social withdrawal Developmental disorders, including autism and Asperger syndrome Depression Severe anxiety Other personality disorders, including avoidant personality disorder (which is distinguished by the fact that people with this disorder desire interpersonal relationships)
Schizotypal	A pattern of eccentric beliefs and behaviors and problems with interpersonal relationships, including the following symptoms: ▶ Lack of close friends ▶ Peculiar behavior or appearance, e.g., wearing strange clothing such as a wizard's robe ▶ Strange beliefs, including believing in magic, telepathy, ESP, etc. ▶ Believing that media such as newspapers or television programs may contain references or messages to oneself ▶ Persistent suspicious or paranoid beliefs ▶ Odd patterns of thought or speech ▶ Unusual perceptual experiences ▶ Narrowed range of emotional expression or expressions that tend to be inappropriate for a situation (e.g., smiling when hearing sad news)	Schizophrenia or other psychotic disorders Other personality disorders, including schizoid and paranoid personality disorder Developmental disorders Drug abuse

Table 13.2	**Cluster B Personality Disorders: Dramatic, Emotional, or Erratic Disorders**	
Personality Disorder	**Symptoms**	**Differential Diagnosis** (conditions with similiar symptoms that may be confused with the disorder)
Antisocial	Pattern of violating the rights of others and often engaging in criminal activity with symptoms that may include ▸ Repeatedly breaking the law ▸ Deceiving others ▸ Impulsivity ▸ Aggressive behavior ▸ Recklessness and disregard for safety of others ▸ Lack of responsibility ▸ Lack of remorse for actions	Conduct disorder or oppositional defiant disorder (in an adolescent) Drug abuse Bipolar disorder Other personality disorders, e.g., narcissistic personality disorder
Borderline	Pattern of instability in relationships, moods, and self-image, with symptoms including ▸ Intense fear of abandonment ▸ Unstable interpersonal relationships ▸ Lack of a stable self-image ▸ Impulsivity ▸ Recurrent self-injurious behavior or suicide attempts ▸ Unstable, rapidly shifting, and intense moods ▸ Frequent feelings of emptiness ▸ Intense anger	Mood disorders, especially bipolar disorder Posttraumatic stress disorder Other personality disorders Drug abuse
Histrionic	Pattern of excessive attention-seeking behavior, including ▸ Feeling uncomfortable in situations where one is not the center of attention ▸ Inappropriately seductive or provocative behavior in interpersonal interactions ▸ Rapidly shifting, exaggerated, and shallow displays of emotion ▸ Being overly dramatic and showy ▸ Preoccupation with physical appearance ▸ Considering relationships to be more intimate than they truly are	Other personality disorders, especially narcissistic or borderline personality disorder Bipolar disorder
Narcissistic	A pattern involving an inflated sense of self-importance and excessive need to be admired, including the following: ▸ Preoccupation with fantasies of unlimited success or power ▸ Extreme sense of entitlement ▸ Lack of empathy ▸ Extreme arrogance ▸ Need for excessive admiration ▸ Frequently feeling envious of others or believing that others are envious of oneself ▸ Grandiose sense of self-importance ▸ Belief that one is special and should only associate with people of similar status	Other personality disorders, especially antisocial, histrionic, or borderline personality disorder Bipolar disorder (particularly during a manic episode)

Adolescents with borderline personality disorder tend to experience extreme and rapidly shifting emotions, including uncontrolled fits of anger. The feeling of emptiness and the intense negative emotions associated with this disorder are often evoked by a perceived abandonment, which may occur after a breakup in a romantic relationship or even when a friend cannot be reached by phone or a trusted therapist is away on vacation. In response to these negative feelings, whether evoked by abandonment or other stressors, a person with borderline personality disorder may have suicidal thoughts or engage in self-injurious behavior, such as cutting, which are also hallmarks of the illness. Impulsive and erratic behavior, including reckless driving, sexual promiscuity, and spending sprees, are also common.

Similar to other personality disorders, borderline personality disorder tends to emerge in late adolescence through early adulthood. Although it may be a lifelong disorder for some, often the symptoms improve somewhat later in life. However, the symptoms of borderline personality disorder usually cause significant suffering and chaos in the affected adolescent. These feelings may pose a significant safety risk because of self-injurious behavior, impulsivity, and a high rate of suicide attempts. Obtaining treatment for the disorder is essential. Borderline personality disorder usually requires a specialized approach to treatment.

Table 13.3	Cluster C Personality Disorders: Anxious and Fearful Disorders	
Personality Disorder	Symptoms	Differential Diagnosis (conditions with similar symptoms that may be confused with the disorder)
Avoidant	Longstanding pattern of social difficulties including ▶ Strong fear of being criticized or rejected by others ▶ Viewing oneself as inadequate or inferior to others ▶ Inhibition in social situations ▶ Avoidance of activities and occupations that require interpersonal contact ▶ Restraint in relationships due to fear of being ridiculed ▶ Avoiding relationships with others unless certain of being liked	Other personality disorders, especially schizoid personality disorder (which is distinguished by the fact that the individual has little interest in relationships and is not concerned by the opinions of others) Anxiety disorders, especially social anxiety disorder and panic disorder
Dependent	Excessive need to be taken care of by others, with symptoms that include ▶ Difficulty making decisions or initiating projects without excessive seeking of advice and reassurance from others ▶ Needing others to assume responsibility for important areas of one's life ▶ Preoccupation with fears about being left to care for oneself	Depression Anxiety Other personality disorders, including histrionic and borderline personality disorder

(continued)

Table 13.3 | **Cluster C Personality Disorders** (continued)

Personality Disorder	Symptoms	Differential Diagnosis (conditions with similiar symptoms that may be confused with the disorder)
Dependent (continued)	▶ Difficulty expressing disagreement with others ▶ Feeling helpless when alone and unable to care for oneself ▶ Going to excessive lengths to seek nurturance from others ▶ Feeling an urgent need for a new relationship as a source of support when a close relationship ends	
Obsessive-compulsive	A pattern of perfectionism and preoccupation with order and control such that it limits one's flexibility, openness, and efficiency. Symptoms include ▶ Preoccupation with details, rules, lists, organization, or schedules such that the major point of an activity is lost ▶ Excessive perfectionism that gets in the way of completing tasks ▶ Excessive devotion to work and productivity ▶ Being overly scrupulous or inflexible about moral issues ▶ Reluctance to delegate tasks out of fear that they will not be done properly ▶ Inability to discard old, worthless belongings ▶ Miserly spending of money both on oneself and on others ▶ Rigidity and stubbornness	Obsessive-compulsive disorder, which differs in the presence of obsessive thoughts and/or compulsive rituals Other personality disorders, including narcissistic and schizoid personality disorder

Other Problems to Consider

All the personality disorders may resemble other forms of psychiatric illness. For example, borderline personality disorder is characterized by dramatic mood swings, impulsive and erratic behavior, and explosive fits of anger that may be mistaken for bipolar disorder. Similarly, adolescents in the midst of a depressive episode may demonstrate several symptoms that resemble those of personality disorders. They may avoid social contact, similar to those with schizoid personality disorder, or rely excessively on others, as in dependent personality disorder. Yet, unlike mood disorders, personality disorders represent stable, longstanding traits in an adolescent. Caution must be exercised in attempting to diagnose a personality disorder in someone who is in the midst of a depression or another acute psychiatric episode, such as psychosis or mania.

Because there may be significant implications for the appropriate course of treatment, it is important for mental health clinicians to distinguish personality disorders from other conditions. For example, medications are often not very helpful in the treatment of borderline personality disorder, but they may be essential in the management of bipolar disorder. In tables 13.1, 13.2, and 13.3 the differential diagnosis for each personality disorder is listed. These are similar conditions that should be considered as possible alternative causes of a teen's symptoms.

Adolescents with personality disorders are also at greater risk for developing other forms of psychiatric illness compared to the general population. Typically, there are high rates of mood disorders (particularly depression) and substance abuse in people with personality disorders. Some people with Cluster A disorders (the "odd and eccentric" cluster) may develop significant psychotic disorders, such as schizophrenia, later in life. The risk of anxiety disorders is increased in many of the personality disorders but is particularly high among people with Cluster C disorders (the "anxious and fearful" cluster). The risk of eating disorders such as bulimia nervosa is also increased in people with borderline or obsessive-compulsive personality disorder.

Treatment

Because personality disorders are a fundamental part of the identity of those who suffer from them, it is not surprising that they are not readily susceptible to change. It usually takes a significant amount of time and effort to treat a personality disorder.

Psychotherapy is the mainstay of treatment for personality disorders. Often, insight-oriented psychodynamic psychotherapy is the method used to address them (see chapter 4 for a discussion of different approaches to psychotherapy). The goal of psychodynamic psychotherapy is to help adolescents gain insight into the unhealthy patterns of behavior in their life and connect these patterns to their past experiences and relationships. In addition, a goal is to foster adolescents' understanding of the other unconscious forces that may drive these behaviors. As adolescents become more cognizant of the patterns that contribute to their unhappiness and build an understanding of the reasons these patterns have developed, their behavior may gradually change. They may learn new defense mechanisms for dealing with stress or develop a more flexible template for interactions with others. Often, the relationship adolescents develop with their therapist is a key component of the change that occurs in this form of therapy.

Interpersonal psychotherapy can help address the difficulties in relationships that are a cornerstone of many personality disorders and often one of the most distressing symptoms for the individual. Skills-based treatments, such as cognitive behavioral therapy (CBT) or social skills training can be helpful in targeting specific symptoms.

Dialectical behavioral therapy (DBT), a type of CBT, has been developed specifically for the treatment of borderline personality disorder, and it appears to be the most effective treatment for this condition. DBT, which is discussed in more detail in chapter 4, integrates the structured, skills-based approach of CBT with elements from Zen Buddhism. In essence, DBT involves learning to observe one's emotions and developing the ability to accept and tolerate strong feelings. DBT includes instruction in coping skills that help teens to manage urges to harm themselves. When an undesired behavior, such as cutting oneself, does occur, the teen performs a "chain analysis" to understand the events that led up to the incident and ways that it could have been avoided, including times when a coping skill could have been employed to help prevent the situation from escalating. DBT typically involves a group therapy component in addition to meetings with an individual therapist. DBT groups help review the use of the coping skills that are part of the treatment.

Medications are usually not very effective in treating personality disorders. Still, in some situations they may be incorporated into the treatment for specific symptoms that may be part of the disorder. Thus, adolescents with antisocial personality disorder exhibit a great deal of impulsive and aggressive behavior. Anticonvulsants or atypical antipsychotics may reduce these behaviors in some patients (see chapter 5 for further discussion of these medications). Medications may also play a role in treating comorbid psychiatric disorders, such as depression or anxiety, which are common in people with personality disorders.

While personality disorders can be challenging to treat, change is possible. Often, the limiting factor is a teen's own willingness to change. Treatment requires an active effort on the part of the adolescent, but unfortunately many adolescents with personality disorders have little insight into their problems. Often the first and most challenging step in treatment is to find a way for teens to recognize the ways in which their own behaviors are creating their problems.

Prognosis

Personality disorders can result in a broad range of outcomes. Some adolescents will experience severe impairment in their school or occupational functions, their relationships, and even their safety. Adolescents with borderline personality disorder may have self-injurious behaviors, suicide attempts, and repeated psychiatric hospitalizations. The behaviors related to antisocial personality disorder frequently result in harm to oneself or others, imprisonment, or even death by violence or accidents. But many people with personality disorder do not experience this degree of dysfunction. In contrast, some personality disorders, such as narcissistic personality disorder, may drive individuals to extremes of behavior that may lead to success in competitive fields such as business, medicine, or the law. However, for many such individuals, successes in the professional realm may be accompanied by longstanding problems with relationships or feelings of unhappiness and dissatisfaction with their lives.

The outcome for a particular individual with a personality disorder depends to a large extent on the nature and severity of the disorder. A person's other strengths, including intelligence and the presence of a strong social support group, also play an important role. The presence of comorbid psychiatric illness, including substance abuse, tends to predict a less favorable outcome.

Overall, personality disorders tend to be longstanding problems even with treatment, and they usually last a lifetime if untreated. That said, borderline personality disorder and antisocial personality disorder often become less severe or even resolve later in life.

Conclusion

In contrast to most other psychiatric disorders, personality disorders persist and become a part of a person's identity. They are marked by inflexible, persistent, and maladaptive ways of behaving and interacting with others. These disorders can range in severity, but in some cases they can cause significant dysfunction in a teen's life, including major impairments in relationships and functioning. Moreover, the adolescent is at increased risk for other psychiatric problems, including mood and anxiety disorders and substance abuse. Some disorders can pose a significant threat to the teen's safety. For example, borderline personality disorder is associated with self-injurious behavior and high rates of suicide attempts. Antisocial personality disorder involves criminal activity, risky behavior, and aggression that frequently results in injury, imprisonment, or death.

Because the personality of an adolescent is still a work in progress, personality disorders are infrequently diagnosed in adolescents. These disorders typically first begin to emerge during late adolescence and early adulthood, as the process of personality development begins to slow. Recognizing these disorders early in their course can allow for more effective intervention, as unhealthy patterns have not yet become too ingrained, and the capacity for positive change may be greater in younger patients.

References and Additional Reading

Elkins, I. J., M. McGue, S. Malone, and W. G. Iacono. 2004. "The Effect of Parental Alcohol and Drug Disorders on Adolescent Personality." *American Journal of Psychiatry* 161: 670–676.

Johnson, J. G., P. Cohen, E. Smailes, S. Kasen, J. M. Oldham, A. E. Skodol, and J. S. Brook. 2000. "Adolescent Personality Disorders Associated with Violence and Criminal Behavior during Adolescence and Early Adulthood." *American Journal of Psychiatry* 157: 1406–1412.

Thatcher, D. L., J. R. Cornelius, and D. B. Clark. 2005. "Adolescent Alcohol Use Disorders Predict Adult Borderline Personality." *Addictive Behaviors* 30: 1709–1724.

Behavior Disorders:
Oppositional Defiant Disorder and Conduct Disorder

Testing limits, taking risks, and challenging authority are normal, albeit trying, aspects of adolescent development. However, for some adolescents these behaviors go too far. Teens may become entranced in a pattern of negative behavior that places them at risk for serious legal, social, or academic consequences. When an adolescent goes beyond the occasional bad decision or argument with parents to a persistent pattern of active defiance, rule breaking, or criminal activities, a psychiatric evaluation may be warranted.

In this chapter, we discuss the behavioral disorders: oppositional defiant disorder (ODD) and conduct disorder. These two related disorders are common in adolescents and account for a significant proportion of convicted juvenile

---

Case Presentation, Part 1

John was a fifteen-year-old boy who was brought in for a psychiatric evaluation ordered by a judge in the juvenile court, where he was facing charges related to breaking into cars to steal GPS devices. When John was six, his father was sent to jail, so he was raised by his mother, who had a history of depression and was not consistently available to him. As a result, she often relied on her parents for assistance with her son.

According to John's mother, he was a very stubborn and argumentative child. He had a bad temper and would have a tantrum when asked to do household chores. Because of behavioral and academic problems, when John was nine, his school recommended that he see a psychiatrist. At that time, he was diagnosed with oppositional defiant disorder and attention-deficit/hyperactivity disorder. A course of treatment ensued, including individual psychotherapy for John and regular meetings between John's mother and the therapist. These were designed to provide her with guidance on effective ways to address John's behavioral problems. Initially, this plan was effective. However, because John seemed to be a little better and his mother was having difficulties making appointments because of her work schedule, John did not continue in treatment.

When John was thirteen years old, he started to skip school frequently, and several times, he was suspended from school for fighting. He repeatedly stayed out late, and he did not tell his mother where he was going. Over the next two years, these problems worsened. John engaged in a number of behaviors that resulted in legal trouble, including shoplifting, making graffiti, fighting, and carrying a knife to school. Ultimately, John was placed on probation through the juvenile court. After he was arrested for breaking into cars and went before the judge, he was ordered to have a psychiatric evaluation.

delinquents. Although these disorders can be challenging to treat, early intervention can lead to significant improvement and prevention of a pattern of repeated criminal behavior that can persist into adulthood.

Symptoms and Warning Signs

While ODD may begin in adolescence, most often the symptoms start earlier. The disorder is characterized by frequent negative and defiant behavior that is not merely the result of a developmental transition but is a pattern that persists for at least six months. According to the DSM-IV, symptoms include frequently arguing with adults, refusing to obey rules from authority figures such as teachers or parents, intentionally annoying other people, and often blaming others for one's own mistakes (see sidebar 14.1). Adolescents with this disorder tend to be angry, resentful, vindictive, and easily annoyed. They often lose their temper and have difficulty managing their anger, with tantrums or angry outbursts. In addition, they may be remarkably stubborn. During an argument, they may prefer to give up privileges or accept punishments rather than submit to authority.

The causes of ODD are not well understood, but it is probably due to a combination of genetic predisposition and environmental influences. Potential risk factors include harsh or inconsistent discipline, childhood abuse or neglect, lack of supervision, and exposure to conflict or violence in the household. Family discord, including divorce, frequent moves or changing of caregivers, and financial stress may also place some vulnerable children at risk for developing ODD.

The symptoms of conduct disorder are more severe and problematic than those of ODD. Some teens who had ODD earlier in childhood progress to conduct disorder during adolescence. Conduct disorder is characterized by a pattern of behavior in which the teen routinely violates rules and the rights of others. The symptoms fall into four main categories: aggression, destruction of property, deceit and theft, and serious rule violations. Symptoms are described in more detail in sidebar 14.2. Because of criminal behavior, many adolescents with conduct disorder become involved with the juvenile justice system.

Similar to ODD, the causes of conduct disorder are not well understood. It is thought to be partly the result of en-

> **Sidebar 14.1** | **Symptoms of Oppositional Defiant Disorder**
>
> ► Arguing with adults, particularly authority figures
> ► Defying rules
> ► Losing one's temper frequently or becoming annoyed easily
> ► Feeling angry or resentful frequently
> ► Often acting in a spiteful or vindictive manner
> ► Annoying others intentionally
> ► Blaming others for one's mistakes or misdeeds

vironmental influences in a child's life. Studies of twins and children raised by adoptive families suggest that some children may have a genetic predisposition toward the disorder. Conduct disorder occurs more commonly in teens living in impoverished urban environments, though it may present in adolescents from any socioeconomic background. Teens raised in a home environment with a high degree of conflict or with absent fathers are also at risk. Conduct disorder is more common in children of parents with substance abuse problems, major psychiatric illness, or serious criminal histories. Parents who are inconsistently available or overly harsh and demanding in their disciplinary approach may also put their children at increased risk. Both ODD and conduct disorder appear to be more common in boys than in girls.

> **Sidebar 14.2 | Symptoms of Conduct Disorder**
>
> ► Aggressive behavior
>   - ► Bullying or threatening others
>   - ► Fighting frequently
>   - ► Using weapons
>   - ► Performing cruelty to animals
>   - ► Perpetrating violent crime, including rapes or muggings
> ► Destruction of property
>   - ► Setting fires
>   - ► Making graffiti or vandalizing property
> ► Theft and deceit
>   - ► Lying to or conning others to get one's way
>   - ► Breaking into houses or cars
>   - ► Shoplifting
> ► Serious rule-breaking behavior
>   - ► Running away
>   - ► Skipping school
>   - ► Breaking the law or violating school rules

Making the Diagnosis

The diagnosis of ODD or conduct disorder is made through a thorough evaluation by a child and adolescent psychiatrist, a psychologist, or another mental health clinician with experience in working with adolescents. Because teens with these problems minimize their symptoms or have little insight into the problem, the teen's own report of symptoms is often less helpful in evaluating these disorders than it is for many other psychiatric disorders. Also, some teens with these disorders will be intentionally dishonest during an evaluation. Thus, gathering detailed information from parents is essential. Important information may also be obtained from school staff, coaches, probation officers, or other adults who have interacted with the teen. This information can help the clinician to develop a more complete picture of the teen's behavior in a variety of settings.

Ultimately, the diagnoses of ODD and conduct disorder are made according to whether the teen's clinical symptoms fit the diagnostic criteria. There are no blood tests or imaging studies that can be used to confirm the diagnosis. Still, there are a number of other psychiatric disorders that are common in adolescents with ODD and conduct disorder, so consideration of these disorders and appropriate screening for their symptoms should be part of the psychiatric evaluation. Further psychological testing is indicated only when the psychiatric evaluation suggests a possible comorbid problem, such as a learning disorder. In this case, testing can help to clarify the diagnostic picture.

Other Problems to Consider

In order to make a diagnosis of ODD or conduct disorder, the clinician must determine if the symptoms the teen is exhibiting are not due to another psychiatric disorder. Since the symptoms of ODD and conduct disorder are similar and even overlap with those of some other psychiatric problems, this may be challenging. Furthermore, there are high rates of comorbid psychiatric illness in teens with these disorders.

Mood disorders share many features with ODD and conduct disorder. Teens with major depression often are very short-tempered, which may lead to arguments with parents. In addition, teens with bipolar disorder may be extremely irritable and argumentative. The impulsivity and increased risk taking that are associated with mania may lead teens with bipolar disorder to run away, stay out all night, drive recklessly, or break other rules. The presence of a major disturbance in a teen's mood along with major disruptions in sleep, appetite, and energy level can help to distinguish mood disorders from disruptive behavior disorders. Furthermore, rule breaking or argumentative behavior that is due to a mood disorder should resolve when the mood symptoms are effectively treated. However, it should be noted that mood disorders frequently occur together with ODD and conduct disorder.

ADHD is another disorder that commonly occurs in teens with ODD and conduct disorder. The symptoms of ADHD overlap with these two behavior disorders. Teens with ADHD may disrupt class and have disciplinary issues. They may act impulsively, talking back to teachers and fighting with peers. Teens with ADHD tend to have a low frustration tolerance, and they may be emotionally temperamental. Still, ADHD can be distinguished from ODD and conduct disorder in that persistent arguing or premeditated and intentional defiance (as opposed to that due to impulsivity or failure to listen) are not features of ADHD and suggest the diagnosis of ODD. Similarly, ADHD does not typically lead to the degree of rule breaking and criminal behavior seen in conduct disorder.

Teens abusing substances may have behaviors that resemble conduct disorder or ODD. For example, they may have changes in their mood and behavior that may make them irritable, argumentative, or aggressive. They may engage in criminal activities, such as stealing, in order to pay for or obtain drugs. If these behaviors occur exclusively in relationship to the teen's drug use, then the diagnosis of conduct disorder or ODD is not appropriate. Still, substance abuse problems commonly occur together with behavioral disorders.

There are other comorbid psychiatric issues that typically occur together with disruptive behavior disorders. These include learning difficulties, Tourette syndrome, and anxiety disorders.

Treatment

Treating disruptive behavior disorders requires a combination of psychosocial interventions. For both ODD and conduct disorder, treatment frequently involves instituting a behavioral plan at home that includes firm limits, rewards for positive behaviors, and consistently enforced consequences for negative behaviors. In particular, teens with conduct disorder require close supervision. This may require enforcing a curfew and monitoring the teen's whereabouts. Parents can work with a therapist to help develop an effective plan that should be repeatedly fine-tuned. As the behavioral plan is being implemented, it is helpful to provide individual psychotherapy for the adolescent. Through therapy, teens may learn more effective ways of expressing themselves, managing their anger, and having their needs met.

Behavioral disorders are often associated with difficulties at home, such as conflict in the family or a parent with a psychiatric or substance abuse problem. Before a teen's behavior will significantly improve, these issues must be addressed. A mental health professional will assist in identifying the kinds of treatment that would be useful. Family therapy or individual psychiatric treatment for a parent may be appropriate.

Unless the teen is suffering from one of the comorbid psychiatric problems previously noted, medications do not appear to be effective for the treatment of ODD or conduct disorder. Yet effective treatment of these comorbid problems, including medications when appropriate, is an essential component of the treatment of a disruptive behavior disorder. If unrecognized and untreated, these problems can further aggravate the behavioral problems. Thus, a teen with conduct disorder and untreated ADHD will be more impulsive and more likely to fight and will probably have academic and disciplinary difficulties.

Treatment of disruptive behavior disorders often involves the school, community-based programs, state and local agencies, and the juvenile justice system. This is particularly true in conduct disorder, for which symptoms are more likely to become manifest in settings outside the home and need to be addressed accordingly.

As an important ally in treatment, schools can establish good communication with a teen's mental health providers and involved outside agencies. Moreover, the school can develop interventions based at school that extend a teen's treatment into that setting. Schools can also provide the structure to supervise a troubled adolescent. With some modifications, the school may be able to enforce the same behavioral plan that is in place at home, providing greater consistency in the teen's experience of rules and consequences. For students with comorbid cognitive or psychiatric problems that affect their learning, schools may offer testing and support through special educational programs. Involvement in school activities, such as sports or after-school programs, can give a teen alternatives to antisocial activity and can offer a sense of connectedness to the community. Involvement in vocational or career mentorship programs can help some troubled adolescents identify positive goals for the future and improve their self-esteem. These interventions can prevent premature school dropout, which can put a teen at further risk for engaging in problematic behaviors.

Community organizations such as the Boys and Girls Club (www.bcga.org) and the United Way (www.unitedway.org) have a range of structured programs, including sports, arts classes, and educational initiatives around gang violence and substance abuse prevention. Involvement in these activities allows adolescents to find healthy interests and connections to peers. As with vocational programs at school, some community organizations offer skills training or mentorship programs that can help teens build a positive vision of their future.

For serious cases of conduct disorder in which parents have difficulty enforcing consequences with an out-of-control teen, the juvenile justice system may be useful. If faced with the threat of legal consequence, difficult teens may be more compliant with rules. In many states, parents can receive assistance from the juvenile justice system on a voluntary basis. Although many parents are understandably reluctant to involve the legal system in their child's life, voluntary involvement with a teen that is on a dangerous path can be useful in preventing more serious criminal activity and legal penalties.

Parents can work with the court to develop a plan that is focused on helping a teen rather than one that is strictly punitive. If a teen is currently in treatment, input from the therapist or psychiatrist in the form of a letter to the judge or discussion with the teen's probation officer may be beneficial. An effective plan may include terms of probation such as participation in psychiatric treatment, attendance at school, adherence to household rules, and mandatory drug screening. For adolescents who are not in treatment, a psychiatric evaluation by a court-appointed clinician may be ordered. Failure to adhere to these requirements may result in the teen's being placed in a residential treatment program, juvenile detention facility, or home incarceration.

State social services agencies, the department of mental health, and local community mental health centers are other agencies that can assist with the treatment of adolescents with disruptive behavior disorders. These agencies may have intensive services, including home visits and integrated treatment of the whole family, that are particularly effective for behavioral problems. A specific form of treatment called multisystemic treatment (MST) is offered through some community mental health centers. This approach is based on the idea that treatment of behavioral disorders involves an intensive approach with the coordinated participation of various systems involved in the teen's life. MST often includes the family, the school, and the juvenile justice system into the treatment.

When an adolescent with a severe behavioral disorder continues to engage in problem behaviors despite intensive treatment efforts, placement in a residential treatment program may be necessary. The duration of placements may vary according to the needs of the adolescent, but they are often for a few months to a year. Such programs engage teens in intensive treatment and remove them from the environment that may be contributing to their problems. The programs are able to provide a level of structure and supervision that is not possible at home. The ultimate goal of a residential program is to return the adolescent home.

Prognosis

Even with intensive treatment, ODD and conduct disorder tend to take months to years to improve. It is important for parents to recognize that treatment is

---

Case Presentation, Part 2

The psychiatrist performing John's court-ordered evaluation diagnosed John with conduct disorder and ADHD; he was also suspected of abusing marijuana. The psychiatrist recommended that John and his mother undergo a course of treatment at the local community health center. The court placed John on probation, and he was ordered to attend weekly therapy sessions and return to school. Additionally, he was to adhere to a new curfew and agree to tell his mother where he was at all times, abstain from use of drugs and alcohol, and submit to random urine drug screens. John was told that he needed to comply with these terms, or he would face the possibility of placement in a juvenile detention facility. To ensure his compliance, he met with a probation officer regularly.

John's psychiatrist prescribed a medication for his ADHD; further testing at school revealed that he had a learning disorder that affected his ability to read. To help address these issues, John was placed on an individualized education plan (IEP) at school. To provide supervision and to assist with his homework until his mother returned home from work, he attended an after-school program.

In individual therapy, John learned ways to control his anger. To help John's mother devise a behavioral plan for managing his behavior at home, she met with his therapist on a regular basis. Through joint meetings with the therapist, she and John also learned to improve communication with each other. On the advice of the therapist, John's mother entered separate treatment at the mental health agency. John began to participate in a basketball league through the local Boys and Girls Club and spent increasing amounts of time there. At the club, he connected with a young man who volunteered as a coach; he was able to engage in conversations often with this individual whom he respected.

Through work with his therapist, John identified an interest in "figuring out how stuff works" and entered a high school vocational program to begin training as an electrician. Over time, John's behavior gradually improved. Occasionally, he would still act out, skipping school, arguing with his mother, or not coming home at the appropriate time. But when this happened, his mother would enforce strict consequences, and John would need to discuss it with his probation officer. Over the next two years, these incidents occurred with decreasing frequency, and his relationship with his mother significantly improved. Ultimately, John graduated from high school and entered a formal training program to become an electrician.

lengthy. They should try not to become discouraged or give up on treatment too hastily. The course of these disorders is variable, but ODD eventually resolves for most adolescents. Left untreated, the symptoms may persist for several years. A significant proportion of people with persistent ODD have a progression of their symptoms and develop conduct disorder.

Teens with conduct disorder are at risk for continued criminal and antisocial behaviors in adulthood. Roughly one-third of adolescents with conduct disorder develop antisocial personality disorder, a psychiatric condition in adults that is characterized by disregard for the rights of others and high rates of criminal activity and incarceration. Other possible negative outcomes associated with both ODD and conduct disorder include teen pregnancy, injuries related to accidents or fights, academic underachievement including school dropout, and legal problems. Teens with these disorders also have higher rates of other psychiatric illnesses, including substance abuse and mood and anxiety disorders.

Several risk factors have been associated with a less favorable prognosis in disruptive behavior disorders. These factors include early onset of the symptoms, presence of comorbid psychiatric problems (including substance abuse), low socioeconomic status, high levels of family conflict, and a family history of antisocial personality disorder. Use of physical discipline by parents also appears to predict negative outcomes in ODD. Teens who have good social skills or who are able to develop positive social relationships appear to have a better prognosis.

Conclusion

The disruptive behavior disorders oppositional defiant disorder (ODD) and conduct disorder are characterized by repeated rule-breaking behaviors. The problem behaviors seen in these disorders go far beyond the normal challenging of authority that is commonly seen during adolescence. Teens with ODD frequently argue with parents and teachers, disobey rules, lose their temper easily, and blame others for their mistakes. Some of these teens will progress to a conduct disorder, which involves a more severe pattern of behaviors that may involve aggression, destruction of property, theft, or serious rule violations including criminal activity.

For an accurate diagnosis, these disorders must be distinguished from other psychiatric problems that can cause similar behaviors, including ADHD, bipolar disorder, and substance abuse. Moreover, teens with ODD and conduct disorder have high rates of other comorbid psychiatric issues and learning problems. Recognition and treatment of these comorbid disorders is a critical component of the treatment.

Although medications may have a role in treating comorbid psychiatric illness, at present there is no good evidence that medications are effective in treating the symptoms of ODD or conduct disorder. Rather, the treatment tends to involve psychosocial interventions. In addition to individual therapy for the teen, involvement of the family is usually indicated as well. Parents can work with a therapist to address related family problems, to improve communication within the family, and to develop a behavior plan involving clear rules and expectations and consistent rewards for positive behavior and consequences for negative behavior. Structure and close supervision are also valuable.

Integrated collaborations with school, community programs, agencies such as community mental health centers, and, when appropriate, the juvenile justice system are often the best approach to addressing disruptive behavior disorders, particularly in the case of conduct disorder. Establishing a coordinated treatment plan involving these institutions and maintaining good communication among all the involved parties are important factors in the success of this approach.

ODD and conduct disorder are challenging to treat and trying for parents. Change often takes a long time. So it is important for parents to stick with treatment. These disorders carry a high risk of negative outcomes for the adolescent, including criminal activity and resultant legal consequences, continuing psychiatric illness, injury from fights or other high-risk activities, and significantly impaired academic and occupational achievement.

References and Additional Reading

Pager, K. A., A. Kazmi, W. P. Gardner, and Y. Wang. 2007. "Female Conduct Disorder: Health Status in Young Adulthood." *Journal of Adolescent Health* 84: e1–e7.

Sanders, L. M., J. Schaechter, and J. R. Serwint. 2007. "Conduct Disorder." *Pediatrics in Review* 38: 433–434.

Van Cleave J., and M. M. Davis. 2006. "Bullying and Peer Victimization among Children with Special Health Care Needs." *Pediatrics* 118: e1212–e1219.

Welte, J. W., G. M. Barnes, M.C.O. Tidwell, and J. H. Hoffman. 2009. "Association between Problem Gambling and Conduct Disorder in a National Survey of Adolescent and Young Adults in the United States." *Journal of Adolescent Health* 45: 396–401.

Eating Disorders

Eating disorders are a group of serious psychiatric problems that have the highest fatality rate of all mental disorders. Though often thought to be a modern problem, behaviors similar to bingeing and purging have been described since ancient Roman times. In the 1880s, *anorexia nervosa* was coined to describe individuals who voluntarily limit their intake and then endure weight loss. By contrast, it has been only in the past thirty years that the term *bulimia* was introduced to describe the bingeing and purging behaviors identified in some women with eating disorders.

In the past forty years, increasingly more adolescents, both male and female, have been diagnosed with eating disorders. Part, but certainly not all, of this increasing prevalence is due to the changing ways that society views body size, shape, and weight. There are other factors that may predispose adolescents to eating disorders. Teens may have family members who have been diagnosed with anorexia. Adolescents in families that have experienced divorce, separation, remarriage, or abuse have a higher prevalence of eating disorders. Teens with other psychiatric conditions including depression, obsessive-compulsive disorder, and addiction are also at higher risk for eating disorders. Impulsive adolescents may be more likely to engage in bulimic behaviors. With the increasing incidence of obesity in adolescents and their parents, dieting or talking about weight loss may contribute to adolescent eating disorders. Perhaps counterintuitively, recessionary times with decreasing home budgets do not directly cause anorexia; conversely, obesity is more likely a result of teens eating less costly and less healthful food.

With these myriad risk factors, eating disorders are very prevalent. Approximately 0.5 percent of adolescent and young adult females fit the DSM-IV definition of anorexia nervosa. Between 1 to 3 percent of females in this age group have a diagnosis of bulimia. For both anorexia and bulimia, the prevalence in males is much lower than in females, but the incidence appears to be increasing.

Anorexia usually begins in adolescence, whereas bulimia usually starts in young adulthood. These disorders tend to occur in teens from upper-middle-class or wealthier families. In the United States, eating disorders are seen much more frequently in Caucasian or Asian adolescents than in Hispanic or African American youth. Broadcasts of American television programs appear central to the recent appearance of eating disorders on the island of Fiji. Moreover, research suggests that exposure to American media may be spurring the onset of eating disorders in areas of India where there had been no such disorders in the past.

Case Presentation: Anorexia

Jenny, a seventeen-year-old girl, was seen in the adolescent medicine division for concerns about a possible eating disorder. Her parents noted that she began to decrease her eating about one year ago, which was shortly after her parents told her that they planned to separate. Five months prior to the doctor visit, she reported having her last menstrual period. There was no family history of eating disorders. They were an upper-middle-class family: the teen's mother was a psychologist, her father was employed in real estate, and her older brothers had successful careers.

The adolescent appeared to be very thin. She weighed 102 pounds, 34 pounds below her ideal weight of 136 pounds, and her height was 67.5 inches. Her blood pressure was low, and her pulse was very slow. She was diagnosed with anorexia nervosa, and she was hospitalized immediately because of her low weight.

After twelve days in the hospital, the teen was transferred to a residential care facility for continuing treatment of anorexia. She spent five weeks at the facility and gained a total of 20 pounds. At that point, she was transferred to a day outpatient program for further care. After several months in the day program, she was discharged. Over the ensuing months, as she tried to attend college classes and maintain an apartment, her weight dropped slowly. She left college and reenrolled in the day and evening treatment programs at her residential treatment facility. For about six months, she saw a therapist and nutritionist every week, and her weight stabilized at 115 pounds. But this weight was too low for her to have menstrual periods.

Unfortunately, she discontinued her therapy program for a two-month period and lost eight pounds. She had also discontinued, without permission, her antidepressant medication. She was readmitted to the residential facility, now two years after her initial diagnosis of anorexia. After two months of residential treatment, she had gained 20 pounds, and her menstrual cycles returned. She was placed in a day and evening program for several months, after which she stepped down to weekly nutrition and therapy appointments, biweekly medical follow-up, and monthly psychiatric visits. Thirty-two months after her initial diagnosis of anorexia nervosa, her weight had stabilized at 134 pounds. She began to date one boy steadily, and she requested oral contraceptive pills. The clinicians felt her anorexia was in recovery.

Symptoms and Warning Signs

Eating disorders are divided into three types: anorexia nervosa, bulimia nervosa, and eating disorders not otherwise specified (EDNOS). There is significant overlap among the types.

Certain behaviors suggest that an adolescent has anorexia. A change in eating habits such as becoming a vegetarian or a vegan or a decision to eat healthfully may be the first sign. Although these changes may not always represent a problem and, indeed, may be a positive step for many teens, eating disorders often start when changes are carried too far. In addition, excessive exercise or difficulty eating in social settings or at family meals may be suggestive of anorexia. Social isolation, deceptive or secretive behaviors, or dressing with extra layers of clothing should raise red flags. Frequent weighing, sometimes up to ten times a

Sidebar 15.1 | **Behavioral Issues That Suggest an Eating Disorder**

- ▶ Isolation from friends
- ▶ Frequent trips to the bathroom after meals
- ▶ Change in bowel-movement habits
- ▶ Increasing school absenteeism
- ▶ More interest in cooking but not eating
- ▶ Changes in eating patterns: cuts food into tiny pieces, takes longer time to eat

day, is very troubling. Many teens with anorexia think about food, body image, and shape more than 50 percent of the time.

Sometimes, anorexia may be suspected at the teen's annual physical examination. There may be a slowdown in growth or weight gain, loss or delay of menstruation, and marked weight loss, which are further clues. The teen's blood pressure and pulse may be too low. With anorexia, the core body temperature may also be below normal.

Bulimia can be more difficult to recognize, as boys and girls afflicted with this problem may not show obvious physical signs, such as weight loss or cessation of growth. Concerning behaviors that may be observed include frequent trips to the bathroom after meals and consuming large amounts of food without obvious weight gain. In addition, teens with bulimia may show some of the behavioral changes that are seen in anorexia. Researchers have shown that some boys with bulimia, but not the majority, are suffering from sexual identity issues, and, on occasion, these boys may show effeminate behaviors.

Eating disorder not otherwise specified (EDNOS) is a category for adolescents whose symptoms do not clearly fit the criteria for anorexia or bulimia. For example, an adolescent may have body-image concerns and fear of weight gain and be very thin, but she may still be menstruating, thus not fulfilling the criteria for the diagnosis of anorexia. Even though a teen with EDNOS may not neatly fit the diagnostic pattern of anorexia or bulimia, these symptoms can be just as severe as for other eating disorders, and they usually warrant the same intensive monitoring and treatment.

The "athletic triad" is an additional problem faced by many adolescents. Though not classified as a mental illness, the pattern of symptoms is similar to problems seen in other eating disorders. Girls with this disorder are usually serious athletes who have lost their periods, have significant loss of bone mineralization, occasionally leading to osteoporosis, and have a pattern of disordered eating. This disorder is seen especially in girls who participate in sports such as ballet and gymnastics for which lean body weight is important for performance.

As a parent, you may observe warning signs, aside from behaviors, that suggest your teen may have an eating disorder. Cessation of menstruation is always worrisome, as it may indicate too low weight. Changes in vital signs, including low pulse or blood pressure, which may cause lightheadedness or faintness, are reasons for concern. Bluish hands and feet and feeling cold when others are warm may indicate low body temperature and poor circulation, other signs of too low weight or body fat. Stress fractures may also occur if bone density has been compromised. A change in bowel-movement habits, particularly constipation, may signal an eating disorder. Tooth decay may be caused by the stomach acid produced by vomiting, and therefore, an increase in the number of cavities raises concern for induced purging. Spending increasing amounts of time in the bathroom after meals decreasing athletic capabilities, and diminishing academic performance may all signal an eating disorder.

Making the Diagnosis

The diagnosis of an eating disorder may be made by an adolescent medicine specialist, pediatrician, psychiatrist, or therapist. Anorexia is a mental illness for which there are medical criteria for diagnosis, so a medical clinician is usually involved in the diagnosis and may also be involved in the treatment of this condition.

To diagnose an adolescent with anorexia, two medical criteria must be met: First, the weight is abnormally low, generally less than 85 percent of expected weight for age and height. Second, there is a loss of menstruation for three consecutive months, assuming the girl has started having periods. If the girl has not started her period, then a delay in onset of menstruation may be a consideration.

Case Presentation: Bulimia

Elizabeth was a college freshman whose parents became concerned about her when she was home over winter break. They noted that Elizabeth was coming downstairs in the evening after her parents had gone to bed and eating huge amounts of food, going through bags of potato chips and large tubs of ice cream. Elizabeth's parents also noticed that she frequently went to the bathroom immediately after meals, always using the upstairs bathroom when the family was downstairs so she could have "more privacy." After a few days, Elizabeth's parents began to suspect that Elizabeth was making herself vomit. They noticed a smell of vomit in the bathroom, found foul-smelling towels hidden in her bedroom, and finally heard her vomiting after one of her evening binges.

When her parents confronted her with their concerns, Elizabeth admitted that she did not feel in control of her eating. She would have a strong urge to snack, then eat a much bigger quantity of food than she intended in a short period of time. Feeling badly about herself afterward and worrying about her appearance, she made herself vomit several times each day. Elizabeth recognized that she had a problem and agreed to go with her parents to see a psychiatrist.

Upon evaluation, Elizabeth was diagnosed with bulimia as well as a mild case of depression. She began a course of treatment with psychotherapy and medication. The psychiatrist notified Elizabeth's primary care doctor, who began meeting with her regularly for monitoring and who educated Elizabeth about the serious health problems that can be caused by bingeing and purging. With time, Elizabeth's symptoms improved, and she began to have a more healthy relationship with food.

The two psychiatric criteria needed to diagnose anorexia include a profound fear of gaining weight, even in an underweight adolescent, and a body-image disturbance. The fear of weight gain may manifest itself as intense anxiety around meals or high-calorie or fatty foods. Individuals with body-image distortion perceive themselves to be overweight, even when they are dangerously thin. They may be preoccupied with specific areas of their bodies that they think are fat. Boys with anorexia should also fit these criteria, with the obvious exception of menstruation. Boys who are trying to make a lower weight class in wrestling are usually not anorexic, but they often have disordered eating.

There are several medical conditions that may mimic anorexia. Pregnancy needs to be excluded as an alternative cause of missed periods. In addition, inflammatory bowel disease such as Crohn's disease or ulcerative colitis or malabsorption due to celiac disease should be considered. These illnesses could cause abdominal pain, vomiting, changes in bowel-movement habits, and weight loss, which may be confused for disordered eating and its consequences. Brain tumors should be excluded in some cases, as they may cause weight loss and vomiting. Endocrinological problems, such as an overactive thyroid, diabetes, and a hormonal condition called Addison's disease, may need to be considered. Tuberculosis and HIV infection can cause profound weight loss and can be a cause of concern for a teen with anorexia symptoms and appropriate risk factors for these illnesses.

Adolescents with bulimia repeatedly eat larger than normal amounts of food in a discrete period, usually in fewer than two hours, than most people would eat in the same time frame. In addition, these teens often have compensatory purging behaviors to prevent weight gain, usually inducing vomiting, using laxatives or diuretics, or exercising excessively. Because teens with bulimia are usually in a normal weight range, there are fewer medical conditions to be excluded when considering the diagnosis. However, bulimia can pose serious medical risks. Some teens with bulimia first come to the physician with a complaint of vomiting blood. Thus, in these cases, rupture of the esophagus, a bleeding ulcer, or esophageal varices (dilated veins around the esophagus) would need to be considered.

Depending on the particular adolescent's clinical presentation, diagnosing a teen with suspected EDNOS or the athletic triad may require some additional testing. Generally, if menstrual periods are missed, pregnancy and other hormonal disorders need to be excluded. Psychiatric evaluation of eating disorders should include consideration of other possible psychiatric disorders that may be mistaken for eating disorders. Most notably, depression should be considered, as it can cause loss of appetite and significant weight loss. Abuse of many substances, including cocaine, heroin, and methamphetamine, may also lead to weight loss and decreased food intake. Sometimes, teens with obsessive-compulsive disorder (OCD) may have obsessions or compulsive behaviors that are focused on food. In these cases, the line between OCD and an eating disorder may be blurred.

Comorbidities

Due to a high likelihood of medical complications and comorbid psychiatric disorders, adolescents with a diagnosis of anorexia, bulimia, or EDNOS are usually seen by a team of medical and psychiatric clinicians. Teens with eating disorders are at increased risk for several psychiatric problems. These comorbid psychiatric issues contribute to the high rate of suicide in those who suffer from eating disorders. Depression is the most common comorbid psychiatric issue in teens with anorexia nervosa, and it frequently occurs in teens with bulimia as well. In anorexia nervosa, depression may, in part, be due to abnormalities in brain and hormonal functioning related to severe malnourishment. Often, depression in a significantly underweight adolescent does not resolve until the teen's nutritional status improves.

Anxiety disorders are quite common in adolescents with eating disorders. Some degree of anxiety around food and weight gain occurs as part of anorexia nervosa, so the diagnosis of a distinct anxiety disorder requires identification of anxiety unrelated to eating issues. Obsessive-compulsive disorder occurs in roughly one-third of patients with eating disorders. The two disorders share many features, including intrusive and distressing thoughts (which in the case of eating disorders relate to body image) and strict behavioral routines performed in response to these thoughts.

Substance abuse is fairly common in teens with eating disorders and is highest in those with bulimia. Possible reasons include low self-esteem, a high degree of impulsivity, an attempt to self-medicate distress, or the use of substances, such as stimulants or cocaine, to suppress appetite.

Many adults with eating disorders are diagnosed with personality disorders. Because it is felt that one's personality is still forming in adolescence, these disorders are diagnosed less frequently in teenagers (see chapter 13). However, it is common for teens with eating disorders to demonstrate strong and potentially impairing personality traits. Teens with anorexia tend to be perfectionists who are often rigid in their thinking and have a strong need to feel that they are in control. Teens with bulimia are frequently impulsive and prone to extremes in their behavior and expressions of emotion. They may have difficulty regulating strong feelings. Low self-esteem and difficulties with trust and interpersonal relationships are common in both disorders.

There are a number of possible medical complications in anorexia and bulimia. Some complications, especially those involving the blood potassium level or heart rhythm, can cause sudden death in teens with an eating disorder. Because of the potential for fatal complications, anorexia has the highest death rate of all mental illnesses.

Research studies have shown that girls and boys with anorexia are at high risk for bone mineralization problems that can lead to osteopenia or the more severe

Table 15.1	Medical Complications of Eating Disorders	
System	**Anorexia**	**Bulimia**
Gastrointestinal	Constipation, decreased intestinal motility	Inflammation or rupture of esophagus, stomach rupture or dilation
Cardiovascular	Slow heart rate, low blood pressure, heart rhythm disturbance	Slow heart rate, low blood pressure, heart rhythm disturbance
Hematologic	Low red count, white count, and platelet count	Bleeding
Endocrine and Metabolic	Delay in puberty, growth arrest, osteoporosis, loss of menstruation, high cholesterol, low potassium and blood sugar	Low potassium and sodium
Renal	Kidney stones	Dehydration
Neurologic	Brain shrinkage, disturbance of peripheral nerve function	Seizures, memory loss, bleeding into the brain
Skin	Dryness, acne, hair loss, or increase in hair	Bleeding under the skin due to vomiting

condition called osteoporosis. Due to low serum estrogen in girls and low serum testosterone in boys, which are both due to diminished body weight and body fat from anorexia, the bones begin to lose mineral density. This is especially profound in the hips and lumbar spine, leading in severe cases to a diagnosis of osteoporosis. These adolescents have significant risk for fracture, especially later in life. Most teens with anorexia for six months or more should have a DEXA (dual energy x-ray absorptiometry) study to determine bone mineralization. Medications may be given to address low bone density.

Treatment

Several general points about treatment for eating disorders are noted in sidebar 15.2.

During the evaluation of a teen with anorexia, the clinician will design a framework for the treatment plan. An initial level of care is determined. These levels include inpatient medical hospitalization, inpatient psychiatric hospitalization, residential care, intensive outpatient care, partial outpatient care, or outpatient care. Sometimes teens require long-term residential care.

Levels of Care

Medical Hospitalization. Some teens are so ill that they need an immediate medical hospitalization for their safety. These hospitalizations tend to range in length from seven to ten days. Sidebar 15.3 outlines the reasons a teen would need to be hospitalized immediately for medical reasons.

The medical hospitalization for anorexia serves several roles: It begins the medical, nutritional, behavioral, and educational components of treatment in an acute and intensive setting. Furthermore, it allows for professionals in medicine, psychiatry, nutrition, and social services to see the teen and the parents. Additionally, complications from refeeding the adolescent are watched for carefully. Specifically, refeeding syndrome may occur during the first week of restoring nutrition, when the body uses up available phosphorous as it makes new protein. This occurs as the adolescent consumes increasing amounts of calories. If the teen is not given supplemental phosphorous, then serious side effects including fluid retention and heart failure can occur. Daily blood phosphorous levels are often necessary to determine if the refeeding syndrome is under way. The hospitalization also allows for careful planning for the next step in the teen's treatment plan.

To accomplish these goals in a coordinated manner, some hospitals have designed a written protocol for the management of adolescent inpatients who have anorexia. These documents define the roles and expectations for the teen, her or his parents, and the team clinicians. It encourages positive behaviors and eating habits. As a contract signed by the teen, the parents, and the clinicians, it necessitates participation

---

Sidebar 15.2 | Important Points about Treatment of a Teen with Eating Disorder

- The earlier the diagnosis is made for an eating disorder and the more aggressive the treatment, the more likely the adolescent's outcome will be favorable
- Eating disorders tend to relapse
- Treatment is long term, expensive, and extensive
- A team of clinicians who communicate with one another is usually the optimal way to treat eating disorders
- Parents should be involved in the treatment

Sidebar 15.3 | Reasons to Hospitalize Adolescents with Anorexia

- Weight less than 75 percent of ideal weight
- Weight loss despite intensive outpatient program
- Food refusal or significant and sudden weight loss
- Low body temperature
- Low blood pressure
- Low heart rate
- Unstable blood pressure and pulse
- Problems with blood electrolytes (such as low potassium or sodium)
- Heart rhythm disturbance
- Suicidal issues

by all parties. Family and clinician meetings are held during the hospitalization not only to address concerns and update the family but also to outline the next steps in treatment.

During the medical hospitalization, the teen's blood pressure, pulse, weight, temperature, and blood chemistry are carefully monitored. When it is appears that the teen is able to eat adequate calories, begins to gain weight, starts to stabilize blood pressure and pulse, and is able to cooperate in treatment, then usually she or he is transferred to residential care. Teens' cooperation does not necessarily come easily or quickly. On occasion, the adolescent tries to play one team member against another team member or the parents against the team.

Inpatient Psychiatric Hospitalization. Inpatient psychiatric hospitalization may be necessary for some teens with eating disorders. In general, this level of care is considered when a teen's psychiatric symptoms are so severe that they pose an imminent threat to the teen's safety, and they cannot be managed safely in a less intensive setting. For example, an adolescent with an eating disorder who is having intense suicidal thoughts and is at high risk of harming herself is likely to require inpatient psychiatric care. It should be noted that many inpatient psychiatric units are not equipped to provide the high level of medical care, including interventions such as continuous heart monitoring or administration of intravenous fluids, that adolescents with severe eating disorders may require. In these situations, adolescents may need to remain on an inpatient medical unit until they are medically stable for transfer to a psychiatric unit. In some areas of the country, there are specialized adolescent "med-psych" units that can provide intensive medical and psychiatric care for adolescents with eating disorders.

Residential Care. Residential care for anorexia is provided in specialized eating disorder treatment centers; however, health insurers vary in their willingness to pay for residential care. Adolescents spend twenty-four hours a day in residential care, often until they gain weight up to their ideal weight or at least to 90 or 95 percent of that weight. This may take weeks or even months.

Group therapy, nutritional sessions, and group meals are commonplace. Daily vital signs and weekly medical checks are often performed. Individual and family therapy may be part of some programs. The treatment is intensive, and the treaters often meet frequently to evaluate the teen's progress. Each residential center has its own goals, which are often customized to the teen. The larger centers have outpatient programs that are part of its operations. When teens reaches their goals, many centers transfer them to a partial hospital program or an intensive outpatient program (IOP).

Many parents worry about having their children in residential programs or other eating disorder treatment programs, fearing that their child will learn unhealthy behaviors from other adolescents in the program. Though this concern should not be taken lightly, the risk of an adolescent developing new problems after exposure to other adolescents needs to be weighed against the serious risks associated with undertreatment of a severe eating disorder. A teen may be just as likely to pick up bad behaviors from peers at school or on the Internet, and the likelihood of one of these behaviors sticking is increased dramatically if the underlying problems contributing to the eating disorder have not been recognized and addressed. A good eating disorder program will maintain a structured, tightly controlled treatment setting where teens are much more likely to contribute to each other's healing than they are to cause new problems.

Partial Hospital Programs. A number of programs provide intensive treatment during the daytime, Monday through Friday, thus allowing teens with anorexia to return to their home at night and to have the weekend for recreation. Group therapy, nutritional counseling, common meals, and medical surveillance continue as well. In order for this level of care to be appropriate, a teen should be in need of intensive treatment but stable enough to be safe at home. In order to benefit from a partial hospital program, a teen should also have some degree of motivation to work on the eating disorder, though some degree of ambivalence about treatment is common.

Intensive Outpatient Programs. These programs are similar to partial hospital programs in that the teen lives at home but receives regular intensive treatment at the program. The primary difference is that an intensive outpatient program normally takes place in the evening, allowing the adolescent to continue participating in school or other daytime activities. A typical intensive outpatient program (or IOP) might be held Monday through Thursday from 3 p.m. to 7 p.m. and include an observed dinner. Individual, group, and family therapy as well as nutritional counseling are all common components of these programs.

Outpatient Care. Outpatient care for an adolescent with an eating disorder is usually organized with a team approach. A teen with anorexia may continue with an outpatient therapist from the residential treatment center or have services from a local therapist. In order to develop healthy eating patterns, overcome obstacles to eating, and promote stable weight gain, most adolescents require periodic visits with a nutritionist. A physician should monitor these adolescents for medical stability and weight gain and perform necessary laboratory testing. Some adolescent specialists offer counseling. When appropriate, a psychiatrist or individual therapist is usually involved to provide psychotherapy and prescribe medications. Family therapy is an important component of the treatment for most teens as well, as family dynamics can play a big role in eating disorders. Often, outpatient care continues for several years.

Long-Term Residential Care. There are facilities that provide residential care to adolescents with both anorexia and bulimia and combine the treatment with

---

Sidebar 15.4 | **Reasons to Hospitalize Adolescents with Bulimia**

▶ Low blood potassium or chlorides
▶ Fainting
▶ Tear in esophagus causing bleeding
▶ Heart rhythm disturbance
▶ Low temperature
▶ Intractable vomiting
▶ Vomiting blood
▶ Failure to respond to outpatient treatment
▶ Suicidality

---

an age-appropriate academic program. Teens admitted to these types of programs have often failed to improve and stay well after going through other levels of care. These programs are quite expensive. However, since an academic education is part of the treatment program, the cost may be subsidized by the teen's school district.

Adolescents with anorexia may enter the treatment system at any point, depending on their medical and psychiatric condition. In general, teens do better, in a prognostic sense, if they receive intensive services for anorexia as early in the disease as possible. Services may continue for years, and relapses are common.

Because most residential care is geared toward girls, boys with anorexia have far fewer treatment options. There are only a few facilities that care for adolescent boys with anorexia. Nonetheless, the levels of care also apply to boys.

Teens with bulimia are often in a safe weight range, but there are certain medical conditions that may require a medical hospitalization for teens with bulimia (see sidebar 15.4). Even though the levels of care outlined for teens with anorexia can apply to teens with bulimia, most often in bulimia, while the acute medical issues are treated, plans are made for the next level of care. For example, a teen with bulimia and low potassium would be admitted to the hospital for correction of the potassium. Then, the teen would return to an outpatient care program. For teens with a history of repeated low potassium levels, it may be desirable to consider residential care for further mental health therapy. The plan is customized to the individual patient. A team approach works well, with the physician monitoring for medical stability, a psychiatrist prescribing medications and possibly delivering therapy, and a nutritionist counseling on appropriate foods. A therapist such as a psychologist or clinical social work trained in the management of adolescents with eating disorders may also be involved.

Medications

Teens with anorexia are usually prescribed a multivitamin, calcium supplements, and vitamin D, the latter two being important for the prevention of osteopenia and osteoporosis. In addition, supplemental phosphorous may be recommended early in treatment when refeeding is initiated, since the body uses extra amounts of phosphorous when weight gain initially occurs. Some teens require stool softeners, gentle laxatives for constipation, and antacids or acid blockers for heartburn.

In combination with other treatments, psychiatric medications may have a role for some adolescents with eating disorders. Medications need to be considered carefully, as the side effects of some medications have the potential to exacerbate some medical complications of an eating disorder, including seizures, cardiac arrhythmias, low blood pressure when standing up (called orthostatic hypotension), lightheadedness, and constipation.

For teens with bulimia, antidepressant medications are often used. These can reduce bingeing and the intensity of the impulse to purge. Of the antidepressants, the selective serotonin reuptake inhibitors (SSRIs; see chapter 5) are generally used first because of their safety and efficacy. Other antidepressants may also be tried. The antidepressant buproprion (Wellbutrin), which is commonly used to treat other disorders, is often avoided in teens with eating disorders because it can increase the likelihood of a seizure. Seizures are more likely if there is an abnormality in the blood chemistry due to purging or restricting food intake.

Thus far, research on the treatment of anorexia nervosa has not found any medications to be truly effective for the disorder. However, comorbid psychiatric disorders are common in teens with anorexia, and medications may play a role in treating these disorders. In order to bring an eating disorder under control, it is important to treat coexisting conditions, such as depression, anxiety, or obsessive-compulsive disorder.

Therapy

Nutritional Therapy. In the hospital, a nutritionist meets with the adolescent with anorexia and performs a detailed interview that concentrates on the teen's eating habits prior to the hospital admission. Furthermore, the nutritionist helps the teen select foods from the hospital menu based on the teen's caloric and nutritional needs. In the hospital, the goal is to achieve a weight gain of about half a pound each day. The nutritionist determines maintenance requirements for weight stabilization, and a calorie count begins with admission. Only food provided by the hospital nutrition services is included in the daily calorie count. The nutritionist also determines the need and amount of supplemental calories each day.

After a teen is discharged from the hospital, nutritional care continues to ensure adequate weight gain on a healthy diet. In residential care, teens usually gain less than half a pound daily; in outpatient care, the goal is to gain one to two pounds weekly. Nutritional counseling is continued during recovery.

Individual Psychotherapy. Individual psychotherapy is the cornerstone of psychiatric treatment for adolescents with eating disorders. Several different treatment modalities may be employed. Cognitive behavioral therapy (CBT; see chapter 4) is an effective and commonly used treatment approach for bulimia and anorexia nervosa. The goal of CBT is to help correct the teen's underlying body-image distortion and preoccupation with weight, food intake, or exercise and to normalize eating behaviors. Adolescents can learn to identify thoughts and feelings that trigger their symptoms and work to correct distorted perceptions or ideas that contribute to the disorder. They are taught coping skills for managing urges to binge, purge, restrict food intake, or exercise excessively.

Psychodynamic psychotherapy (discussed in detail in chapter 4) is also commonly used in the treatment of eating disorders. In eating disorder treatment, the goal of psychodynamic psychotherapy is to guide teens toward an understanding of the meaning that the eating disorder symptoms have in their life. Exploring teens' current and past relationships, particularly within the family, is one way to achieve this understanding.

Regardless of the specific approach to therapy, psychoeducation is an important element of psychotherapy for the treatment of eating disorders. Insight is often lacking in youth with eating disorders, and denial may be strong. Thus, therapists of all theoretical orientations help build teens' insight into the problem and recognize the toll it is taking on their life in order to motivate them to work toward improved health.

Family Therapy. Family dynamics often play a large role in eating disorders. That is not to say that parents are to blame for the problem; the development of an eating disorder is the result of many different factors, both biological and psychological. However, it is often the case that patterns of interaction that have developed within the family over years play a part in perpetuating the illness, despite everyone's best intentions. Moreover, eating disorders place families under a great deal of stress. Parents may feel overwhelmed and not know how to respond, and siblings may feel angry, worried, confused, or even jealous of all the attention the teen with the disorder seems to attract.

With the importance of family factors in the illness, it is not surprising that family therapy appears to be one of the most effective interventions for adolescents with eating disorders. Thus, it is a critical component of the treatment for many teens.

One form of family treatment, called the Maudsley method, after the hospital in London where it was developed, has demonstrated very favorable results for adolescents with anorexia nervosa. This treatment empowers parents to play an active role in helping the teen restore a healthy weight. Parents are trained to use techniques to encourage their teen to eat. Such techniques may include rewards for good behaviors and limit setting; criticism and punishments are generally not used in the Maudsley method. Control over eating is handed back to the adolescent when she or he is ready. A great effort is made during the treatment to avoid assignment of blame and to focus instead on helping parents find positive solutions for the problem. More information about the Maudsley method is available at www.maudsleyparents.org, including a listing of treatment centers that use this approach.

Even when intensive family therapy does not seem to be the best approach for a particular family, the family's active involvement in the treatment is still essential for success. This may take many forms, including meeting with the teen's treatment team to discuss how best to help the teen at home.

Group Therapy. Group therapy is another important component of the treatment plan for many adolescents with eating disorders, as part of both residential treatment programs and outpatient treatment. Teens may take comfort in talking with peers who are struggling with similar issues and may offer support to one another through the group. More structured groups may provide education about eating disorders and related issues, such as nutrition, or teach skills for managing the illness.

Prognosis

A number of studies have evaluated the long-term outcome for the treatment of anorexia. About half of people undergoing treatment for anorexia do well, 30 percent do reasonably well, and 20 percent do poorly. Unfortunately, in the case of anorexia, there is a 5 to 10 percent mortality rate. Although many of these deaths are related to medical complications of the disorder, anorexia is associated with a high rate of suicide as well. Studies have shown that early diagnosis and aggressive treatment give rise to a better long-term outcome.

Pro-Eating Disorder Information

There are sites on MySpace, Facebook, and elsewhere on the Internet that actively promote eating disorders through a support network. These so-called pro-ana and pro-mia sites work against the advice and counseling given by the treatment team to adolescents afflicted with eating disorders. The sites share dieting techniques, advise how to hide weight loss from clinicians, and teach methods of inducing purging such as vomiting. These sites validate, glamorize, or normalize eating disorders, especially anorexia, even though anorexia and bulimia are illnesses. As a result, teens who view these sites may have further misconceptions about their illness, which impedes treatment and recovery.

Conclusion

Anorexia and bulimia are very serious mental illnesses that afflict adolescents, and they can have significant medical complications that can include death. These disorders may start insidiously, and teens may try to hide the fact that they have an eating disorder.

Teens with an eating disorder need early diagnosis and aggressive treatment by a multidisciplinary team including a psychiatrist or therapist, nutritionist, and primary care physician or adolescent medicine specialist. Treatment can take place in a variety of venues, and the participation of family in treatment can be key to the teen's recovery. Unfortunately, eating disorders are often chronic, and in the worst-case scenario, they can last a lifetime.

References and Additional Reading

American Psychiatric Association, Work Group on Eating Disorders. 2006. "Practice Guideline for the Treatment of Patients with Eating Disorders." 3rd ed. Arlington, VA: American Psychiatric Association.

Becker, A. E. 2004. "Television, Disordered Eating, and Young Women in Fiji: Negotiating Body Image and Identity during Rapid Social Change." *Culture, Medicine, and Psychiatry* 28: 533–559.

Fisher, M. E. 1995. "Eating Disorders in Adolescents: A Background Paper." *Journal of Adolescent Health* 16: 420–437.

———. 2006. "Treatment of Eating Disorders in Children, Adolescents, and Young Adults." *Pediatrics in Review* 27: 5–16.

Goldstein, M. A., D. B. Herzog, M. Misra, and P. Sagar. 2008. "A 19-Year-Old Man with Weight Loss and Abdominal Pain." *New England Journal of Medicine* 359: 1272–1283.

Herzog, D. B., D. L. Franko, and P. Cable. 2007. *Unlocking the Mysteries of Eating Disorders.* New York: McGraw-Hill.

16 Obsessive-Compulsive Disorder and Tic Disorders

Obsessive-compulsive disorder (OCD) and tic disorders have similarities. In both cases, an adolescent's sense of self comes under assault as he or she experiences thoughts or urges that do not seem to make sense and feel impossible to control. OCD is characterized by bizarre, disturbing, intrusive thoughts or images and repetitive behaviors that are difficult to resist, while tic disorders, such as Tourette's disorder, involve sudden, repetitive, habitual movements or vocalizations known as tics. As with OCD, most teens with tic disorders recognize the problem and wish that they could stop. Unfortunately, they just cannot help themselves.

Tic disorders and OCD frequently occur together. Both disorders have a broad range of severity, from a few mild symptoms that are not too uncommon even in the general population to a severe and debilitating illness. They are believed to be caused by similar underlying mechanisms, with abnormal functioning of the basal ganglia in the brain. Some experts maintain that the symptoms of OCD and tic disorders represent different ends of the spectrum of a single common underlying illness.

Case Presentation

Jeff, a fifteen-year-old boy, and his mother consulted an adolescent medicine specialist for what the teen called "recurring obsessive thoughts." The teen continually thought of harming members of his family or engaging in sexual activities with them. No physical harm took place, but he reported that he was not able to carry out his usual activities. Jeff was immediately referred to a general psychiatrist, who felt he was prepsychotic.

The teen was placed on an SSRI medication; however, because of the medication's potential side effects, his mother insisted that he stop taking it. At the time, Jeff had a documented streptococcal infection and was treated with antibiotics. The adolescent was referred to a psychiatrist specializing in OCD, who diagnosed him with that disorder. He also saw a rheumatologist, who diagnosed the symptoms and behavior as a complication of streptococcal infection called PANDAS (pediatric autoimmune neuropsychiatric disorder associated with streptococcal infection).

Over several years of coordinated treatment with adolescent medicine, child psychiatry, and rheumatology Jeff's obsessive thoughts slowly diminished. He required long-term antibiotics, psychiatric medications (introduced at a later date), and psychotherapy. His academics improved during high school, and he was symptom free during his freshman year in college.

As these disorders can engender shame, social isolation, poor self-esteem, and academic struggles, they have the potential to cause significant distress for teenagers. It is important to recognize and treat OCD and tic disorders as well as manage their secondary effects.

Obsessive-Compulsive Disorder

Obsessive-compulsive disorder is a common and potentially disabling psychiatric illness that frequently begins in early adolescence. It is characterized by the presence of either obsessions, which are intrusive and persistent thoughts, or compulsions, which are distressing, unnecessary behaviors that are repeatedly performed to ward off an obsessive thought or bad event. It is estimated that approximately 2 to 4 percent of children and adolescents suffer from the disorder, although greater numbers may have some symptoms of OCD that are not sufficiently severe to warrant the diagnosis. OCD is the subject of media fascination, with portrayals in popular television shows such as *Monk,* about a detective with the disorder, and movies such as *As Good as It Gets,* starring Jack Nicholson as an obsessive-compulsive misanthropic writer. The public perception of OCD has been influenced by prominent public figures, perhaps most notably the aviator, film producer, and business tycoon Howard Hughes, who was believed to have suffered from the disorder. OCD is part of everyday speech, as people frequently joke about their "OCD" when obsessively double-checking a paper for errors or insisting that things be arranged on a shelf in a particular way.

While media portrayals and public perception of the disorder capture some of its elements, they are not entirely accurate, and most people are not aware of the range of ways that OCD can manifest itself in people's lives. The lack of awareness can contribute to a delay in diagnosis. Moreover, children and adolescents frequently have difficulty expressing their OCD symptoms, making it more difficult to recognize and differentiate OCD from other psychiatric problems. As noted in the case presentation, OCD symptoms may occur entirely within the mind of the adolescent, without obvious external manifestations. And fear of being viewed as "weird" or "crazy" may lead adolescents to avoid talking about their obsessive thoughts and hide their compulsive behaviors, so that the adults in their life may not be aware of the problem.

What Causes OCD?

The cause of OCD is not completely understood, but in recent years, scientists have begun to make some headway in understanding the disorder. Although environmental factors may play a role, OCD appears to be a biologically based illness. It tends to run in families, suggesting a genetic component, though there are many patients with OCD who do not have any relatives who have the disorder. Brain imaging studies and other converging lines of evidence have implicated dysfunction in an area of the brain called the basal ganglia. The basal ganglia are a group of structures located deep within the brain that connect broadly to many other brain areas. They are involved in a number of brain functions, including attention, movement, emotion, and filtering sensory stimuli. It appears that patients with OCD have abnormal patterns of connection between the basal ganglia and other areas of the brain. Some studies have shown that these abnormal patterns normalize when patient's symptoms are successfully treated.

Another related hypothesis involves the brain chemical serotonin. Serotonin is a chemical messenger produced in many areas of the brain, including the basal ganglia. There is some evidence that abnormalities in serotonin transmission in certain parts of the brain, including the basal ganglia, are related to OCD symptoms. This hypothesis is supported by the fact that many of the medications used to treat OCD act on serotonin transmission.

Some children and adolescents have been found to develop OCD and other psychiatric problems after they have had an infection with the group A streptococcus bacteria, a common cause of infection in children and the cause of strep throat, a ubiquitous infection with which most parents are quite familiar. The vast majority of children who have strep throat do not have any lasting effects, particularly if the infection is treated with antibiotics. But in rare circumstances, symptoms of OCD develop shortly after the onset of the infection. In addition to OCD symptoms, some children and adolescents experience other problems, which may include tics, attention issues, moodiness, or abnormal movements. This phenomenon of psychiatric or neurological symptoms related to infection with group A streptococcus is referred to as PANDAS, which stands for pediatric autoimmune neuropsychiatric disorders associated with streptococcal infections.

Children whose OCD symptoms are related to PANDAS typically have an exacerbation of their symptoms when they have another bout of strep throat. Thus, it is important to inform your child's doctor if your child's symptoms seem to have begun or to have worsened after a sore throat or fever, as it may influence the approach to treatment. It has been theorized that OCD symptoms and other problems associated with PANDAS are caused by antibodies that the body makes to fight off the streptococcus bacteria. PANDAS is still incompletely understood, and it remains an area of active research.

Symptoms and Warning Signs

Although OCD can begin later in life, it most frequently emerges between the ages of seven and twelve. Both obsessions and compulsions are often present together, but it only takes one or the other to make the diagnosis.

Obsessions are frequently experienced as unwanted thoughts that are disturbing to the individual. Unlike psychosis, in which strange thoughts or sensory experiences tend to be perceived as real, obsessions in OCD are generally recognized by sufferers as coming from their own mind. Teens with OCD usually know that their obsessions are irrational. Nonetheless, the obsessions tend to be quite intrusive, difficult to control, and often quite bizarre. Adolescents with OCD may fear that they will do something bad to a loved one, despite the fact that they do not want to and that the very thought of it is upsetting to them. Similarly, obsessions may take the form of transient, intense, and often grotesque imagery of something terrible happening, such as of a parent's being badly injured.

Often obsessions center on the dirty, the horrifying, or the taboo. Preoccupation with germs and excessive concern about picking up germs, such as by touching doorknobs or counters, is a common obsession. Teens may come to view certain objects or places, such as a backpack, the kitchen, or a parent's car, as being "contaminated," and they may go to great lengths to avoid contamination. Socially unacceptable activities are often fertile ground for obsessions. Teens may fear that they will swear in church or act in a sexually inappropriate manner in school. Some teens become preoccupied with the concern that they might be sexually "perverted" despite no evidence to support this notion. Thoughts of this kind are disturbing to a victim of OCD at any age, but to an adolescent who is not yet secure in his or her identity, they can induce a profound sense of shame.

Preoccupation with exactness and symmetry is another common feature of obsessions in OCD. A sensation experienced on one side of the body, such as brushing one's hand against the wall or stepping on a crack in the sidewalk, may produce a strong urge to reproduce the sensation in exactly the same way on the opposite side of the body. Things in the house or related to school may need to be arranged or performed "just right," and teens with OCD sometimes take excessive amounts of time to get things exactly right. For example, they may put on and take off their socks and shoes countless times until they feel "just right" and then spend just as much time tying and retying their shoelaces. Adolescents with OCD may devote hours to checking and rechecking their homework assignments or repeatedly rewriting and erasing their work. While this degree of care may sound like a potentially beneficial quality, often it becomes impairing. Because of the obsession to get things just right, teens may be unable to complete their work

Obsessive thoughts are frequently related to compulsive behaviors. Compulsion behaviors are performed in order to protect against the fear associated with the obsession. Thus in response to a fear of germs, an adolescent may engage in excessive hand-washing. Teens may bathe repeatedly, aggressively scrub surfaces with bleach, or engage in other behaviors to "decontaminate" themselves or their environment. Checking behaviors are another common form of compulsion that is related to an obsessive fear. So, teens may need to return repeatedly to the house to check that the door is locked. They may continuously verify that family members are okay or seek reassurance that others are not upset with them.

Compulsive behaviors often do not have any logical connection to the matter the individual is trying to prevent. Rather, they may appear to be an extreme form of superstition. A teen may have a specific way of entering a doorway or have a ritual of tapping her fingers on a table in a specific pattern in order to prevent something bad from happening. If she does not do it exactly right, she may be compelled to repeat the process. Usually, teens are able to recognize that this behavior does not make sense, but they feel they cannot stop themselves and become very anxious when they do not perform the compulsive behavior.

Compulsions may also appear in the form of mental acts, as opposed to physical actions. People with OCD may count or say a prayer, phrase, or word to themselves over and over. As with other compulsions, the object of these mental acts is to protect against something bad happening or to drive away an obsessive thought.

Parents may recognize some of these symptoms in their own behaviors or in those of people they know and wonder whether OCD is running rampant. Most of us have a few obsessive-compulsive traits. We may have a lucky object that we wear or carry when we feel we need it. Many people prefer things to be arranged in their homes in a very particular way. Others worry that they have left the oven on and find that they go back several times to check. Obsessive-compulsive symptoms exist along a spectrum, from a few harmless symptoms to a debilitating condition. What separates the large numbers of people who have some of these traits from the smaller numbers who meet the criteria for a diagnosis of OCD is the degree of impairment and suffering that these symptoms cause.

In those teens with OCD, symptoms can result in a great deal of distress for themselves and their families. Obsessive thoughts are disturbing and anxiety provoking, and teens may have a difficult time focusing on anything else. Compulsive rituals may consume large amounts of time. Teens may be late for school and activities, and their school performance frequently suffers. OCD often affects an adolescent's social life, as embarrassment about compulsions or fear of contamination at a friend's house lead to increasing isolation. Sometimes the symptoms of OCD can be so severe and impairing that the victim is unable to leave the house or adequately care for him- or herself. Excessive cleaning or hand-washing can cause severe skin breakdown, which, ironically, increases the risk of infection. When obsessions or compulsions affect a teen's healthy functioning, it is time to obtain a psychiatric evaluation.

Making the Diagnosis

Determining whether an adolescent is suffering from OCD requires a thorough psychiatric evaluation by a child and adolescent psychiatrist or another mental health clinician, such as a clinical psychologist. The diagnosis of OCD is made clinically, meaning it is based on symptoms rather than on results of a test or other diagnostic procedure. Nonetheless, neuropsychological testing sometimes plays a role in the evaluation, particularly in cases that are unusual or complicated. By using standardized symptom checklists as well as projective measures, which may help identify patterns and tendencies in an individual's thinking, neuropsychological testing can help confirm the diagnosis or identify other psychiatric difficulties that may be exacerbating the situation.

The psychiatric evaluation for possible OCD should involve screening for other comorbid psychiatric conditions. In addition, as part of the evaluation, a detailed medical history should be obtained. Occasionally if a teen's medical history suggests a possible medical problem that may be contributing to the symptoms, some additional laboratory testing may be required. For example, if your doctor suspects PANDAS, tests related to streptococcal infection, such as a throat swab or levels of antibodies against the streptococcal bacterium, may be indicated.

Other Problems to Consider

Differential Diagnosis: What Else Might Be Wrong?

Several psychiatric disorders have symptoms that can resemble OCD, and they should be considered by the psychiatrist as possible diagnoses in the evaluation of suspected OCD. Other anxiety disorders, such as generalized anxiety disorder and phobias, can appear similar to OCD. Thus, teens with generalized anxiety disorder may be fearful in a number of different situations. They may worry that someone will break into the house or that something bad will happen to their family, which may also occur in OCD, are common. These fears may lead to checking behavior and frequent need for reassurance from parents that everything is okay. Similarly, teens with phobias may have intense fear of a specific object, such as spiders, and may go to great lengths to avoid them. While these symptoms may resemble OCD, a psychiatrist can distinguish the disorders by asking detailed questions about the nature of the worries. In OCD, obsessions have a different character than the worries of other anxiety disorders. They are more intrusive and often more irrational in nature. A teen with generalized anxiety may fear that his parents will be involved in a car accident, whereas a teen with OCD may feel that he has to repeat a sequence of numbers in his head a specified number of times to prevent anything bad from happening. The presence of compulsions also helps distinguish OCD from other anxiety disorders.

In some cases, OCD can be difficult to distinguish from psychotic disorders, such as schizophrenia. As in OCD, psychotic teens may experience intrusive thoughts or images. They may have odd, irrational fears and may engage in unusual behavior. However, in psychotic disorders, teens generally have little insight that the thoughts they are experiencing are exaggerated or irrational, whereas adolescents with OCD are able to recognize their thoughts as strange, even though they still act on them. In addition, psychotic disorders often involve auditory hallucinations and disorganized patterns of thinking and speaking, whereas these symptoms are not typically seen in OCD.

Tic disorders, such as Tourette's, share many features with OCD and often occur together with OCD. In a tic disorder, the patient typically feels an overwhelming urge to make a particular movement or noise or utter a particular word or phrase. This may be similar to compulsive behavior. But in contrast to OCD, teens with a tic disorder do not feel they need to perform the behavior to stop something bad from happening. Rather, performing the behavior simply relieves, temporarily, the urge to complete the behavior. For example, an adolescent afflicted with a tic disorder may crack his knuckles to relieve the feeling that he needs to do so. However, he is not doing it to prevent something bad from happening.

OCD needs to be distinguished from personality characteristics that can resemble the disorder. Just as with adults, some teens tend to be more rigid, particular, and perfectionist. They may be overly focused on being in control and may like things to be done in a certain way at the expense of flexibility. They may be preoccupied with rules, to-do lists, or staying organized. In an adult, when these personality traits are so extreme that they begin to interfere with one's life, the condition is recognized as a personality disorder called obsessive-compulsive personality disorder (see chapter 13). Although this disorder is generally not diagnosed until adulthood, when one's personality is more fully formed, these traits may be evident in adolescence. People who have this disorder may have such extreme perfectionism that they have trouble finishing a task, and, as a result, their school or job performance may suffer. They tend to be miserly with money and very focused on work over other values. People with these strong personality traits often have difficulties in their social and romantic relationships. Despite some superficial similarities, personality traits such as these can be distinguished easily from OCD by the absence of true obsessions and compulsions.

Several medical conditions can cause symptoms similar to OCD or even lead to OCD. The most common medical condition related to OCD is PANDAS. Brain injury from head trauma or carbon-monoxide poisoning can also lead to OCD symptoms. OCD is also very common in adolescents with Prader-Willi syndrome, a genetic disorder that involves developmental delay, characteristic facial features, and a tendency to hoard food and eat excessively.

Comorbidities

There are several other psychiatric problems that commonly occur in adolescents with OCD. Identification of any coexisting disorders is essential because failure to recognize and address an additional problem may make the effective treatment of a teen's OCD more difficult.

Mood disorders, such as depression and bipolar disorder, are among the most common comorbid psychiatric conditions in adolescents with OCD. It has been shown that more than 60 percent of adolescents with OCD also suffer from major depression (Geller 2006). This is probably an indication of the severe stress and social isolation that OCD can cause, although there also may be common genetic or biological factors at work. Mood disorders may interfere with adolescents' willingness to seek help for OCD symptoms and their ability to adhere to treatments.

OCD is categorized as an anxiety disorder, and anxiety disorders are known for their tendency to occur in clusters. Thus, it is not surprising that other anxiety disorders, such as generalized anxiety, phobias, and social anxiety, are very common in adolescents with OCD. These problems have the potential to amplify the negative impact that OCD has on a teen's life.

Tic disorders are believed to be closely related to OCD. The symptoms of tic disorders can resemble those of OCD. It is thought that similar abnormalities in brain functioning, with a particular focus on the basal ganglia, underlie both OCD and tic disorders. As mentioned earlier, some researchers even believe that OCD and tic disorders represent two ends of the spectrum of a common underlying disease process. Tic disorders, which include Tourette's disorder and related conditions, are very common in adolescents with OCD. Adolescents with OCD are at greater risk of having attention-deficit/hyperactivity disorder (ADHD) and learning disorders. These conditions often manifest themselves before the onset of OCD. When they occur together, they can compound school difficulties. Other conditions that have been associated with OCD in adolescents include pervasive developmental disorders, oppositional defiant disorder, and trichotillomania (a disorder of excessive, compulsive hair pulling or skin picking). Rates of OCD may also be increased in adolescents with eating disorders such as anorexia nervosa.

Treatment

The treatment plan for adolescents with OCD depends to some extent on their symptoms and their individual needs. For mild cases that are not causing too much disruption in a teen's life, a watch-and-wait approach is reasonable. On the other hand, when OCD symptoms are having a negative impact on development or healthy functioning, then further intervention is indicated. Treatment usually involves psychotherapy, medications, or a combination of the two. While therapy alone may be tried for mild cases of OCD, the combination of therapy and medications is more powerful than either treatment alone. Education and guidance for the family are often an important part of the treatment. Finally, recognition and treatment of any comorbid psychiatric disorders, such as depression, ADHD, or tics, helps to improve a teen's response to treatment.

Psychotherapy

Cognitive behavioral therapy (CBT) is the psychotherapy that appears to be most effective in the treatment of OCD. In brief, the therapist helps the teen to identify and challenge inaccurate beliefs and change patterns of behavior. CBT is useful in reducing symptoms of OCD and helping adolescents learn to manage their illness. It also lowers the risk of relapse.

How does CBT work? In OCD, an unhealthy cycle develops when teens begin to avoid certain places or things that they associate with obsessions. So consider a teenage boy who has intrusive, disturbing thoughts about germs and catching an illness from places, such as the kitchen, which are "loaded with germs." Accordingly, he may avoid going into the kitchen, since entering the kitchen may trigger obsessive thoughts about germs. Avoiding the kitchen brings temporary relief from these thoughts. As time passes, the obsessive thoughts spread to other areas. Other rooms in the house may start to seem contaminated as well. These areas are then avoided too. This process may continue until the teen is avoiding much of the house, the school, and just about everywhere else, leaving him feeling very anxious in most places and trapped within an increasingly narrow pattern of avoidance.

Compulsions frequently play into this cycle as well. A compulsive behavior may bring about temporary relief from an obsession. For example, if the teen enters a room in the house that is seen as contaminated, he may then engage in excessive hand-washing and other compulsive rituals, such as counting or tapping, in order to decontaminate himself and feel less anxious. Just as with avoidance behavior, the relief from obsessive thoughts that compulsions bring tends to be short-lived. Before long, the obsessions return, often stronger than they were before. The teen may try to counter them by engaging in compulsive behaviors more intensely or for longer periods of time, such as washing his hands repeatedly and aggressively. Once again, this behavior brings relief that is only temporary, and the cycle continues.

One of the goals of CBT is to help teens recognize these cycles and break them. This may be accomplished through a technique called exposure and response prevention (ERP). The principle of ERP involves overcoming avoidance: expose the teen to a trigger of his obsessions, and then help him refrain from engaging in compulsive behaviors in response to the thoughts. Relaxation techniques, such as breathing exercises, may be used to help the teen manage the anxiety that is associated with obsessions. With gradually increasing exposure to triggers that are increasingly anxiety provoking, the obsessive thoughts associated with these triggers begin to diminish, the teen's anxiety wanes, and the teen learns more effective strategies for managing obsessions than avoidance and compulsive behaviors.

As an example of what ERP might look like in practice, consider the same teenage boy, who has obsessive thoughts about germs, avoids doorknobs and certain rooms in his house that he sees as contaminated, and engages in excessive hand-washing and other compulsive behaviors in response to his obsessive thoughts. Early on, the therapist gathers information from the teen about his obsessions and compulsions. In so doing, the therapist may recognize the cycles described and help the teen understand how his current pattern of behavior provides only fleeting relief while making his overall problem worse. The therapist may ask the teen to list things that trigger his fear of germs, and the list may include items such as doorknobs, water fountains, and the kitchen. The teen is asked to rank these items according to how much anxiety is provoked.

After explaining the process and outlining the plan for the teen, the therapist exposes him to his triggers, starting with the ones that are the least anxiety provoking and gradually working up toward the more feared triggers. The teen may be asked to hold onto a doorknob in the therapist's office. Rather than giving in to the urge to wash his hands after doing this, the teen instead is encouraged to use relaxation techniques that the therapist has taught him and to observe what happens to his anxiety level with time. Soon, the teen recognizes that if he resists the urge to perform a compulsion, his anxiety level comes down on its own, even while he is holding the doorknob. The teen then builds up to more challenging tasks. He may hold the doorknob for increasing amounts of time or work up to doorknobs that seem more germ ridden, such as the one on the restroom door. He may be given homework, such as spending increasing amounts of time in the kitchen without washing his hands afterward. These homework assignments often require involvement by the parents, who can offer help and encouragement.

Through CBT with ERP, many teens with OCD are able to gain control of their symptoms. Obsessions and urges to perform compulsions may continue, but therapy can reduce the intensity of these experiences and minimize the impact that they have on the adolescent's life. As teens' OCD symptoms decrease with repeated exposure to triggers, the focus of therapy shifts to helping them learn to maintain progress on their own and to recognize and manage potential relapses, which may occur, particularly in times of stress. CBT may consist of eight to twelve weekly sessions with homework assignments for the teen in between, but some adolescents may require more prolonged treatment. Teenagers often return periodically for "refresher" sessions to brush up on their skills for managing their illness.

Other forms of psychotherapy, including psychodynamic psychotherapy, have been tried in the treatment of OCD. The evidence from scientific studies is strongly in favor of CBT in reducing OCD symptoms. Once their OCD symptoms have been brought under control, adolescents who have other comorbid psychiatric issues such as depression may benefit from ongoing psychotherapy with an approach other than CBT. In addition, the other approaches may be useful in mitigating the harmful secondary effects of OCD on an adolescent's self-esteem and interpersonal relationships. As a result, the treatment for an adolescent with OCD is not a one-size-fits-all approach. Rather, it should involve a plan that takes into account the specific needs of the individual.

Family Treatment

Since OCD usually has an impact on the whole family, in addition to individual treatment, family involvement is often a very important component of psychotherapy for adolescents with OCD. Other family members may be involved in rituals or other compulsive behaviors: a teen may ask her parents to wash her clothes repeatedly or insist parents return to the house on the way to school to check that the doors are locked. Refusal to participate in the teen's rituals may provoke intense, prolonged, anxiety-fueled blow-ups. Most parents find themselves going along with the adolescent's demands, as their own will to resist is no match for the determination of a teen with OCD. That said, demands tend to increase with time, and it is difficult for parents to know where to draw the line.

Family involvement may include education for parents and siblings about the illness and help in dealing with the strain the disorder places on a family. Parents can obtain guidance on managing the symptoms at home and can learn to reinforce the work that the teen is doing in therapy.

Medications

Along with CBT, medications are the most effective treatment for OCD. Medications can significantly reduce the frequency and intensity of obsessions and decrease urges to engage in compulsions, making it easier for teens to use the techniques learned in therapy to manage their symptoms. In some adolescents, medication may entirely eliminate OCD symptoms.

The medications most effective in OCD treatment are the selective serotonin reuptake inhibitors (SSRIs), and because of their relative safety and demonstrated efficacy, these are the first-line treatment. SSRIs include the medications fluoxetine (Prozac), sertraline (Zoloft), citalopram (Celexa), escitalopram (Lexapro), and paroxetine (Paxil). One of the SSRIs, fluvoxamine (Luvox), is used almost exclusively to treat OCD.

There is no evidence that one SSRI is more effective than the others. The choice of a particular medication may be based on slight differences between them or in their side effects and duration of action. Fluvoxamine, sertraline, and fluoxetine tend to be used most often in adolescents because there are more data to support their use in this population. The doses of SSRIs that are effective in treating OCD tend to be higher than those used to treat depression or other anxiety disorders. SSRIs tend to take at least a few weeks and up to ten weeks before they begin to reduce OCD symptoms. After a medication is started, continued improvement in symptoms may occur over two or three months. For this reason, it is important to be patient and to give a medication sufficient time to allow for results.

SSRIs are safe and well tolerated by most patients. Common side effects include headache, dizziness, upset stomach, changes in appetite, dry mouth, and constipation. Some adolescents feel slightly drowsy while taking SSRIs, and others may feel restlessness or have difficulty sleeping. Although SSRIs reduce anxiety in most people, they may make some people feel more anxious.

In rare cases, SSRIs can cause dramatic changes in mood or behavior, such as inducing a manic episode. There is also some evidence that SSRIs may increase the risk of suicidal thoughts in some teenagers, although there is some controversy around this issue. Close monitoring by the prescribing doctor is essential for the safe use of these medications in teenagers.

When SSRIs are not effective, an older medication called clomipramine is sometimes used. Clomipramine is a member of the class of medications called tricyclic antidepressants. It inhibits the uptake of serotonin in the space between cells, increasing serotonin transmission in the brain. It is important to note that clomipramine has the potential to cause more serious side effects than SSRIs. Among its more concerning side effects, clomipramine sometimes can cause a heart rhythm disturbance. These changes can usually be detected on an electrocardiogram (ECG or EKG). Monitoring with ECGs before and during treatment is recommended for adolescents taking clomipramine. Although cardiac problems associated with clomipramine are relatively uncommon, there are a number of more frequent side effects, including upset stomach, dry mouth, constipation, drowsiness, dizziness, blurry vision, and tremors. Clomipramine is also more dangerous in overdose than SSRIs. An overdose on clomipramine can cause seizures or death.

In cases of OCD that do not respond to the usual treatments, other medications may be added. Benzodiazepines, a group of antianxiety medications that includes the drugs lorazepam (Ativan), clonazepam (Klonopin), and diazepam (Valium) are sometimes used in this way. These medications can be quite effective in lowering anxiety and thus may have some benefit in OCD when added to an SSRI or clomipramine. They may also be used when an adolescent has another comorbid anxiety disorder, such as generalized anxiety disorder. Still, the use of benzodiazepines in the treatment of adolescents with OCD has not been studied extensively. Furthermore, these medications can have side effects that limit their use in teenagers, including drowsiness and impaired attention. They also can be habit forming and have the potential to be abused by teens who take them in order to get high. For these reasons, benzodiazepines are not generally a first-line treatment for OCD.

In some studies in adults, the antipsychotic medications haloperidol (Haldol) and risperidone (Risperdal) have shown some benefit in treatment-resistant OCD. They are added to more standard medication treatments, such as SSRIs or clomipramine. But these medications have significant side effects and have not been studied well in adolescents with OCD.

In the relatively rare cases of OCD that appear to be related to PANDAS, treatment with antibiotics may be warranted. In some cases of recurrent streptococcal infections and OCD exacerbations, prophylactic antibiotic treatment over a longer period of time can prevent infections from occurring.

When medications have brought OCD symptoms under control, most parents wonder how long the medications should be continued. Although it is clearly not desirable to have an adolescent on medication for longer than is necessary, OCD symptoms frequently recur when medications are tapered. The sooner they are stopped, the greater the risk of relapse. As a result, most psychiatrists recommend continuing medications for at least a year after symptoms have been brought under control. When the decision is made to stop the medication, it is best done by gradually lowering the dose under the close supervision of a psychiatrist, who can monitor for signs of relapse. It is advisable to initiate tapering the medication at a relatively low-stress time in the adolescent's life, such as over summer vacation. When medications are stopped, treatment with CBT can help reduce the risk of relapse.

Other Interventions

For adolescents whose OCD symptoms are affecting their academic functioning, school-based interventions may be appropriate. In public schools, interventions may be formalized through a 504 plan or an individualized education plan (IEP). It may be useful for the therapist and parents to provide education for teachers about the disorder and practical advice about how to help a teen break out of a compulsion when he or she is "stuck." Close, regular communication between the school and a teen's parents can help identify potential problems or relapses. Some adolescents with OCD may also need the school to allow more time for some assignments. As transitions can be difficult for adolescents with OCD, schools should be more flexible about tardiness and allow more time for them to go from class to class.

In severe cases of OCD, adolescents may be unable to function. They may refuse to leave the house, neglect their hygiene, or become so stuck in a series of compulsive behaviors that they are unable to do anything else. In these circumstances, the adolescent may require more intensive treatment outside the home, at a day treatment program, a residential treatment program, or an inpatient psychiatric unit. Hospitalization may also be required for teens when other comorbid psychiatric disorders are out of control and posing a safety risk.

When more intensive treatment is required, it is best to locate a facility that has experience in treating OCD. An adolescent's therapist or psychiatrist can help parents decide which treatment program would be most effective.

Prognosis

OCD in adolescents can take a somewhat variable course. It appears that roughly 40 percent of people who are diagnosed with OCD during childhood and adolescence will have complete remission of their symptoms and are free of OCD in adulthood. An additional 20 percent will have some mild symptoms that are not sufficiently severe to warrant the OCD diagnosis. The rest will continue to have the disorder into adulthood.

Several factors have been identified that help predict the prognosis for a teen with OCD. The presence of other comorbid psychiatric problems is associated with an OCD that is more resistant to treatment and more likely to persist into adulthood. Teens whose symptoms began at an earlier age or who require psychiatric hospitalization at some point in their lives are more likely to have chronic OCD symptoms. A high degree of family conflict can also worsen prognosis.

OCD that is not adequately treated can have a significant, lifelong impact. The illness itself can be debilitating, and, even in relatively mild cases, the repercussions can be pervasive in nearly every aspect of a teen's life, including occupational achievement and interpersonal relationships. Yet, with appropriate treatment, most teens with OCD are able to deal with the illness and proceed with the important developmental tasks of adolescence.

Tic Disorders and Tourette's Disorder

Tics are sudden, repetitive, habitual movements or vocalizations. Though they are often described as involuntary, they are a bit like having an itch that you want to scratch very badly. You can hold off for a while if you really need to, but the urge grows stronger and stronger until you give in. Tics involving muscle movements are called motor tics. Common motor tics include shoulder shrugging, eye blinking, grimacing, head jerking, and facial muscle twitching. More complex motor tics, including gestures or whole body movements, may also occur. Vocal tics include simple grunting noises, throat clearing, coughing, or yelping sounds and coprolalia. Coprolalia are vocal tics that may involve obscene statements.

During childhood, tics are very common, with estimates that 10 to 20 percent of children are affected. They tend to be intermittent and worsen during times of stress. They do not usually cause much distress and usually resolve on their own without treatment over a period of weeks to months. Transient tics of this nature may also occur during the adolescent years.

On the other hand, tics may persist and evolve with other symptoms that disrupt a teen's life. When tics persist for over a year, a chronic tic disorder may be present. While estimates vary, these disorders occur in roughly 1 percent of all children and adolescents, affecting boys much more often than girls. Tics that cause a teen distress or last for an extended time warrant further evaluation.

Symptoms and Warning Signs

Diagnoses involving tics are categorized according to the type of tic—namely, motor or vocal—as well as by their duration. Chronic motor tic disorder is defined by the exclusive presence of motor tics on a frequent basis over at least a year. Similarly, when vocal tics occur often over a period of a year or more without the presence of motor tics, the diagnosis of chronic vocal tic disorder may be established. Tourette's disorder (which is also referred to as Tourette syndrome) is characterized by the presence of both vocal and multiple motor tics over a period of a year or more, although these symptoms may occur consecutively rather than at the same time. The diagnosis of transient tic disorder is used to describe tics that occur frequently for a period of over four weeks but less than a year.

Tics may wax and wane; they typically evolve over time, with old tics disappearing and new ones arising. They may decrease during focused activities involving fine movements, including sports or playing a musical instrument. Tics may be triggered by fatigue, excitement, boredom, anxiety, or particular sensations (for example, wearing a shirt with a tight collar or hearing someone else clear his throat). Some medications have the potential to exacerbate tics. In particular, stimulant medications that are used to treat ADHD may cause significant worsening of tics, sometimes turning a barely noticeable tic into a serious problem. When this occurs, the problem is usually reversed shortly after the medication is stopped.

Tic disorders range in severity from a mild annoyance to a severe disturbance in a teen's life. For self-conscious adolescents, they can be a source of embarrassment. Over time, this may lead to social isolation and poor self-esteem, which in turn places a teen at risk for a host of problems, including drug abuse and depression. Tics can be very distracting and may interfere with school performance. This can be compounded by the presence of a learning or attention problem. Because some tics involve obscene gestures or statements, unless teachers and staff are well informed about the problem, a teen may end up in trouble at school.

In addition to the secondary impact of tics on social and academic functioning, they can also cause direct harm to a teen. Repetitive muscle movements may cause neck or back pain and in severe cases may lead to orthopedic injury or nerve problems. Tics sometimes involve self-injurious behavior as well, such as hitting oneself or biting the lips or the inside of the cheek. Moreover, cases of more complex tics involving behaviors such as cutting or aggression toward others have been described.

Making the Diagnosis

Child and adolescent psychiatrists, as well as pediatric neurologists, have the background to evaluate tic disorders. The primary component of the evaluation is a thorough clinical assessment, including close observation of the patient. Because other psychiatric disorders are common in teens with tic disorders, a complete evaluation and screening for these other issues is a critical part of the assessment. It is important to notify the doctor of any current or past medications your child has taken and any possible association between medications and worsening symptoms.

Because tic disorders tend to run in families, a family history of medical, neurological, and psychiatric illness should be part of the evaluation. A medical history is essential also to rule out possible medical causes of tics or other psychiatric or neurological problems that may be similar in appearance to tics. Depending on this history, further medical or neurological work-up may be necessary. Normally, the diagnosis of a tic disorder is made based solely on a doctor's evaluation, without need for further testing.

Other Problems to Consider

Differential Diagnosis: What Else Might Be Wrong?

Although tics can usually be easily differentiated from other problems, particularly if they are observed by the clinician, there are several other conditions that may be confused with tics. A number of different neurological conditions produce abnormal involuntary movements. Movement disorders can be due to brain abnormalities caused by trauma, genetic conditions, or abnormalities in metabolism. The movements associated with neurological problems may include tremors, jerks (called myoclonus), writhing motions (called chorea or athetosis), or sudden flailing or throwing movements (called ballismus). Neurological disorders that may be responsible for these movements include Huntington's disease, Wilson's disease, seizures disorders, and specific forms of head injury. If a teen's symptoms are not typical or if there are elements of the teen's medical or family history that suggest a possible neurological problem, further evaluation by a pediatric neurologist may be indicated.

In some cases of OCD, compulsive behaviors can be difficult to distinguish from tics. Both tics and compulsions are repetitive, problematic behaviors performed in response to strong urges. To complicate matters further, OCD and tics frequently occur together. Nonetheless, it is important to make this distinction, as it has implications for treatment. Whereas simple tics that involve quick muscle movements such as shoulder shrugging or eye blinking are easily recognized, with more complex tics the distinction between tics and compulsions is more difficult to delineate. In these challenging cases, the best way to make the distinction is through working closely with a clinician who is experienced in treating these disorders.

Teens with developmental disorders, such as the autism spectrum, may demonstrate particular patterns of movement, such as flapping of the hands, that psychiatrists refer to as "stereotypies." The repetitive nature of these movements makes them difficult to distinguish from tics, which also occur more frequently in people with autistic-spectrum disorders.

Several medications, in addition to stimulant medications to treat ADHD, are known to worsen tics or even cause tics in some susceptible patients. These include antihistamines, certain antidepressants, seizure medications, and some prescription pain killers. Furthermore, some drugs of abuse, including cocaine and amphetamines, have the potential to trigger tics.

Comorbidities

As in OCD, adolescents affected with a tic disorder are at increased risk to be diagnosed with other psychiatric disorders, including ADHD and learning disorders. Many teens with tic disorders have some obsessive-compulsive symptoms without meeting full diagnostic criteria for the disorder.

Depression and anxiety frequently occur in teens with tic disorders. This is partly due to the stress that tics create. When anxiety occurs together with tics, an unhealthy cycle can develop in which the anxiety exacerbates tics, which in turn leads to increased anxiety. Migraine headaches and conduct disorder have also been shown to be more common in teens with tic disorders.

Treatment

Because tics often resolve without treatment, a watch-and-wait approach to managing them is often best. However, when a tic disorder is persistent and causes significant distress for an adolescent, treatment may be warranted, including medication, psychotherapy, or some combination of both. Because existing treatments have limited efficacy for many people, treatment of tic disorders can be challenging. Most often, the goal of treatment is not to stop all tics but rather to reduce the frequency and intensity of tics to a more manageable level. As with OCD, comorbid psychiatric disorders are very common in tic disorders and have the potential to worsen tic symptoms and interfere with treatment. Thus, identification and management of other problems is an important component of successful treatment of tics.

Psychotherapy

The most common form of psychotherapy used to address tic disorders is behavioral therapy, a therapeutic approach that involves identifying behaviors that contribute to a psychiatric problem and learning to modify these problem behaviors or replace them with healthy behaviors. For treatment of tics, a specific form of behavioral therapy called habit reversal training (HRT) has been shown to be effective. The first step of HRT involves awareness training to help teens learn to identify triggers for their tics and to notice cues that tell them when the urge to perform a tic is first starting to develop. In order for teens to become more aware of the movements, HRT may involve performing tics in front of the mirror or on a video. Some teens keep a journal monitoring frequency of tics throughout the day.

After becoming more aware of the tics, the teen is taught to perform another voluntary action in response to the urge to perform a tic. The voluntary action that is chosen is one that is less problematic and more socially acceptable than the tic but that uses the same muscles, making it impossible to perform the tic. For example, a teen with an eye-blinking tic might be instructed to gently close his eyes for a few seconds and then reopen them in response to the sense that a tic is coming on. A teen with a tic involving hand gestures may practice doing something else with her hands that prevents the tic motion. Once these competing responses are learned, they are practiced to make them come more easily in a time of need. The teen may practice them while imagining being in a situation where tics frequently occur, such as in the classroom.

Because tics are often exacerbated by stress, relaxation exercises and other stress reduction techniques are another important aspect of behavioral therapy. As tics improve, therapy may shift to identifying and correcting patterns of avoidance, such as teens' having dropped out of activities they once enjoyed because of self-consciousness.

Maintaining self-esteem and navigating social relationships are critical to healthy adolescent development, and these tasks may be disrupted by a tic disorder. So, in addition to treating tics themselves, psychotherapy may be useful for teens in addressing the secondary effects of the disorder on their life. In this regard, several different approaches to psychotherapy may be effective, including cognitive behavioral therapy (CBT), psychodynamic psychotherapy, and interpersonal psychotherapy (IPT).

Medications

Careful use of medications by an experienced physician, usually by a child and adolescent psychiatrist or a pediatric neurologist, may be part of the treatment for tics. The medications that are often used as first line in the treatment of tics are clonidine (Catapres) and guanfacine (Tenex). Both these medications, which are categorized as "alpha-1 agonists," work through a similar mechanism that leads indirectly to decreased release of a brain chemical called norepinephrine. Norepinephrine plays many different roles in the nervous system, including mediating the fight-or-flight response under anxiety-provoking conditions. Exactly how or why these medications work for tic disorders is not well understood. Both these medications also have the advantage of treating some of the symptoms of ADHD, which is very common with tic disorders. Still, they are not typically viewed as first-line treatments for ADHD.

Clonidine and guanfacine have similar side effect profiles. Sedation is common with both medications, though it is more pronounced with clonidine. Other frequent side effects include constipation, dry mouth, low blood pressure, and lightheadedness. Blood pressure and pulse should be monitored for teens taking either of these medications. Adolescents with underlying heart problems may be at increased risk of an arrhythmia on clonidine or guanfacine. If an adolescent's medical or family history indicates the possibility of such a problem, an electrocardiogram (ECG or EKG) may be obtained before and sometimes during treatment to help ensure that the medication can be safely used.

When clonidine and guanfacine are not effective, antipsychotic medications may be considered. These medications work by blocking a certain type of receptor for a brain chemical (neurotransmitter) called dopamine. The newer antipsychotic medications, called atypical antipsychotics, tend to be used over the older typical antipsychotics. This is because the side effects of atypical antipsychotics tend to be less severe than those of the typical antipsychotics. Of the atypical antipsychotics, risperidone (Risperdal) is a popular choice, as it has proven efficacy and has greater potency in blocking dopamine receptors than do others in this class.

Though atypical antipsychotics may be safer than the older medications, they do have numerous side effects. These include weight gain, increased risk of diabetes and other metabolic changes, sedation, and changes in the heart rhythm.

Older antipsychotics are also effective in treating tic disorders and may be used when other treatments have not achieved desired results. Medications in this group that may be used to treat tics include haloperidol (Haldol) and pimozide (Orap). These medications have potentially severe side effects and thus should be used only under close supervision by a physician experienced in their use.

Other Treatments

In addition to managing the tics themselves, it is important to address the secondary effects that this disorder can have on a teen's academic and social functioning. An adolescent with a tic disorder needs to receive appropriate support at school. The type of support will vary according to the needs of the individual teen.

Prognosis

For many adolescents with tic disorders, symptoms resolve or improve significantly in early adulthood. The prognosis depends in part on the specific diagnosis, with chronic motor or vocal tic disorders having a more favorable prognosis than Tourette's disorder. Roughly two-thirds of children and adolescents with chronic motor or vocal tic disorders have significant symptomatic improvement by adulthood, compared to approximately half of children and adolescents with Tourette's disorder. The presence of other psychiatric conditions is another important factor in determining prognosis. Teens with comorbid disorders such as ADHD or OCD have a less favorable prognosis, with higher likelihood of chronic symptoms and a greater degree of impairment from their symptoms.

Those adolescents with tic disorders that continue into adulthood are at risk for a number of adverse effects, including impaired academic and occupational functioning. Adults with Tourette's disorder have been shown to have a higher rate of unemployment than that for the general population. Social difficulties are common as well, as the embarrassment associated with tics can cause some adolescents to become more isolated and to avoid intimate relationships. Even teens with tic disorders that resolve prior to adulthood can suffer negative consequences that outlast the tics themselves. Providing treatment and support for teens suffering from a tic disorder can help minimize this risk.

Conclusion

OCD and tic disorders are often viewed as two ends of a common underlying illness. The two problems commonly occur together and are believed to have similar underlying mechanisms. Furthermore, both OCD and tics involve an assault on one's sense of self, with intrusive thoughts or overwhelming urges that may be paradoxically recognized as products of one's own mind while nonetheless seeming strangely foreign. These disorders can be extremely disturbing and can cause significant impairment for adolescents, whose sense of self is still developing. Proper treatment is essential to minimize the negative impact these disorders can have on a teen's development. An important aspect of treatment is the recognition and management of other co-occurring psychiatric conditions, as both OCD and tic disorders have high rates of comorbidity, including risk of ADHD and learning disorders. The presence of comorbid disorders can interfere with treatment of the primary problem.

References and Additional Reading

Geller, D. A. 2006. "Obsessive-Compulsive and Spectrum Disorders in Children and Adolescents." *Psychiatric Clinics of North America* 29: 353–370.

Marsh, T. L. 2007. *Children with Tourette Syndrome: A Parents' Guide.* Bethesda, MD. Woodbine House.

Stewart, S. E., D. A. Geller, M. Jenike, D. Pauls, D. Shaw, B. Mullin, and S. V. Faraone. 2004. "Long-Term Outcome of Pediatric Obsessive-Compulsive Disorder: A Meta-Analysis and Qualitative Review of the Literature." *Acta Psychiatrica Scandinavica* 110: 4–13.

Swain, J. E., L. Scahill, P. J. Lombroso, R. A. King, and J. F. Leckman. 2007. "Tourette Syndrome and Tic Disorders: A Decade of Progress." *Journal of the American Academy of Child and Adolescent Psychiatry* 46: 947–968.

17   Reactions to Stress, Loss, and Illness

Under the best of circumstances, adolescence is a stressful time. The rapid developmental changes coupled with the shifts that occur in an adolescent's family and social relationships may be challenging to manage. Some teens face the additional burden of managing a major stressor in their lives. Academic difficulties and traumatic events such as sexual abuse are discussed in other chapters. In this chapter, we review some of the more common forms of significant stress in the life of an adolescent: loss of a loved one, parental divorce or separation, and chronic medical illness. It is important to understand a general approach to gauging a teen's reaction to stress and determining when to seek help from a mental health professional.

Factors Related to Adolescents' Responses to Stress

The response of adolescents to stresses in their life can vary widely and is related to several factors. The nature, severity, and duration of the stressor are obviously important factors. A teen's age and developmental level are important determinants. Younger teens may have a harder time verbalizing their emotions; they are more likely to develop physical symptoms, such as headaches or stomachaches. Younger teens have less ability to think in abstract terms, which may become apparent in stressful situations, as a younger adolescent may express an overly simplistic explanation for a problem. For example, in a divorce a younger teen may be more likely to assign all the blame to one parent, whereas a more mature adolescent may be capable of a nuanced understanding of circumstances. That said, it is important to note that adolescents of all ages frequently regress psychologically in the face of stress and think and behave more like a younger teen.

The psychological characteristics of a particular teen also play a key role in determining his or her response to stress. Some teens are more laid-back and are able to roll with the punches, but others are more sensitive. Teens may be overly internalizing. They may attribute stressful events around them to their own actions and may blame themselves for problems, even for things that are not in their control. Others are excessively externalizing, seeing problems with everyone else but never taking responsibility.

Psychologists use the term *defenses* to refer to ways that an adolescent handles psychological distress or inner conflict. Some teens have healthier, more effective

Case Presentation

Mary was thirteen years old when her grandfather, with whom she was very close, died suddenly of a heart attack. Mary was devastated when she heard the news, and in the weeks that followed, her parents became worried about her. She appeared sad, crying often and talking about missing her grandfather. Before her grandfather's death, Mary seemed to spend all her free time hanging out at the mall with her friends and had little interest in being with her parents; but after his death, she spent much more time at home and became "clingy" with her mother. She began playing and sleeping with her childhood dolls. She often had difficulty sleeping, and she had vivid, realistic dreams in which her grandfather was still alive. On a few occasions, Mary told her mother that she felt as if her grandfather was in the room with her.

In addition, Mary seemed more absent-minded and forgetful. She had always been an A and B student, but she now began bringing home tests and quizzes with Cs and Ds. One afternoon, Mary came home early from school with a stomachache; she then started to cry inconsolably and could hardly speak. Mary's mother learned that Mary had forgotten about a major term paper that her English teacher had assigned the previous month. It was due in two days. Mary was overwhelmed, thinking that there was no way she would be able to do it and that she would probably fail the class.

Mary's parents, who had already been quite concerned about her, called their pediatrician to discuss what was happening. The pediatrician reassured Mary's parents that Mary's recent behaviors were not unusual for someone her age who is grieving the loss of a loved one. He encouraged her parents to continue to provide support for her but asked them to check in with him again in a couple weeks and to call sooner if things seemed to be worsening.

The following day, Mary's mother contacted the school and spoke with Mary's guidance counselor and English teacher and explained the situation. Mary's English teacher agreed to give Mary an extension on the paper. Mary's father helped her design a schedule for completing the paper. That night, over dinner at Mary's favorite restaurant, Mary and her parents shared fond memories of her grandfather. Mary and her mother decided to put together a scrapbook with photos and mementos of her grandfather. Over the following weekend, Mary's friends called to ask her to go to the mall. Mary said she did not want to go and had too much work to do, but Mary's parents gently encouraged her to go. She went and had a good time, laughing with her friends.

For many weeks, Mary continued to feel sad about her grandfather. Her grades that quarter were down a bit from her usual performance. But over several months, she returned to her usual self. Her sleep improved, and she spent more time with friends, placing her dolls back in the closet. When Mary met with her pediatrician a few weeks after her mother had initially called, she said, "I still miss my grandfather, but I know he'll always be with me, and I'll always have my memories of him."

defenses than other teens. Healthy defenses include using humor and channeling one's distress into a more productive enterprise, such as sports or the arts. Less healthy responses include denial, in which a problem is ignored, or projection, in which negative feelings are unconsciously attributed to others. Resiliency, a positive attribute, involves the capability of being adaptable in the face of stress. Unfortunately, some teens have a narrow range of responses to stressful situations and use the same strategies repeatedly, regardless of whether they are well suited to the situation. Ignoring something and moving on is a useful approach in handling the occasional insults made by a classmate. However, it is not an appropriate strategy for managing stress caused by a chronic illness such as diabetes, when ignoring the problem may have significant health consequences. An adaptable and resilient teen will find ways of handling stress that are suited to the situation. Of course, the effectiveness and flexibility of one's psychological defenses depends in part on one's developmental level, as the defenses continue to mature during adolescence, but they also vary with the psychological makeup of the teen.

There has been a growing appreciation of the biological factors that play into an adolescent's responses to stress. Teens with a family history of psychiatric illness may be biologically predisposed to develop a psychiatric problem such as depression. Recently, specific genes have been identified that place some adolescents at risk for a psychiatric illness when faced with life stressors. It is possible that at some time, genetic testing will be able to identify those who are at greatest biological risk for mood and anxiety disorders.

Family and cultural factors play a large role in determining a teen's response to stress. Families have different patterns of managing and expressing emotion, and this is often culturally influenced. A family that is overly reserved in their emotional expressions may make it difficult for a teen to show that he or she is suffering. Conversely, families that are highly emotionally expressive may present challenges for teens, particularly when negative emotions are displayed. Studies of young people with schizophrenia have shown that those living in families with a high degree of expressed negative emotions tend to have a less favorable prognosis.

Finally, one of the most important factors in determining a teen's response to stress is the presence of a good support system. Parents obviously play a key role in an adolescent's support network. Still, parents should not be surprised if their teen turns to others in time of need. As part of the normal developmental process of becoming independent and psychologically separating from one's parents, teens may increasingly rely on peer support. They may also seek out other trusted "parent substitutes" for advice and comfort, including teachers, coaches, or the parents of their friends. Teens should have someone (or preferably a group of people) they trust and to whom they can turn. Teens who lack an adequate support group are at greater risk of developing psychiatric problems or negative behaviors, such as substance abuse.

Common Responses to Stress

When faced with a threatening situation, humans are biologically and evolutionarily programmed to have an automatic response termed "fight or flight." One either stays and confronts the situation or quickly flees. The heart beats faster and stronger, breathing becomes more rapid, blood is shifted away from digestive organs and into muscles, and the pupils of the eyes dilate. This response is coordinated by the release of hormones, including cortisol and adrenalin. In modern life, this response may be problematic. When a stressor is not a hungry predator but rather a difficult problem at home or school that does not go away, the body's stress response persists. Being on biological overdrive for a long period of time may lead to exhaustion as well as the physical manifestations of chronic stress, including muscle tension, stomach upset, and disturbances of sleep and appetite. Excessive release of stress hormones, such as cortisol, can have negative effects including suppression of the immune system and possible increased risk for depression.

Parents may notice several behavioral changes in a teenager who is under stress. Related to the physiological responses, temporary changes in sleep and appetite patterns are common, with some teens experiencing a decrease in appetite and others overeating. Restlessness is common. Teens may have nervous energy, shifting in a chair at dinner or biting fingernails. Others become fatigued more easily and retreat to their bedroom. Concentration may suffer during a time of stress, and a teen may appear more distractible, spacey, or forgetful. Moodiness and irritability are also common signs of stress.

In most cases, an adolescent's reaction to stress is transient. Either the stressful situation passes, or the adolescent learns to adapt to it and his or her behavior returns to normal. Most adolescents show remarkable resilience in their ability to handle the difficulties that life presents. One of the most important elements to help a teen weather difficult times is family and friend support. There are several ways in which parents can help support a teen to manage stress. These strategies are listed in sidebar 17.1.

Signs of Difficulty Managing Stress

Although most teens are able to manage the stresses in their lives and return to their normal behavior, in some situations a stressful situation will sow the seeds for a more serious problem. Teens who lack an adequate support network, have poor coping skills, or have an underlying predisposition toward psychiatric illness may be particularly vulnerable to stress. Teens who are faced with more than they are able to handle alone may turn to unhealthy behaviors or develop psychiatric symptoms, including mood or anxiety disorders. Signs that a teen is struggling and may need further evaluation and assistance are listed in sidebar 17.2.

On occasion, it is a matter of degree that determines the difference between a healthy response to a stressful situation and a reaction that warrants input from a mental health professional. At times, parents need to trust their own instincts in determining when an adolescent's response to a stressful event is more severe or has lasted longer than would be expected. When there are warning signs present or a parent senses that something is not right, it is time to seek an evaluation

---

Sidebar 17.1 | Approaches That Parents Can Use to Help an Adolescent Manage Stress

- ► Be clear that you are available and concerned
- ► Create opportunities for your adolescent to open up if she or he feels ready to do so
- ► Encourage your teen to avoid isolation and to make use of other supports, e.g., spending time with friends, talking to a trusted teacher or coach
- ► Support the adolescent's involvement in healthy activities, such as sports
- ► Involve the school in providing support for the teen when appropriate, e.g., making sure the school is aware of a major crisis in a teen's life or requesting extra time for an assignment during a time of crisis
- ► Endorse healthy ways to manage stress, including taking breaks for fun activities, exercise, listening to music, relaxation exercises, creative outlets
- ► Try to maintain usual routines and expectations to the greatest extent possible
- ► Encourage healthy habits (e.g., a regular sleep routine, a healthy diet, avoiding excessive caffeine intake and junk food)
- ► Offer practical help and talk through problem-solving strategies, e.g., helping the teen break down a large, overwhelming school project into smaller, more manageable steps
- ► Avoid excessive criticism
- ► Join with the adolescent in learning and practicing stress management skills, e.g., joining and going to the gym together, learning breathing exercises, taking a yoga class
- ► Be on the lookout for warning signs of a larger problem or unhealthy responses to stress

---

from a mental health professional. If a parent questions whether this is the correct step, it may be useful to talk with the teen's pediatrician.

Specific Causes of Stress

Loss

Adolescence is frequently a time when many people first experience a major loss in their lives. Younger children may not fully comprehend the concept of death, but by early adolescence most teens have developed a mature understanding of death as an irreversible event that happens to all living things. Adolescents' emotional responses to death are often similar to those of adults. However, adolescents may lack the life experience and psychological maturity to help them manage these intense emotions. As a result, the support of parents and adult role models is of great importance to teens coping with loss.

The feelings and experiences associated with loss can be complex. Sadness and longing for the loved one are common. Teens may have guilt, feel responsible for the death, or regret how they acted toward the departed. Anger at the unfairness of the loss or due to a feeling of abandonment is also common and may emerge in the form of irritability with friends and family. Anxiety is commonly seen. For teens who have never experienced a significant loss, a death may provoke an acute awareness of their own mortality and existential questioning about the meaning of their existence.

Another common response includes intrusive thoughts about the loved one. These may take the form of vivid dreams in which the loved one is still alive. Some adolescents have strange experiences, such as thinking they see the loved one on the street or in a passing car. Hallucinations that are intrusive, persistent, or frightening are not common and suggest a need for further evaluation.

In the famous book *On Death and Dying*, the psychiatrist Elisabeth Kubler-Ross described five stages of grieving experienced by those suffering a loss or anticipating their own death:

1. *Denial*: in which the individual has difficulty accepting the reality of the loss
2. *Anger*: in which the individual has feelings that the event is unfair or that it should not have happened
3. *Bargaining*: in which the individual may wish to make "deals with God," wishing for more time with the loved one, such as, "If only I could see him one more time, I would never do anything to get in trouble again"
4. *Depression*: in which the individual experiences deep sadness about the loss
5. *Acceptance*: in which the individual comes to terms with the loss

Although this work was based on adults, adolescents may experience this same process. These stages do not necessarily occur in order or unfold according to a predictable timeline. It is a common misconception that there is a clearly defined "normal" response to loss. In fact, there is a tremendous amount of variability in

---

Sidebar 17.2 | Warning Signs of an Adolescent under Stress

- ► Evidence of drug or alcohol abuse
- ► Prolonged (i.e., more than just a few days) withdrawal from family and friends
- ► Dramatic and/or persistent decline in school performance or attendance
- ► Leaving activities, such as sports, that were once enjoyed
- ► Acting-out behaviors such as running away, fighting, skipping school, breaking the law
- ► Severe sadness or anxiety leading to inability to function, e.g., not being able to get out of bed, poor hygiene
- ► Extreme irritability or explosiveness
- ► Frequent or severe physical symptoms for which no medical cause can be identified
- ► Self-harm, such as cutting
- ► Talk of suicide or other signs of suicidal thinking, e.g., giving away one's possessions, talking about "going away for awhile," statements about joining a lost loved one or making someone "sorry for what they have done"

how people of all ages respond to the death of a loved one. Cultural differences also contribute to the diverse ways that grief may be expressed.

Despite the great variability in "normal" responses to bereavement, teens who appear to be having a great deal of difficulty managing or who are exhibiting any of the warning signs described in sidebar 17.2 should be considered for psychiatric evaluation. Adolescents who have experienced a significant loss are at risk for developing depression, substance abuse, or other psychiatric difficulties. Risk of suicide is increased particularly when the loss involved suicide. These teens may benefit from a course of psychotherapy.

Frequently, when a teen is grieving, a parent is grieving the same loss. As hard as it may be to find the strength to be supportive in a difficult time, the support of parents is critical to a teenager coping with loss. For some parents, providing this support to their adolescent is in itself therapeutic. Because teens are masters of appearance, and may falsely appear to be "together," it is important not to underestimate how a teenager is affected by a tragic event. Because of denial or fear of being a burden on others, many adolescents will hide their feelings about a loss, particularly when it occurs in the family.

Encourage your teen to talk about his or her feelings. Be nonjudgmental. Teens' reactions may seem irrational, scary, or even selfish, such as worrying about how a death will affect their own life and plans, but it is important for them to be able to express these thoughts. If a teen does not want to talk, it is best not to push too hard but to make it clear that you are available to talk if and when he or she feels differently. Teachers, coaches, school counselors, and friends' parents often play an important role in providing support for grieving teens as well.

Sharing memories of a loved one, including funny stories and happy times together, can aid the grieving process. Teens may fear that the loved one will be forgotten. Gathering keepsakes and photos into a scrapbook or some other form of memorial can give comfort.

Parental Divorce or Separation

With about half the marriages in the United States ending in divorce, this event is frequently a stressor for adolescents. Although most teens whose parents divorce go on to lead healthy lives, divorce during childhood and adolescence is a risk factor for a number of emotional and behavioral problems. Teens' reaction to divorce will depend on their developmental level, psychological vulnerability, relationship with their parents, and the level of conflict in the family before, during, and after the divorce.

Because divorce is a major disruption in the adolescent's life, it may trigger a complex set of emotions. Sadness, feelings of loss, and a longing to return to the way things used to be are common reactions. Many teens feel anger, which may be directed at one or both parents. Teens may align themselves with one parent, placing an undue share of the blame on the other parent. Or adolescents may feel guilty, blaming themselves for their parents' problems. Anxiety too is common. Teens may worry about what life will be like after the divorce or what their peers will think about their family.

Behaviorally, teens may show a wide range of responses to divorce. They may become withdrawn and isolative, or they may act out, becoming more argumentative and rebellious. School performance may dip temporarily during the process. Teens become "parentified," becoming protective of younger siblings and acting mature beyond their years. Parents should be aware that this sudden maturity is a false veneer, behind which hides deep insecurity and a sense of powerlessness.

Studies have shown that a teen's immediate reaction to separation and divorce does not necessarily predict the long-term effects. Thus, teens who have significant behavioral problems at the time of the divorce do not necessarily have significant problems later in life. Conversely, many of those who do not seem particularly distressed during a divorce may have evidence of negative psychological effects several years later. It is important for parents to do their best to minimize the impact of divorce on their children, even when there are no noticeable signs of distress.

One of the first steps in helping children cope with divorce is informing them about the separation or divorce. Ideally, both parents should be present for the initial discussion. The best approach is to provide a clear, consistent message that offers a straightforward explanation for the divorce and does not place blame on any one individual. Adolescents are often most interested in the concrete implications of divorce, and this should be addressed. For example, teens will wonder whether the divorce will affect their current living arrangement, their proximity to their friends, or the time they spend with their parents. If these issues are not yet resolved, as is often the case, the teen may at least be told what the temporary arrangement will entail. Parents should reassure the children that the divorce is not their fault and that they are not losing either of them as a parent.

Perhaps the strongest finding in research on divorce outcomes is that children's exposure to hostility and conflict is a major predictor of negative outcomes. This includes prolonged legal battles. Although strong negative feelings are common in divorce situations, usually both parents have the best interests of their children at heart. Parents frequently disagree about what is best for the children, but it is clear that shielding the children from arguments and trying not to let them get caught up in the conflict are among the best measures that parents can take for their children. With this in mind, parents should work together to find some middle ground on parenting issues. When this proves difficult, involvement of a family therapist or a parent coordinator may be beneficial.

For adolescents whose parents are divorcing, maintaining a positive relationship with both parents has been shown to be a good predictor of healthy psychological adjustment in adulthood. In most cases, it is in the teen's best interest for a parent to allow the teen to have the opportunity for a good relationship with the other parent, including having access to that parent. Similarly, parents should avoid criticizing the other parent in the presence of children, as this may undermine the relationship or make a teen feel uncomfortable.

Divorce is a major stressor not only on the children but on the entire family. It is not unusual for parents who are under stress to turn to their adolescent children for support. This has the potential to force the adolescent into the role of friend and confidant and fuel further anxiety or confuse the family roles, potentially undermining the parent's authority. Parents should obtain the support they need from friends, family, and if necessary, a mental health professional.

Finally, parents should be aware of warning signs that their teen is having difficulty managing the stress related to divorce. For teens who appear to be struggling or who are exhibiting any of the warning signs described in sidebar 17.2, parents should consider an evaluation by a mental health clinician. Occasionally, a course of psychotherapy can help adolescents accept their parents' divorce, work through their feelings, and maintain a positive relationship with both parents. Family therapy can reduce conflict or address other upheavals that have resulted from the divorce.

Chronic Medical Illness

Many teens pass through adolescence with a chronic medical illness such as diabetes, cystic fibrosis, colitis, or epilepsy. The normal developmental processes that occur during the adolescent years can present unique challenges for managing such an illness for both teens and their parents. Even adolescents who have been coping well with a chronic illness throughout childhood may start to experience difficulties when they reach their teenage years.

The desire to be part of a peer group and avoid seeming "weird" or different can make an illness that much more difficult to bear, particularly in younger adolescents, for whom these feelings are most intense. A teen's urge to take risks often comes into direct conflict with the need to manage the illness. For example, adolescents with diabetes who experiment with alcohol can suffer significant negative health consequences, as large amounts of alcohol can lead to dangerous fluctuations in blood sugar. Lack of compliance with medical treatments or recommendations may be further fueled by a sense of invulnerability and a tendency not to consider long-term consequences, which are typical characteristics of adolescents' thinking. Parents' efforts to oversee the medical care of their teenagers may conflict with the teen's emerging desire for independence and autonomy.

There are a few strategies that parents can employ to help them face the dual tasks of assuring their teen's physical health and helping him or her cope with the psychological effects of the illness. First, parents should avoid treating their adolescent like a younger child. Feelings of guilt and concern often cause parents of medically ill teens to be overprotective. Such an approach can breed resentment in an adolescent who is longing for independence, and this may lead to acting out and noncompliance. A preferred approach is to show respect for your teen and allow him or her to participate in discussions about medical care. This includes being open and honest with your teen about what is wrong and the implications of the illness. When appropriate, allow your adolescent to have input into decisions. He or she should not have the final say, particularly when making a decision that can seriously compromise his or her health; but it is your teen's body, and his or her opinion should be taken into consideration.

When it comes to the ongoing management of an illness, an adolescent should be allowed the opportunity to demonstrate responsibility and should be given increasing amounts of freedom. For example, many parents struggle with their teen to be certain that medications are being taken as prescribed. Parents rightfully want to ensure that their child is taking the medication, but teens may become annoyed by their parents' micromanaging them and asking repeatedly if they have taken the dose. To avoid these problems, parents can tell their teen that if he or she takes the medication as prescribed every day for a week, then they will stop asking about it. In the meantime, using daily pill organizers and keeping track of pill counts can help parents double-check that the medication is being taken as prescribed, without making an independently minded adolescent feel smothered. Allowing a teen to assume responsibility for managing an illness not only reduces the risk of rebellion but prepares the teen to transition to being responsible for his or her own medical care.

Avoidance of an overprotective approach must be balanced by the need to maintain firm limits. It should be made clear that, though teens can earn some responsibility, the parents are still the boss. Moreover, while a teen's input is always respected, certain fundamental aspects of medical care are not open for negotiation. Thus, an adolescent may be allowed to have input as to when a medical appointment is scheduled (e.g., not on a day that would cause him to miss a basketball game), but there is no debate about the fact that the teen must attend the appointments. Compliance with treatment is not an area to compromise.

Similarly, parents should not try to compensate for their child's illness by letting things slide more than they would (or do) with a child who is healthy. Relaxing rules and consequences for teens who are medically ill does them a disservice, as appropriate limits are essential to healthy development. Inconsistencies in the enforcement of rules can create problems if there are other children. Expectations for behavior should be maintained for an adolescent with a chronic illness, except when the illness has a direct impact on the teen's ability to meet the expectation.

Since teens have a developmentally normal drive to take risks, an effective strategy for many parents is to channel that drive. Parents can help teens learn the difference between healthy risks that have the potential to allow opportunities for growth (e.g., trying out for a sports team, asking out the object of a crush, starting a band) and unhealthy risks (e.g., using drugs, having unprotected sex, stopping one's medications). Parents can then encourage their teen to take the healthy risks and discourage the unhealthy ones. This approach is preferable to suppressing the drive to take risks altogether, which may only create more drama around the forbidden fruit of risk.

Trips to medical appointments can provide unexpected opportunities to connect with your teen. This connection can be amplified by creating a pleasant ritual around the trip that softens the blow of the appointment and gives the teen a chance to talk. The ritual may involve a stop on the way for lunch at a favorite restaurant or an ice cream cone from the hospital cafeteria. During the car ride, allow your teen to choose the radio station or play his or her music on the car stereo rather than listening to headphones. This allows the possibility of conversation and, as music is an important form of expression for many adolescents, may offer both a window into the teen's emotional world or a jumping-off point for discussion by asking about what is playing.

When an adolescent has a chronic illness, parents should be his or her advocate, particularly in the school setting. Parents should work with school staff to assure that there are appropriate supports in place to help the teen manage the illness. Talk to your teen about the challenges he or she faces as a result of the illness and problem solve together to devise solutions. It may help to imagine yourself in your child's shoes going through the school day. For example, teens with ulcerative colitis often have frequent bouts of sudden diarrhea, which may cause them to live in fear of having to use the student bathroom. Permission to leave class quickly and use the staff bathroom can save a great deal of shame and anxiety.

Parents should be aware of warning signs that their adolescent is having difficulty coping with an illness. Signs of distress are listed in sidebar 17.2. Teens with chronic medical illness are at risk for developing mood and anxiety disorders, and parents should have a low threshold for seeking a consultation from a mental health provider. For some teens, psychotherapy can help them cope with their illness, and it may improve their compliance with medical treatment. There are support groups, activity programs, and summer camps for teens suffering from particular illnesses. These activities can help maintain teens' self-esteem and help them to feel less isolated due to their illness.

Evaluation and Treatment

The evaluation for an adolescent who is having difficulty managing stress should include screening questions for psychiatric conditions, such as mood or anxiety disorders. As in any psychiatric assessment, evaluation of a teen's safety is also important.

When an adolescent is experiencing emotional or behavioral problems that appear related to an identifiable stressor but cannot be diagnosed as major depression, generalized anxiety, or other significant psychiatric disorder, a diagnosis of adjustment disorder may be made. This term refers to emotional or behavioral symptoms (in response to a stressor) that cause significant distress or impairment in functioning and are out of proportion to what would normally be expected.

Several interventions may be useful for adolescents who are suffering from adjustment disorder or who are otherwise having difficulty managing the stresses in their lives. Individual psychotherapy can be extremely helpful. A variety of theoretical approaches, including psychodynamic psychotherapy, cognitive behavioral therapy, and interpersonal therapy, may be employed. (See chapter 4 for further discussion of these approaches.) Therapy can strengthen adolescents' defenses and assist them in learning new ways to manage stress. It can provide support and a place to think through problems. Therapy can improve relationships, allowing an adolescent to manage social stressors and develop a healthy support system. Specific skills, including relaxation exercises such as deep breathing or guided imagery, may be useful.

When family conflict is a part of the problem, family therapy may be effective. If bullying is occurring at school, then interventions there are likely to be needed. Many teens find participation in a support group beneficial. Groups may include teens with a variety of problems or may center on a particular issue. There are groups such as Alateen for the adolescent children of alcoholic parents or hospital-based support groups for adolescents with chronic illness. These groups allow teens to have a safe place to express feelings and to take comfort in learning that they are not the only one grappling with a major problem. Similarly, community activities, including sports and programs such as the Boys and Girls Club, can decrease social isolation and give adolescents an outlet for feelings related to the stressors they are facing.

If adolescents become acutely stressed, they can try relaxation techniques (see sidebar 17.3). These are simple to do and may bring relif.

Sidebar 17.3 | A Simple Relaxation Exercise for Adolescents

► Find a quiet, comfortable place and sit or lie down in a comfortable position, allowing all your muscles to relax.

► Take a deep breath, and on the exhale let your eyes gently close.

► Take another deep breath through your nose slowly over a few seconds, gradually filling your lungs with air. Allow your abdomen to expand as you breathe in, so that you are breathing with your belly (your diaphragm, the large muscle that lies beneath the lungs) and not your chest or shoulders.

► At the peak of the inhalation, hold your breath for a second or two and then gently release the breath, slowly exhaling.

► Repeat this process of breathing in and out. If you wish, you may imagine that with each inhalation you are breathing in a sense of calm and that with each exhalation you are breathing out any tension or anxiety that is left in your body.

► As you are breathing, scan your body for any areas that may be holding tension, such as a tightened fist, clenched jaw, or hunched shoulders, and gently release this tension as you exhale.

Case Presentation

Joe was sixteen years old when he was diagnosed with diabetes. Although he was popular at school and a good student, Joe had always been a sensitive boy, and his parents were worried about how he would handle the diagnosis. Initially, he appeared to take it in stride. He learned to check his blood sugar and to administer injections of insulin. At school, however, Joe was self-conscious about having to go to the nurse's office before lunch to check his blood sugar, and he would complain to his parents that it "isn't fair." His parents noticed that he was frequently eating foods not on his diet, and he was hiding candy in his room.

Soon, Joe became increasingly sullen and withdrawn. He spent more time in his room, and his grades began to drop. He occasionally wore the same clothes day after day and showered less frequently. When his parents tried to talk with him about his diet, he was irritable. He resented their efforts to help him manage his diabetes, saying, "I'm not an idiot. I can do it myself." But blood tests confirmed that his diabetes was not well controlled; the doctor gave Joe and his parents a strict warning about the potential consequences of high blood sugar.

Joe began to hang out with a different group of friends, whom he did not bring to his home. One night he was caught drinking by the police. His parents searched his room and found beer cans hidden under his bed. Finally, Joe's parents decided to talk to him together. They knocked on his door. Joe shouted, "Don't come in!" and when his parents opened the door, they found him sitting on his bed cutting himself.

Joe's parents called his pediatrician and discussed the events. The doctor arranged for Joe to see a child and adolescent psychiatrist who was affiliated with the diabetes clinic. After a thorough evaluation, Joe was diagnosed with major depression. The psychiatrist recommended a course of individual psychotherapy for Joe as well as a support group for adolescents with diabetes. He also discussed concerns about Joe's drinking.

Initially, Joe was reluctant to participate in these interventions, but his parents told him that if he went, they would shorten his two-month grounding for the drinking incident to one month. Joe agreed to participate, and he grew to like his therapist. Joe talked about his anger about having diabetes and all the ways that it affected his life. The therapist helped Joe learn strategies for managing these feelings. Periodically, the therapist met separately with Joe's parents to help them learn ways of providing support for Joe at home. In the group, Joe was initially quiet, but soon he began to relate to the other kids. Eventually he talked about his own experiences, and he offered advice to the group members when they were facing similar problems.

Joe's parents supervised him more closely and, at all times, insisted on knowing where and with whom he was going. They checked in with him when he arrived home. On several occasions, when they smelled alcohol on his breath, he was grounded.

Over time, Joe's mood improved, he stopped drinking, and he became less sullen. His sense of humor returned. He stopped cutting. Six months after he entered therapy, Joe surprised his parents by bringing home a report card with straight As. His parents asked him how he did it, and Joe told them with a smile, "Well, I'm going to need to buckle down if I'm going to get into medical school. Someone's got to figure out a better way to deal with diabetes. It might as well be me."

Conclusion

The reaction of adolescents to stressful events including loss of a loved one, divorce, and chronic disease varies. Developmental age, innate psychological makeup, family and cultural background, and support network are factors that can influence a teen's reaction to stressful life events. Adolescents who are more resilient may deal with stress more effectively. It is important to know warning signs when teens are not managing stress effectively and when to obtain help from a mental health professional. Parents can employ strategies to help their adolescent cope with stressful situations.

References and Additional Reading

Bryner, C. L. 2001. "Children of Divorce." *Journal of the American Board of Family Practice* 14: 201–210.

Kubler-Ross, E. 1969. *On Death and Dying.* New York: Macmillan.

Richardson, S., and M. P. McCabe. 2001. "Parental Divorce during Adolescence and Adjustment during Early Adulthood." *Adolescence* 36: 467–489.

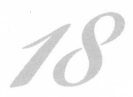 # Reactions to Trauma

Every year, many adolescents are confronted with a traumatic event. Trauma can take many forms, including witnessing or being a victim of natural disasters, accidents, sexual abuse, or violence including dating or relationship violence. Traumatic events may be sudden and short-lived, such as an accident, or they may be ongoing, such as suffering from repeated physical abuse from a caregiver.

Although trauma is difficult to quantify, it appears that rates of exposure to traumatic events during adolescence are high and may exceed rates of exposure during adulthood. In 2007, the National Youth Risk Behavior Survey, a poll of high school students in the United States conducted by the Centers for Disease Control, indicated that close to 8 percent of students surveyed reported that they had been threatened or injured by a weapon on school property at least once during the past year (http://www.cdc.gov/healthyyouth/yrbs). Up to one in three adolescent girls in the United States is a victim of physical, emotional, or verbal abuse from a dating partner. In one study, over 40 percent of adolescents in a sample population were found to have experienced a trauma such as rape, assault, or sudden severe injury prior to the age of eighteen. Adolescents who are confronted with these events are at risk for having significant psychiatric difficulties, including acute stress disorder and posttraumatic stress disorder (PTSD). However, not all adolescents who live through traumatic experiences develop these problems. In this chapter, we discuss adolescents' reactions to trauma, the symptoms and warning signs of the psychiatric disorders that can result from exposure to trauma, and the prevention and treatment of these disorders.

Sidebar 18.1 | Symptoms That Adolescents May Develop after a Traumatic Event

- Shock and disbelief about the event
- Feelings of fear or anxiety
- Anger, including revenge fantasies involving the perpetrator
- Sadness and episodes of crying
- Shame or guilt about what happened
- Changes in sleep patterns or appetite
- Nightmares, including nightmares about the event

- Physical symptoms, including muscle aches, headaches, or stomach upset
- Difficulty concentrating
- Feeling a decreased sense of personal safety or feeling a lack of control
- Brief periods of feeling numb or detached
- Regression, i.e., acting younger than normal
- Acting more clingy or dependent on parents

Case Presentation

Michael was seventeen years old when he and his best friend were in a motor-vehicle accident. Michael broke his leg; his best friend, Allen, was killed. Michael was the driver of the car, which skidded off an icy road into a tree. In the days following the accident, Michael appeared to be in a state of shock and seemed somewhat detached emotionally. His parents noticed that he often appeared to be "in a daze" or that he would "space out" when people were talking to him, often missing what they said.

Over the next several weeks, Michael began to have difficulty sleeping. He had frequent realistic nightmares about the accident. He would awaken in a cold sweat and have trouble falling asleep again. Michael became increasingly isolated, pushing away his family and friends, and he stopped playing the guitar, which he used to love.

Michael was very irritable with his parents and his friends, snapping at them often. He had explosive, angry outbursts in which he would become very upset over seemingly minor things. His parents noticed that he seemed quite nervous and jumpy, giving a start when there was a loud noise. Michael seemed fearful not only of driving a car but also of riding in one. He stopped driving altogether and began to walk to school.

His parents became even more concerned when they learned that he had failed three classes. When they tried to talk to him about it, Michael broke down crying, saying, "I just can't take this anymore. It should have been me that died, not Allen. I don't deserve to live."

Upon hearing this, Michael's parents arranged an evaluation with a psychologist who had a history of working with adolescents who had experienced trauma. The psychologist recommended that Michael begin therapy. Initially, Michael avoided talking about the accident and was somewhat resistant to going to the sessions. However, as he became more comfortable, he began to verbalize more openly. He told the psychologist that he was having thoughts about the accident that would pop into his head all day and that he could not make them go away. On a few occasions, he even felt as if he were back in the car with Allen as it was about to crash.

The psychologist diagnosed Michael with PTSD. Concerned that Michael was also suffering from depression, he referred him to a child and adolescent psychiatrist, who agreed with the diagnosis of PTSD as well as comorbid depression. Michael was started on fluoxetine (Prozac) to help with his mood and anxiety and continued seeing his therapist weekly. With time and ongoing treatment, his symptoms gradually improved, and his parents thought he began to seem like himself again.

Common Reactions to Trauma

Adolescents may display a broad range of reactions in response to a traumatic experience. Trauma is, by definition, an experience that is far outside the range of normal human experience. Thus, intense emotional and behavioral responses to this experience are not necessarily pathological. In the aftermath of trauma, an adolescent may demonstrate any combination of the symptoms noted in sidebar 18.1. In addition, school failure, disengagement from school activities, loss of friends, disinterest in hobbies, and onset of binge drinking may be symptoms of partner violence.

After a traumatic event, these symptoms may last for weeks or even months. It is difficult to establish a timeline that can be considered a "normal" recovery time. Teens' individual response will depend on many factors, including the nature of the trauma, their developmental level, their overall psychological functioning, and the support that they receive. With time, teens who are recovering in a healthy way will show gradual improvement in these symptoms. Before long they will be able to return to their old routines and engage in the same kinds of activities that they did before the trauma. Teens who do not show a pattern of improvement over time may require the assistance of a mental health professional to help them recover.

Support for Traumatized Adolescents

Support from parents and other concerned adults in a teen's life is an important component of recovery after a trauma. The first step is taking the necessary steps to assure the teen's safety and to prevent further trauma. For example, if a teen has been assaulted and is being threatened in an ongoing way at school, the police and school staff should be notified, and a plan should be devised to protect him. In cases of suspected physical or sexual abuse in the home, the state social services agency should be notified immediately. The adolescent may need to be removed from the home.

Once an adolescent's safety is assured and the risk of further trauma has been curtailed, the focus shifts to helping an adolescent cope. The most important activity that parents and other adults in a teen's life can do is to listen in a supportive way. Teens should not be forced to talk before they are ready, but it is essential that they know that they are loved and that there are people available who care about them. It is very therapeutic to be together as a family.

When a teen is ready to talk, it is important to listen in an accepting, nonjudgmental way. Trauma can trigger a variety of emotions. Adolescents should be allowed to express the full range of what they are feeling. Parents should validate whatever feelings an adolescent may have about an event, and they can help clarify the facts and gently correct any distorted ideation.

A traumatic event disrupts a child's sense of safety in the world. Part of the recovery process involves restoring that security. One way to do this is by returning to familiar, predictable, comforting routines as soon as possible. These routines may include school, sports, activities, and time with family or friends. Adequate amounts of sleep and a regular schedule are essential for coping with stress. Most adolescents need nine and a quarter hours of sleep nightly. For families without set routines, it may be helpful to create some that are fun and low-key, such as a weekly family pizza and a movie night.

For many adolescents, a traumatic event removes their feeling of being in control of their lives and their environment. This may be particularly difficult for adolescents, who often are struggling to develop their own sense of autonomy and efficacy in the world. Although parents may have a natural instinct to nurture or even baby teens after a trauma, they should allow teens to express their opinion and make their own choices when appropriate.

Each teen has his or her own way of managing stress. Adolescents recovering from trauma should be encouraged to do the healthy things that work for them. For some, this may mean spending more time with family. For others, it may mean time with friends or a boyfriend or girlfriend. Exercise, art, writing, watching movies, and listening to or playing music are all common outlets. Teens who still have not found an outlet may need gentle encouragement to explore and positive reinforcement for their efforts. This may mean asking a teen if she would enjoy joining a local pool facility or reminding a teen how a poem he wrote for English class was well received. Finding healthy ways to manage stress reduces the chances that teens will turn to unhealthy means, such as self-harm, substance abuse, or risk-taking behaviors.

To allow for a healthy recovery, it is important to reduce other stressors in an adolescent's life. While returning to usual routines and enjoyable activities, such as sports, is generally helpful for teens, it is also important to ensure that they are not overscheduled. Teens may need more downtime after a traumatic event. Dropping an elective class or an extracurricular activity or asking for an extension on a school project may reduce their stress. Parents who have been through a trauma with their adolescent should be certain that they are taking care of their own mental health. Sometimes, the family should seek professional assistance.

For adolescents who have suffered a serious injury as a result of a traumatic event, an essential aspect of reducing stress is managing any associated pain. Studies of children and adolescents who have suffered severe injuries such as burns have shown that good pain control can significantly reduce the risk of further psychiatric problems. Injured and traumatized teens may be overwhelmed and have difficulty advocating for themselves. Thus, parents may need to speak to medical providers to be certain that they are aware of any discomfort in their teen. For adolescents who are so severely injured that they are unable to communicate, other measures such as heart rate and blood pressure can be used to help identify physical discomfort.

Finally, parents and other involved adults should check for signs that a teen is having difficulty recovering from a trauma. Concerned parents should not delay in bringing their child for a psychiatric evaluation, as timely treatment can ensure a significant difference in recovery time and save a great deal of suffering. And if teachers or other adults in an adolescent's life notice issues, it is important to bring them to a parent's attention.

> **Sidebar 18.2 | Signs That an Adolescent Is Having
> Difficulty Recovering from a Traumatic Event**
>
> ▸ Frequent, disturbing flashbacks or reexperiencing the traumatic event
> ▸ Intrusive, unwanted thoughts about the trauma or inability to stop thinking about it
> ▸ Constantly feeling unsafe or on edge
> ▸ Startling easily
> ▸ Intense distress at matters that remind one of the trauma
> ▸ Feeling or seeming numb or abnormally detached from one's environment
> ▸ Avoiding things, places, or people that remind one of the trauma
> ▸ Persistent loss of interest in activities
> ▸ Inability to function, e.g., poor self-care or persistently poor attendance in school
> ▸ Social withdrawal and isolation
> ▸ Persistent feelings of sadness, anger, or anxiety that do not improve with time
> ▸ Engaging in risky behavior, e.g., sexual promiscuity, going into dangerous neighborhoods late at
>   night, driving recklessly
> ▸ Evidence of alcohol or other substance abuse
> ▸ Belief that one will die at a young age
> ▸ Suicidal thoughts, frequent thoughts about death, or self-injurious behavior, e.g., cutting oneself

Warning Signs

Psychological problems resulting from trauma can manifest themselves in different ways. Signs that an adolescent is having difficulty recovering from a traumatic experience and may benefit from a psychiatric evaluation are noted in sidebar 18.2. In addition to watching for these signs, parents should follow their instincts. If in doubt, talk with your child's pediatrician or a school counselor. A teen's safety should always be the first priority. Suicidal statements or attempts should always be taken seriously and are a sure sign that an evaluation is needed. If there is doubt as to an adolescent's immediate safety, an urgent evaluation at an emergency room or crisis center should be arranged.

Risk Factors

Not every adolescent who is exposed to a traumatic event will develop psychiatric difficulties. Certain risk factors have been identified that make problems such as posttraumatic stress disorder more likely to occur. These risk factors can be divided into three categories: factors relating to the traumatic event itself, factors relating to the adolescent exposed to the event, and the adolescent's social environment.

The events associated with the development of PTSD involve a threat of death, serious injury, or violation of one's physical integrity and linked to intense fear and helplessness. It is not surprising that more severe and terrifying events are more likely to cause psychiatric difficulties, with exposure to physical violence carrying a particularly strong risk. In addition, the risk for PTSD is related to the teen's relationship with the victim of the trauma. Witnessing an event that threatens or harms a loved one is more likely to result in PTSD than witnessing one that happens to a stranger. Events that pose a threat to adolescents themselves or cause them direct harm have an even greater risk. Trauma that is repeated, such as recurrent physical or sexual abuse at home, poses greater risk of PTSD and other negative psychiatric effects than a single traumatic episode.

Children who have behavioral or emotional problems, such as an anxiety disorder, prior to a traumatic event are believed to be at greater risk of developing PTSD. Previous trauma exposure and high levels of psychosocial stress are also associated with greater risk. Although boys have been found to have higher rates of exposure to traumatic events, there is some evidence to suggest that girls may have higher rates of PTSD onset after such an exposure. However, results of studies in this area are difficult to interpret, and there is some controversy over this finding.

Finally, an adolescent's family and community environment play an important role in his risk of developing PTSD. Adolescents in families with high levels of discord, frequent moves, inconsistency, and conflict are at increased risk. Teens living in communities that have suffered a severe disruption, such as a natural disaster, are at increased risk. In contrast, communities that offer an outpouring of support after such an event can be protective. Access to trusted supports, including adult role models, and mental health services can help at-risk teens recover without lasting psychological damage.

Making the Diagnosis

Acute Stress Disorder

Acute stress disorder is a name given to a set of symptoms that may occur in the weeks immediately following a traumatic event. The symptoms of acute stress disorder are described in sidebar 18.3. To make the diagnosis of acute stress disorder, the symptoms must begin within four weeks of the traumatic event. By definition, the disorder may last no longer than four weeks. The symptoms must resolve within this time period. If the symptoms persist for longer than four weeks, most often the diagnosis of PTSD is made.

The symptoms of acute stress disorder include dissociation, which is a disturbance in a person's normal consciousness or perception that may occur during a traumatic event or in its aftermath. During an episode of dissociation, adolescents may feel strangely detached from the events happening around them. They may sense that events are not real but rather are taking place in a dream. This is called "derealization." They may also experience "depersonalization," which is a

> ### Sidebar 18.3 | **Symptoms of Acute Stress Disorder** (adapted from the DSM-IV)
>
> If an adolescent has been exposed to a traumatic event that involves threat of death, serious injury, or violation of physical integrity involving him- or herself or others, associated with feelings of fear, helplessness, or horror, the following symptoms, beginning within four weeks of the traumatic event and lasting no longer than four weeks, are signs of acute stress disorder:
>
> ▸ During or after the event the person experiences "dissociation," which may include feeling numb or detached from one's surroundings, feeling that things are not real, feeling detached from one's body, or being unable to remember some aspects of the trauma
> ▸ Reexperiencing symptoms, which may include intrusive thoughts or memories about the trauma, recurring nightmares, or flashbacks in which the event seems to be happening again
> ▸ Avoidance symptoms, in which the individual goes to great lengths to avoid thoughts or reminders of the trauma, feeling emotionally numb or unable to experience pleasure, becoming withdrawn and socially isolated, giving up formerly pleasurable activities, or having a sense that one will have a shortened future (e.g., will not live a long life or will not have a productive or meaningful life)
> ▸ Increased arousal, including difficulty sleeping, irritability, anger outbursts, feeling on edge, being constantly on the lookout for danger, or startling easily

feeling of detachment from one's body or sense of self, as if one is floating above the room looking down on oneself. Dissociation is often seen with traumatic events, and by itself it does not necessarily indicate a psychiatric problem. It is a type of psychological defense mechanism. However, when dissociative episodes recur following a trauma, they can be a source of distress and dysfunction.

Posttraumatic Stress Disorder

Posttraumatic stress disorder is defined by a characteristic pattern of symptoms that occurs in response to a traumatic event. These symptoms, which are described in detail in sidebar 18.4, fall into three general categories: (1) reexperiencing, in which the individual has unwanted and intrusive memories, dreams, or flashbacks related to the trauma; (2) avoidance, in which the individual tries desperately to avoid places, thoughts, conversations, or other things that might remind him or her of the trauma; and (3) hyperarousal, which involves a state of heightened anxiety and sensitivity to potential threats in the environment. Before the diagnosis of PTSD can be made, these symptoms must be present for at least one month.

Though these feelings are not part of the criteria for diagnosis, PTSD tends to be associated with intense feelings of guilt, shame, and worthlessness. Many victims of trauma blame themselves for the events that happened to them. For those who have lived through a trauma that took the lives of others, these feelings may emerge in the form of "survivor guilt," in which people feel that they did something wrong by surviving the event or that they should have been the one to die. These feelings can significantly amplify the distress of those suffering from PTSD and must be addressed in treatment.

Other Problems to Consider

Differential Diagnosis: What Else Might Be Wrong?

Several other psychiatric disorders that may result from a traumatic event have symptoms that resemble acute stress disorder and PTSD. Depression and bipolar disorder can cause similar patterns of behavior, including social withdrawal, loss of interest in activities, lack of pleasure in things that one previously enjoyed, irritability, and explosive outbursts. Mood disorders can be distinguished from

---

Sidebar 18.4 | **Symptoms of Posttraumatic Stress Disorder** (adapted from the DSM-IV)

If an adolescent has been exposed to a traumatic event that involves threat of death, serious injury, or violation of physical integrity involving him- or herself or others, associated with feelings of fear, helplessness, or horror, symptoms in each of the following areas, lasting at least one month and causing significant distress or impairment, are signs of PTSD.

- ▶ Reexperiencing
  - ▶ Intrusive thoughts or memories about the trauma
  - ▶ Recurring nightmares related to the incident
  - ▶ Flashbacks in which the person believes the event is occurring again
  - ▶ Intense distress or physical reaction (e.g., rapid heartbeat, sweating, etc.) in response to reminders of the event
- ▶ Avoidance
  - ▶ Avoiding thoughts, feelings, or discussions related to the trauma
  - ▶ Avoidance of people, places, or activities related to the trauma, e.g., the place where it occurred
  - ▶ Inability to remember some major aspects of the event
  - ▶ Decline in interests or participation in usual activities
  - ▶ Experiencing feelings of detachment or being isolated from others
  - ▶ Limited expression of emotions or seeming unable to experience positive feelings
  - ▶ Sense that one's future is shortened, e.g., not expecting to live a long life or to have a productive future
- ▶ Increased anxiety or arousal
  - ▶ Major difficulties sleeping
  - ▶ Irritability or anger outbursts
  - ▶ Difficulty concentrating
  - ▶ Frequently acting on edge or looking out for danger, even in seemingly safe situations
  - ▶ Exaggerated startle response

PTSD by the absence of reexperiencing phenomena, such as flashbacks or intrusive thoughts about the trauma, as well as by the absence of avoidance behavior that is specific to matters related to the trauma.

PTSD and acute stress disorder are classified as anxiety disorders. Other anxiety disorders, such as panic disorder and generalized anxiety disorder, share features with the posttraumatic reactions. As with PTSD and acute stress disorder, other forms of anxiety disorder cause a feeling of being unsafe and on edge. Adolescents with anxiety disorders may go to great lengths to avoid triggering their anxiety. For example, teens who have panic attacks in crowded areas often begin to avoid these places. The relationship of the symptoms to a traumatic event and the presence of reexperiencing symptoms may help to distinguish acute stress disorder and PTSD from other anxiety disorders.

Psychiatric disorders including borderline personality disorder, substance abuse, and psychotic disorders such as schizophrenia can have symptoms that resemble PTSD or acute stress disorder. A thorough psychiatric evaluation may distinguish these conditions based on the pattern of symptoms that is present, but in challenging cases psychological testing may be helpful. Urine screening for drugs of abuse will help to identify substance abuse, although it does not rule out the possibility that PTSD is also present.

Comorbidities

PTSD commonly occurs with other psychiatric disorders. These disorders may precede the onset of PTSD, making the adolescent more vulnerable to developing the disorder, or they may begin later, with PTSD. Identification of coexisting psychiatric disorders is an important aspect of the PTSD evaluation, as failure to recognize and treat these disorders can impede recovery.

Major depression is one of the most common comorbid psychiatric disorders that occurs in teens with PTSD. Anxiety and substance abuse disorders are also very prevalent in adolescents with PTSD. Attention-deficit/hyperactivity disorder (ADHD) has been found to be more common in adolescents with PTSD. Increased risk for behavioral disorders such as oppositional defiant disorder and conduct disorder has been shown for adolescents with PTSD, particularly in males. PTSD that is associated with sexual abuse during childhood or adolescence is thought to increase the risk of developing borderline personality disorder later in life.

Evaluation for Trauma-Related Concerns

Evaluation for concerns about possible acute stress disorder, PTSD, or other psychological effects should be performed by a child and adolescent psychiatrist, a clinical psychologist, or another mental health professional with appropriate training and experience. As with most psychiatric disorders, the diagnosis is made primarily on the basis of the history of symptoms gathered by the mental health clinician conducting the evaluation.

The clinician should offer the opportunity for parents or caretakers accompanying the adolescent to speak to the clinician in private. Allowing for private discussion is always helpful in the psychiatric evaluation of adolescents, but it is particularly important in cases of trauma. Adolescents who have been traumatized may not feel comfortable discussing the event with the clinician, especially in the first meeting. If a teen is suffering from PTSD, he or she may not recall all aspects of the event or may try to avoid talking or thinking about it.

It may be helpful for the clinician to gather additional information about teens' symptoms from other important people in their life, including teachers and the school counselor. In cases of trauma, extra care must be taken to protect the adolescent's confidentiality. Parents and the clinician need to strike a balance between the adolescent's confidentiality and the potential value of the additional information. Most often, the clinician will speak to other important people in the teen's life without disclosing the reason for the evaluation.

Trauma can contribute to the development of other psychiatric problems including depression or anxiety. Thus, an evaluation for trauma-related concerns should involve a complete medical and psychiatric history. Teens who have undergone trauma or loss are at increased risk for attempting suicide. As a result, it is important to assess the adolescent's safety, including questions about suicidal thoughts and suicide risk factors.

Usually there is no role for blood tests, brain imaging, or other medical tests in making the diagnosis of acute stress disorder or PTSD. But there are some exceptions. For example, a traumatic event that involved serious head injury may warrant further testing to rule out brain damage or seizures as potential causes of the teen's symptoms. In cases of suspected PTSD that are unusual or difficult to distinguish from other possible psychiatric disorders, psychological testing may be helpful. Psychological testing is discussed in more detail in chapter 3.

Treatment

The approach to treating acute stress disorder and PTSD should be customized to the needs of the adolescent. An approach that integrates several kinds of treatment is most effective.

Psychotherapy

Individual psychotherapy is the cornerstone of treatment for posttraumatic disorders and should be a component of the treatment plan for any adolescent who is suffering from PTSD. There are several different approaches.

Cognitive behavioral therapy (CBT) has the most evidence to support its use in the treatment of PTSD. CBT for trauma focuses on identifying and correcting distorted thoughts related to the trauma, such as having an exaggerated perception of potential threat in situations or believing that a traumatic event was one's own fault. Through the therapy, teens learn more accurate and adaptive ways of interpreting and thinking about situations in their life. At the same time, the behavioral component of CBT seeks to teach coping skills for managing stress and overcoming avoidance behavior. Sometimes, the therapy will include gradually increasing exposure to thoughts that the adolescent is avoiding. Relaxation exercises, such as deep breathing, are often incorporated into CBT to help adolescents learn to reduce their anxiety when confronted with reminders or thoughts about the trauma.

Psychodynamic psychotherapy is commonly used to treat PTSD. In this approach, the emphasis is on working through painful feelings and memories associated with the trauma and exploring the connection between the event and the teen's current and past experiences and relationships. Psychodynamic psychotherapy can help adolescents identify patterns in their lives, including potentially unhealthy ways that they manage negative feelings. For example, many teens who have suffered a traumatic experience rely on defense mechanisms to cope. These include repression, in which unwanted memories are driven out of the conscious mind in order to avoid experiencing them, and disavowal, in which the person does not acknowledge the toll that the traumatic event has taken on his or her life. Through psychodynamic psychotherapy, teens may come to realize the ways in which the use of these defenses contributes to perpetuating their distress. Thus, they learn to come to terms with the negative memories and emotions, integrating these experiences back into the fabric of their lives.

Eye movement desensitization and reprocessing (EMDR) is a relatively new, specialized technique that may be incorporated into the treatment of PTSD. Used in adults, EMDR shares many features with CBT. During EMDR, the patient is asked to focus on a negative image and thought, such as reminders of the traumatic event, while performing back-and-forth eye movements guided by the therapist. This process is repeated until the patient experiences a decrease in the distress related to the thought and image. Then, the same eye movements are performed in conjunction with a positive thought that the patient and the therapist have identified as what they want to replace the negative one with. In addition to eye movements, other sensory stimuli such as auditory tones may be used in the treatment. At present, EMDR has not been well studied in adolescents, and its use in adults is the source of some controversy. While there is some evidence to suggest that it is beneficial, findings have been somewhat mixed. Some studies have suggested that the eye movements are not necessary and that other aspects of the treatment are responsible for its therapeutic effect.

Nonetheless, with further study, this technique may have potential benefit for some adolescents with PTSD.

Regardless of the theoretical background of the therapist, empathy and support are essential ingredients for the treatment. In the wake of a trauma, teens often need practical guidance. The therapist can help teens think through and address concrete problems in their life and reduce stress during their recovery.

For teens and their parents, an essential component of psychotherapy for trauma-related difficulties is education. Many adolescents with PTSD symptoms do not understand what is happening, which only adds to their stress. Education helps teens to make sense of the feelings that they are experiencing, realize that they are not alone, and find hope that things will improve. Education for parents enables them to understand what to expect and how best to support their teen during treatment and recovery.

Other Psychosocial Interventions

Involving an adolescent's family in the treatment of trauma-related difficulties improves the chances for success. Parents reinforce strategies that the teen is learning in therapy, such as relaxation exercises or coping skills. In addition, they address problem behaviors, such as excessive risk taking, that may be associated with trauma. Family therapy can be useful for families that are under stress or in cases in which the entire family has experienced a trauma.

Since group therapy can help teens feel less isolated, work through their feelings, and feel good about helping others with similar problems, this type of therapy can be beneficial for some adolescents suffering from PTSD. Skills-focused groups reinforce coping strategies that are being learned in individual therapy. However, before group therapy is begun, careful thought should be given to how an individual adolescent is likely to respond. Strong expressions of anger or shared accounts of traumatic experiences by other members in the group may trigger anxiety or reexperiencing symptoms for some teens. Moreover, trauma can also be associated with feelings of shame, and some adolescents may feel uncomfortable talking about their experiences in a group setting.

Following a disaster in a community, school or community-based interventions can be used to help reduce the development of PTSD and identify at-risk adolescents for further evaluation and treatment. Two government-funded agencies, the National Child Traumatic Stress Center and the National Center for PTSD, have developed a "psychological first aid" approach to responding to a traumatic event in a community. The manual describing this approach is available online through the U.S. Department of Veterans Affairs website, at http://www.ptsd.va.gov/professional/manuals/psych-first-aid.asp. This approach, which offers recommendations specific to adolescents, involves clarifying the facts about what happened, providing education about posttraumatic reactions and

PTSD symptoms, encouraging expression of feelings about the event, and teaching practical problem-solving techniques. While school-based interventions can be very effective, it is important that they be undertaken with guidance from experienced mental health professionals to avoid inadvertently causing more psychological distress for those involved.

Medications

Medications are frequently used in the treatment of adolescents with PTSD. They are especially useful when there is a significant comorbid mood or anxiety disorder, when the PTSD symptoms are particularly severe and impairing, or when the symptoms are not responding to psychotherapy.

In PTSD, medications are usually limited to treating comorbid psychiatric disorders, such as ADHD or depression, or to targeting particular symptoms, such as a major sleep disturbance, rather than treating the disorder itself. Thus, the range of medications that may be used is fairly broad, and the medications that may be recommended for a particular adolescent will depend on the symptoms that are most problematic. Because symptoms of anxiety and depression are common in adolescents with PTSD, the selective serotonin reuptake inhibitors (SSRIs) are often used. SSRIs are relatively safe and are effective in treating symptoms of both anxiety and depression. SSRIs are discussed in more detail in chapter 5.

Adolescents with PTSD are at high risk for developing problems with substance abuse. Thus, it is important for parents and doctors to exercise caution and close supervision when teens are using medications with high potential for abuse, such as benzodiazepines (e.g., lorazepam, diazepam, or clonazepam), to treat PTSD.

Prognosis

The long-term outcome for adolescents with PTSD has not been extensively studied. Evidence from research with adults has shown that in over half of PTSD cases, complete recovery occurs within three months. But the course of the illness is extremely variable. For many adolescents, PTSD can continue for years. In such chronic cases, the symptoms often have a tendency to wax and wane, with periods of worsening alternating with periods of remission.

Several factors can help guide the prognosis. The presence of comorbid psychiatric disorders, particularly substance abuse disorders, is associated with a greater likelihood of a more severe and more chronic course of illness. Factors related to the trauma influence prognosis: less favorable outcomes are associated with traumatic events that were severe or repeated or that directly threatened the affected teen. Factors associated with a more favorable prognosis include good social support networks and access to psychiatric care.

Conclusion

A small but significant number of adolescents will face a traumatic event during their teenage years. A traumatic experience can have a powerful psychological impact, particularly when it occurs during this vulnerable period of psychological development. At the time of the trauma, feelings of shock, horror, and helplessness are common. Some adolescents may have strange feelings of being detached from reality. In the aftermath of the traumatic event, there may be significant changes in an adolescent's feelings and behavior that do not necessarily signify a psychiatric disorder. These changes may include feelings of anger, sadness and worry, developmental regression, difficulty sleeping, and a tendency to eat too little or too much. It may take some time for a teen to recover from a trauma, but with time these disturbances should stop.

During recovery, teens needs significant support from their parents and other important figures to help process the event and restore their feelings of safety. Parents must be aware of warning signs that suggest their child is having difficulty recovering and may need outside help. Parents who notice these warning signs or have concerns about how their child is handling a traumatic event should seek a mental health evaluation immediately.

Acute stress disorder and posttraumatic stress disorder are psychological consequences from exposure to a traumatic event. They have similar patterns of symptoms and are distinguished primarily by their time course. Acute stress disorder is diagnosed in the immediate aftermath of a trauma, whereas PTSD symptoms must be present for at least a month before the diagnosis is established, and PTSD may persist for several months or years.

The major symptoms of acute stress disorder and PTSD fall into three categories: reexperiencing symptoms, avoidance symptoms, and increased arousal. In evaluating an adolescent who has undergone trauma, it is important to distinguish between PTSD and other psychiatric problems, such as anxiety and depression, that may be exacerbated by stressful life events. It is also essential to screen for comorbid disorders that frequently occur in adolescents with PTSD, including mood and anxiety disorders, substance abuse, conduct disorder, oppositional defiant disorder, and ADHD.

Treatment for PTSD typically involves a combination of approaches, and the treatment plan should be customized to meet the needs of the individual teen. Psychotherapy is the cornerstone of PTSD treatment, but medications are commonly used. Medications that address symptoms of anxiety and depression, particularly SSRIs, are often helpful.

The prognosis for adolescents with PTSD varies. Although most teens will recover, for others PTSD is a chronic condition that may remit and relapse for years. The prognosis is influenced by the nature of the trauma, the characteristics of the adolescent who has experienced the trauma, and the availability of social support after the event. By providing support, recognizing warning signs, and obtaining the necessary assistance for teens who are struggling, parents can help traumatized adolescents recover and lead healthy lives.

References and Additional Reading

Davis, L., and L. J. Siegel. 2000. "Posttraumatic Stress Disorder in Children and Adolescents: A Review and Analysis." *Clinical Child and Family Psychology Review* 3: 135–154.

Giaconia, R. M., H. Z. Reinherz, A. B. Silverman, B. Pakiz, A. K. Frost, and E. Cohen. 1995. "Traumas and Posttraumatic Stress Disorder in a Community Population of Older Adolescents." *Journal of the American Academy of Child and Adolescent Psychiatry* 34: 1369–1380.

Miller, E. In press. "Adolescent Relationship Violence in Clinical Settings: Challenges for Identification and Intervention." In *MassGeneral Hospital for Children Adolescent Medicine Handbook,* ed. Mark A. Goldstein, M.D. New York: Springer.

Shaw, J. A. 2000. "Children, Adolescents and Trauma." *Psychiatric Quarterly* 71: 227–243.

Stoddard, F. J., and G. Saxe. 2001. "Ten-Year Research Review of Physical Injuries." *Journal of the American Academy of Child and Adolescent Psychiatry* 40: 1128–1145.

19 Dangerous Behavior: Suicide, Self-Injury, and Violence

An adolescent's safety is the first priority for parents, teachers, and mental health professionals. Although most psychiatric treatments take time, when adolescents' safety or the safety of those around them is at risk, urgent intervention may be required. Adolescents are particularly prone to engage in dangerous and lethal behaviors. And unfortunately, they are at increased risk for suicide.

Suicide, self-injury, and violence are all complex behaviors with multiple causes. So there is no single approach to addressing these problems that will work for every adolescent. Nonetheless, there are steps that parents can take to help maintain the safety of their teens and their families. A successful approach to addressing safety concerns involves understanding the factors that are driving the behavior and dealing with them in every relevant aspect of a teen's life, including home, school, and the community.

Suicide

Parents of a teen with mental illness cannot help but worry about the possibility of suicide. Developmental factors place adolescents at high risk for suicide. At a time when their impulse control and psychological defenses are not yet mature, teens are struggling with issues related to identity, sexuality, societal expectations, and social relationships. In the United States, following accidents and homicide, suicide is the third leading cause of death among adolescents. According to a 2007 survey conducted by the Centers for Disease Control, approximately 15 percent of U.S. high school students report having seriously considered suicide in the past twelve months, and 7 percent report having attempted suicide during this time. For teens with psychiatric illness, the risk is even higher.

Preventing Suicide

The good news is that parents and other concerned adults can help prevent teenage suicide. Most adolescents who commit suicide are suffering from an identifiable psychiatric illness. Perhaps the most important thing that can be done to reduce adolescents' suicide risk is to be aware of their problems and obtain treatment as early as possible. Proper psychiatric treatment and other interventions, such as school and social supports, are critical to maintaining the safety of an at-risk teen.

Recognizing factors associated with increased risk of suicide is another important part of suicide prevention; the risk factors for adolescent suicide are listed in sidebar 19.1. The presence of these factors does not necessary mean that an adolescent will attempt suicide, but they may be used to identify teens at higher risk. It is important for teens at increased risk to have a psychiatric evaluation. If a teen is already in treatment, parents should explore with the child psychiatrist or therapist how to reduce their teen's risk.

Interventions to reduce an individual's risk of suicide can take many forms, and mental health providers, schools, and parents play a critical role. Mental health providers may recommend more intensive treatment, such as increased frequency of therapy appointments or admission to a day treatment or residential program. They may also advise other treatment options, such as group or family therapy. Suicide risk may additionally be addressed through the judicious use of medications to treat the symptoms of anxiety, depression, insomnia, or agitation. When the risk of suicide is high and imminent, an adolescent may require psychiatric hospitalization.

Sidebar 19.1 | **Risk Factors for Adolescent Suicide**

- History of past suicide attempts
- Presence of psychiatric illness, with particular risk for adolescents with mood disorders, such as bipolar disorder and major depression disorder, and psychotic disorders, such as schizophrenia
- Male gender: although females attempt suicide more frequently than males do, completed suicides are much more common in males
- Insomnia, restlessness, agitation, or impulsivity
- Aggressive behavior
- Drug or alcohol abuse
- Family history of suicide
- Easy access to means of suicide, such as having unsecured firearms in the home
- Exposure to suicide, including a recent suicide in the community, a suicide attempt by a friend, or media coverage of a suicide by a public figure
- Recent loss or stressful event, e.g., a romantic breakup, parents' going through a divorce, the death of a loved one, or legal problems
- History of being physically or sexually abused
- Feelings of hopelessness or worthlessness
- Homosexuality in nonaccepting environment
- Poor communication or relationship problems with parents
- Isolation or lack of social support
- Little involvement in school, work, or other activities

Schools can help reduce suicide risk by assessing whether a teen is receiving appropriate services. Academic failure due to unaddressed learning disorders contributes to stress, low self-esteem, and feelings of hopelessness. Students with psychiatric illness may need additional support to help manage the stresses of school. Students who have recurrent suicidal thoughts may benefit from an established safety plan that is developed with input from parents, outpatient mental health providers, and the student. This plan may include how to respond if safety concerns arise at school. Adolescents with severe emotional disturbances may be better served in a therapeutic setting, where they are able to receive the support they need and avoid isolation and alienation.

In addition to interventions for individual students, some schools offer schoolwide programs aimed at preventing suicide. There is controversy about the extent to which such programs are useful. Some studies have shown no benefit to these programs; other studies find that they appear to have the unintended effect of increasing suicide rates. The reasons for this finding are unclear, but it may be that discussing suicide and its risk factors in some way normalizes the idea for some teens, making it seem to be a viable solution for their problems. Thus, school-based prevention programs should be instituted with caution. Structured programs that have been studied and proven to be safe and effective in other schools are preferable. It also appears that programs based on early identification of and intervention with at-risk students, such as those with depression, behavioral problems, or substance abuse, may be effective.

Youth suicide is known to have a "contagion effect." After there has been a suicide in the community, there is an increased risk of additional suicides. In some cases, this is due to "suicide pacts" or the distress caused by the loss of a friend. However, the likelihood of suicide in the community increases even among teens who did not know the victim. As with school-based suicide prevention efforts, the measures taken by a school or community to respond to a suicide should be instituted after careful consideration. Public memorials to a suicide victim may glorify the act of suicide in the eyes of other students. Students who are depressed and isolated may feel that suicide would gain them the attention and sympathy of the entire community.

These concerns do not imply that schools should ignore a suicide. After a tragic event, students and school staff need support and an opportunity to express their grief. However, it is important to find ways of doing so that will not cause further harm. Consultation with experts or review of evidence-based guidelines can help schools determine appropriate responses.

Steps for Parents to Keep Teens Safe

Parents play the most important role in the prevention of adolescent suicide. The steps that parents can take to reduce a teen's risk of suicide are summarized

---

Sidebar 19.2 | **Steps Parents Can Take to Reduce Suicide Risk**

► Pay attention to signs of distress, and seek help for potential psychiatric, academic, and social problems
► Lock unloaded guns in a secure location, and keep ammunition in a separate secure location
► Consider locking up household medications, including over-the-counter medications, for teens who are at high risk
► Try to maintain good communication and a positive relationship with your teen
► Convey love and acceptance of your teen, separating disapproval of certain behaviors, e.g., substance abuse, from rejection of the teen
► Do not ignore remarks about suicide, and do not be afraid to ask a teen if he or she is depressed or having suicidal thoughts if you are worried
► Be aware of risk factors (sidebar 19.1) and pay attention to warning signs (sidebar 19.3) for suicide
► Obtain help immediately if you are concerned about your teen's safety

---

in sidebar 19.2. Because guns are the most common means employed by teens who successfully commit suicide, being involved in over half of completed suicides, keeping the home a safe place is one of the most effective measures to prevent suicide. Gun safety measures include locking and securing guns. Guns should be stored unloaded, and ammunition should be kept in a separate secure location.

Still, overdosing on medication is the most common means employed by all teens who attempt suicide. For high-risk teens, parents should secure all medications in the household. Suicide is often an impulsive act that is performed in a moment of intense distress. When easy access to possible means of suicide is removed, the impulse may pass before the teen is able to act. So raising the threshold of effort required to commit suicide reduces the likelihood that it will occur.

Teens' relationship with their parents is another important factor in determining suicide risk. As noted in sidebar 19.1, poor communication and difficulties between teens and their parents place them at risk of suicide. It is critical for parents to try to maintain a positive relationship with their teen, even under challenging circumstances. Listen to your teen in an open, accepting, nonjudgmental way. When a teen is engaging in negative behaviors, such as substance abuse, clearly state that it is the behavior, not the teen, that is being condemned. Teens who perceive that they are seen as failures or who feel rejected by parents are more likely to commit a desperate act such as suicide. Similarly, teens who identify themselves as homosexual or bisexual are at increased risk of suicide, particularly when they feel that they will not be accepted by their family, friends, or community.

Some families have a difficult time discussing negative feelings, such as expressions of intense sadness. Because the idea is threatening for them, many parents try to avoid topics such as suicide. Similarly, parents may be worried about their child's safety but be afraid to ask their child about depression or suicide. They think that talking about these topics might make them more likely to happen. Most often, the opposite is true. Depression and suicidal thoughts do not usually go away when they are ignored. Teens who are unable to share their suffering with a parent are more likely to feel isolated and alone, and these are feelings that can contribute to a suicide attempt.

Finally, parents should be aware of the warning signs of teenage suicide, which are listed in sidebar 19.3. Although some of these signs are nonspecific and may simply indicate that a teen is suffering, they may also signal that a teen is actively contemplating suicide, particularly when several of them are present. If you have concerns about your child's safety, it is essential to obtain help as soon as possible. If you suspect that your child may be at risk of harming him- or herself, but you are not certain, consider contacting your child's psychiatrist or pediatrician to discuss the best course of action. If you feel that your child is in immediate danger, your child should be closely supervised until an urgent psychiatric evaluation at an emergency room or crisis center is arranged. To ensure the safety of teens who are actively suicidal or out of control, they may need to be transported to an emergency room via ambulance.

Sidebar 19.3 | Warning Signs for Adolescent Suicide

- Dramatic changes in personality or behavior
- Changes in eating or sleeping habits
- Worsening symptoms of depression or the appearance of psychotic symptoms
- Neglect of hygiene or personal appearance
- Increase in dangerous, self-destructive, or risk-taking behavior, e.g., running away, driving recklessly, drinking alcohol to excess
- Withdrawal from family and friends
- Giving away or disposal of valued possessions, including items with sentimental value
- Talk about death or suicide, including comments that may be veiled (e.g., talking about "going away" or saying, "Well, you won't have to worry about me much longer"), vague (e.g., "I don't see the point anymore"), or sound like joking (e.g., laughing and saying sarcastically, "Well, maybe I should just kill myself then")
- Preoccupation with thoughts about death or with suicide of others, e.g., visiting websites discussing suicide or excessive focus on suicide of a public figure
- Restlessness, aggression, or insomnia
- Expressions of guilt, worthlessness, or hopelessness (e.g., talking about being a bad person)
- Decreased concentration or dramatic decline in academic performance
- Suddenly appearing cheerful or relieved with no clear reason after a period of significant depression

Self-Injury

Self-injurious behavior is a fairly common occurrence in adolescents with psychiatric illness, and it seems to be on the rise. These behaviors are often symptoms of great distress in teens and can be very upsetting to parents, who do not know how to interpret or respond to them. Self-injury can take many forms. Superficially cutting oneself, which is frequently done on the forearms, is the most common form of self-injury in teens. Other common forms include burning oneself, such as with a lighter or a lit cigarette, banging one's head against the wall, and punching walls or windows.

Reasons for Self-Injurious Behavior

Teens engage in self-injurious behavior for complex and varied reasons; these acts, such as cutting, do not necessarily indicate suicidal thoughts. Often, self-injury represents an attempt to soothe oneself and obtain relief from negative feelings. Teens may turn to cutting or other forms of self-injury as a way of coping, albeit a maladaptive one. Some teens who harm themselves say that the behavior allows them to focus on the physical pain and displace their emotional distress. Frequent cutters say that it calms them or gives them relief from feelings of depression or anger. Physiologically, this feeling may be due to the release of endorphins, brain chemicals associated with the suppression of pain and a feeling of calm and well-being.

To some teens, self-injury is a form of communicating to others that they are suffering. This may occur when adolescents try to express themselves verbally and feel that their parents are not listening or paying attention. Or self-injury may take place when the suffering involves an issue, such as sexual abuse, that the teen feels too ashamed to express. While adolescents frequently try to hide their self-injurious behavior, those who use it as a form of communication may cut in front of parents, allow their wounds to be discovered, or otherwise make others aware of what they are doing. Sometimes, teens will carve into their skin a word that expresses their feelings. For example, an adolescent with an eating disorder may carve the word "fat" on her arm. A teen who is depressed and isolated may write "alone."

By nature, adolescents are risk takers, and risk does serve a useful role in development. It can drive a teen to explore new friends, interests, and points of view. Still, for some teens, particularly those with low self-esteem, the risk-taking urge does not find an outlet in healthy activities. Rather, it can emerge through harmful behaviors, including self-harm. For these adolescents, self-injury may feel dangerous and forbidden and take on a romantic appeal. Avoiding detection and hiding the evidence may add to the mystique.

Peer influence can play a role in promoting self-injurious behavior. For some teens, particularly those who feel socially isolated or who have limited social skills, cutting may allow them to feel connected to peers who engage in this behavior. A sense of connection to peers who also self-harm may take place online, as there are websites and online discussion groups devoted to this topic. These types of sites may allow teens who cut to feel that they are part of a community.

Cutting is more common in certain adolescent subcultures, including teens who identify themselves as Goth or emo, which have their own characteristic styles of clothing and music. Some adolescent subcultures have a preoccupation with morbid themes, intense emotionality, and expressions of suffering. Many teens are able to explore these subcultures safely without engaging in harmful behavior, but vulnerable adolescents in these subcultures may find unhealthy ways of expressing their troubles or practice harmful behavior to feel more connected to the group.

Risk Factors for Self-Injury

Several factors place a teen at risk for cutting or other forms of self-harm (see sidebar 19.4). Psychiatric illness is the most important of these risk factors. Self-injury is associated with several underlying psychiatric disorders, including mood disorders, anxiety disorders, eating disorders, psychotic disorders, conduct disorder, and posttraumatic stress disorder. Self-injury is often seen in people who have borderline personality disorder, which may begin to emerge during adolescence (see chapter 13). Teens with OCD may injure themselves in an attempt to rid themselves of intrusive thoughts. Teens with developmental disorders, such as autism, may engage in behaviors such as head banging, biting, or hitting themselves.

Certain aspects of teens' individual psychological makeup may make them more vulnerable to self-injury. These include high levels of impulsivity, poor social skills, low self-esteem, and limited coping skills. Furthermore, self-injurious behavior has been shown to be associated with other risk-taking behaviors, such as substance abuse and unprotected sex.

Demographic factors related to self-harm include a history of neglect, physical or sexual abuse, and a family history of suicide or self-injury. Although it was previously believed that females engage in these behaviors more frequently than males do, some experts

---

Sidebar 19.4 | Risk Factors for Self-Injurious Behavior

- ► Underlying psychiatric illness
- ► Low self-esteem
- ► Impaired social skills
- ► Immature or rigid psychological defenses
- ► Impulsivity and risk-taking behavior, including substance abuse
- ► History of abuse or neglect
- ► Family history of suicide or self-injurious behavior

now think that the phenomenon occurs just as often in males. However, it is more likely to be identified in females.

How to Address Self-Injurious Behavior

Before self-harm can be addressed, it needs to be recognized. As previously noted, while some teens may injure themselves in front of parents in an attempt to communicate their distress, most often they are secretive. Teens are frequently ashamed of the behavior or fearful of how others will react. Thus, it is helpful for parents to recognize warning signs of self-injury, which are described in sidebar 19.5. When a parent becomes aware of self-injurious behavior, it is best to address it directly with the teen. This may be uncomfortable, but it is important for teens to know that their parents are concerned and wish to open a dialogue.

A psychiatric evaluation is generally indicated when a problem with self-injury has been identified. If the problem is mild—perhaps one or two episodes of very superficial scratches—and the teen appears to be doing well, then it may be reasonable to take a watch-and-wait approach. Teens may experiment with the behavior, decide it is "stupid," and not continue. However, parents should know that the self-harm that they see may be the tip of the iceberg. There may be other behaviors that the teen is hiding. Moreover, self-injury is similar to addictions and substance abuse. It is easier to stop when it is treated early in its course, before the pattern is ingrained. Thus, parents should have a low threshold for seeking a professional opinion.

An evaluation of self-injurious behavior is usually completed as an outpatient. Although these behaviors do not commonly represent suicidal thoughts, in some instances, they are associated with suicidal thinking and other safety concerns.

Sidebar 19.5 | Warning Signs of Self-Injurious Behavior

▶ Frequent cuts, burns, or other injuries that are unexplained or explained by unlikely excuses
▶ Appearance of cuts with a more regular, deliberate appearance than typical accidental injuries, e.g., a series of parallel straight lines on the forearm or round burn marks from cigarettes
▶ Several cuts in the same part of the body in different stages of healing
▶ Attempts to hide injuries, e.g., wearing long-sleeve shirts or long pants in warm weather or covering cuts with armbands
▶ Finding razor blades, box cutters, or knives in the teen's room
▶ Change in interests, with preoccupation with music, clothing, movies, or websites that have dark, morbid themes
▶ General signs of psychological distress, including depressed mood, social withdrawal, changes in behavior, lack of motivation, and decline in school performance

An urgent safety evaluation, such as at an emergency room, may be necessary if the self-injurious behavior is escalating and out of control, if it has potential to cause serious harm, or if it is associated with other serious signs of a severe psychiatric problem, including threats of suicide or dramatic changes in behavior.

If an adolescent has cutting behaviors, then the psychiatric evaluation should be thorough and include an examination of possible underlying psychiatric disorders. It should include an assessment of the teen's overall safety, including suicidal thoughts. Following the review, the psychiatrist or therapist should propose a treatment plan for addressing the problem.

An adolescent's pediatrician should be aware if the teen is regularly engaging in self-harm. A medical evaluation may be needed for deep cuts, which may require suturing and dressing and possibly a booster immunization of tetanus. If there is infection, antibiotics may be indicated. Teens who punch walls may sustain a boxer fracture of their hand and may require x-ray studies.

Just as there is no single reason why teens engage in self-harm, there is no one-size-fits-all solution. The treatment plan will depend on the underlying psychiatric problem as well as the psychological, social, academic, and family factors that may be driving the behavior. For many adolescents, self-harm resolves when the underlying condition, such as depression, is treated. For others, the problem is like an addiction and may require specific treatment.

Dialectical behavioral therapy (DBT) is one of the most effective treatments for adolescents who engage in self-injurious behavior. DBT is a structured treatment that is similar to cognitive behavioral therapy. It helps adolescents learn to tolerate strong emotions and build coping skills so they are able to deal with distress without resorting to harmful behaviors. When a teen does engage in an unhealthy behavior such as cutting, a DBT therapist may ask him or her to perform a "chain analysis." In this process, the therapist and the teen review in detail the events that led up to the behavior. Together, the therapist and the teen identify ways in which the teen could have acted differently and prevented the behavior.

Even when DBT is not employed, treatment may incorporate some of the same elements, including coping skills and exploring the triggers for self-injury. If teens are able to develop coping skills, the urge to cut or otherwise harm themselves may pass after a few minutes. Coping skills may include talking to a parent or other support, deep breathing, yoga, exercise, listening to music, writing, drawing, or even taking a shower. Other teens need physical sensation when they experience the urge to harm themselves. Benign actions that may be substituted for the harmful ones include wearing a rubber band around the wrist that can be snapped or holding an ice cube in one's hand.

Parents can help to prevent teens' self-harm by discarding or securing as many of the sharp objects in the household as possible. Those that are not used frequently, such as box cutters, safety pins, or knitting needles, should be placed in a locked drawer or cabinet. Those objects used on a regular basis, such as scissors or kitchen knives, can be kept in a central location. Parents should periodically check to see if anything is missing.

Teens who cut or burn themselves may stash their favorite instruments in their rooms or elsewhere in the house. Or adolescents may carry the objects around with them in their purse or backpack. Part of keeping your teen safe and making it harder for him or her to cut or burn is to remove these objects. This may be a difficult undertaking, as teens who are ambivalent about stopping the harmful behavior are unlikely to surrender these objects willingly. Still, it is best to give teens the opportunity to turn the objects over to you. After teens have cut themselves, part of the discussion should include asking them what instruments they used. Tell your teen that you would like him or her to give you the instruments. For those teens unwilling to turn over these items, a search of their belongings may be necessary. It is important to weigh the violation of adolescents' privacy with the need to maintain their safety. Parents may wish to discuss this issue with the adolescent's therapist.

Ultimately, there is no quick fix for self-injurious behaviors. As with most psychiatric problems, it takes time and dedication to treatment before the problem resolves. This may be frustrating for parents. Teens who have been engaging in relatively minor forms of self-harm or who have engaged in the behavior for shorter periods of time are more likely to improve sooner. Sometimes, teens stop self-injury almost immediately after entering treatment. After they know that their problems are being addressed, they are able to discontinue these behaviors. For others, it may take years for the behavior to come under control, with periods of remission and relapse in times of stress. The good news is that the vast majority of adolescents who self-harm manage to overcome this problem before they reach adulthood. Teens who have or develop chronic psychiatric conditions, including borderline personality disorder, pervasive developmental disorders, schizophrenia, or chronic mood disorders, are at greater risk of having self-injurious behavior persist into adulthood.

Violent Behavior

Although most teens are not violent, violent and aggressive behavior reaches a peak during adolescence. This is probably related to developmental factors, including rapid physical, emotional, and hormonal changes, growing independence from parents, shifts in social relationships, and high levels of risk taking and impulsivity. Violence during adolescence can encompass a broad range of behaviors, from shoving in the school halls to use of deadly weapons, and it can occur for a broad variety of reasons.

Sidebar 19.6 | Risk Factors for Teen Violence

- ▶ History of violent behavior in the past
- ▶ Substance abuse
- ▶ Male gender
- ▶ History of exposure to violence, including physical abuse or witnessing domestic abuse
- ▶ Poor school performance
- ▶ Delinquent behaviors, such as truancy, shoplifting, or other crimes
- ▶ Untreated psychiatric illness, especially with symptoms of restlessness, agitation, impulsiveness, and angry or irritable mood
- ▶ History of brain injury or cognitive impairment
- ▶ Poor relationship with parents
- ▶ History of harsh discipline by parents, including physical discipline
- ▶ Lack of parental supervision
- ▶ Little connection to school or community
- ▶ High degree of violence in the school or community
- ▶ Association with delinquent peer group
- ▶ Gang involvement

Risk Factors

Violence is usually the result of a complex interplay between various factors in the teen's life (see sidebar 19.6). These include environmental, family, and individual dynamics. Addressing an adolescent's violent behavior requires an understanding of the particular combination of forces that are driving the behavior and taking appropriate measures to address them. Treating one aspect of the problem, such as trying to address individual factors through psychotherapy, without addressing the others, such as appropriate family and community interventions, is unlikely to be successful.

Violence and the Media

An area of concern for most parents is teens' exposure to violence in the media, including movies, television shows, and video games. Teens' exposure to violent media has grown exponentially in recent decades with the rise of cable television, increasingly sophisticated (and graphic) video games, and the Internet. But for all the attention that has been paid to the question of whether exposure to violent media increases the risk of violent behavior, there continues to be a great deal of controversy among experts in this field.

The relationship of media violence and adolescent violent behavior is difficult to study. Exposure to violent media is hard to quantify. In addition, adolescent violent behavior is relatively uncommon and difficult to use as an outcome measure in a study. Researchers try to measure violent thoughts, although these are also difficult to quantify. Even if it could be shown that violent thoughts and actions are clearly associated with watching violent media, it is not always clear that there is a causal relationship. It seems likely that youth who have a predisposition toward violent behavior may migrate toward violent imagery when they watch television or choose a video game. This does not necessarily mean that the imagery caused the violent behavior. It may actually be the other way around.

Existing studies of this issue have shown conflicting results, which may in part be due to differences in the ways these studies were designed. Overall, when results from multiple studies are combined in what is called a "meta-analysis," it appears that watching violent media does cause increases in short-term aggressive thoughts and behaviors. But when exposure is repeated, it is not clear whether these short-term increases are sustained. It also seems that not all adolescents are affected equally by exposure to media violence. There is some evidence that teens who have other risk factors may be more susceptible.

Based on this conflicting and uncertain evidence, a parent should set reasonable limits on an adolescent's "screen time" (time in front of the television or computer). In general, it is a good practice to be aware of what your teen is viewing. Pay attention to the ratings given to video games in which your child expresses interest. Titles rated "M" (for mature) are deemed appropriate for players seventeen and older, though many younger teens play these games. More importantly, try to obtain a sampling of your child's media diet. For example, watch your child play a new video game, and try to watch at least one episode of the television shows that your child enjoys. It is helpful to talk to your teen about the game or show. Consider asking what he or she likes about it and what he or she thinks about the violence that is portrayed.

Parents should not be afraid to set reasonable limits on the violent media content that their children are allowed to watch, since vulnerable teens may be more susceptible to the effects of this violence. Thus, stricter limits may be appropriate for teens who have a history of a major psychiatric or developmental disorder, have difficulty distinguishing fantasy from reality, or have a past history of aggressive behavior or other risk factors for future violence.

Violence and Psychiatric Illness

The causes of violence are complex, and violent behavior in an adolescent is not necessary a sign of psychiatric illness. Most adolescents suffering from psychiatric illness are not violent. However, psychiatric illness may place some teens at greater risk for violent behavior. Symptoms such as agitation, restlessness, insomnia, and increased impulsivity may cause an at-risk adolescent to commit a violent act. When a psychiatric disorder is one of the factors involved in a teen's violent or aggressive behavior, it is important to obtain help for the problem as soon as possible.

Certain psychiatric disorders, such as conduct disorder, are associated with a greater risk of violent or aggressive behavior than others are. Adolescents with substance abuse disorders are another high-risk group for violence. This violence may occur due to the lack of inhibition that can result from intoxication, as well as the agitation and restlessness that can occur with withdrawal from some substances. There may be underlying risk factors, such as poor social support and a delinquent peer group, that place a teen at risk for both violence and substance abuse.

Teens with bipolar disorder, particularly when they are in a manic or mixed mood state, are often explosive and impulsive. Consequently, they have the potential to become violent. Adolescents with psychotic disorders may also become violent under certain circumstances, especially if they experience paranoid delusions. Youth with cognitive impairments and significant developmental delay may demonstrate aggressive behavior related to a high level of impulsivity or difficulty finding productive ways of having their needs met. Finally, there is some evidence to suggest that ADHD may be associated with increased aggressive behavior, as teens with the disorder may act without thinking. When aggressive behavior is accompanied by other warning signs of psychiatric illness or occurs with little provocation, a thorough psychiatric evaluation is warranted.

How to Address Violent Behavior

The best approach to violence is to prevent it from happening (see sidebar 19.7). In addition to seeking psychiatric help when a teen shows signs of struggling, parents should work to make their home a violence-free zone. By teaching young children that aggressive behavior is not acceptable, you can begin this process well before adolescence. Throughout childhood, set firm and consistent limits on aggressive behavior, and enforce consequences, such as loss of privileges or time-outs. Adolescents are better equipped to deal with overwhelming emotions if they have already learned ways of coping with anger. Teaching young children practices such as counting to ten or separating themselves from a frustrating situation until they calm down helps them learn to regulate themselves.

Children learn by modeling. Physical discipline, such as spanking, is associated with higher levels of violent behavior later in life. Similarly, violent or aggressive behavior in the home, regardless of whether the victim is the child, a spouse, or someone outside the family, predisposes a child to violence during the adolescent years.

When compared to adults, teens may not have the same biological capacity to manage aggressive impulses and make good decisions in a time of high emotion. Evidence from brain imaging studies has shown that the frontal lobe, the part of the brain just behind the forehead that helps to control impulses and evaluate decisions (among other important roles), is not yet mature. Parents should

---

Sidebar 19.7 | **Steps to Address Teen Violence**

- ▸ Prevent violence beginning in early childhood by
    - ▸ Modeling a nonviolent household
    - ▸ Limiting exposure to violent video games, movies, TV shows, etc.
    - ▸ Teaching nonviolent ways of dealing with anger
- ▸ Address underlying psychiatric issues or substance abuse problems by bringing your teen for an evaluation
- ▸ Consider potential educational problems, such as an unrecognized learning disorder, that may be contributing to the violence, and arrange for school evaluation and intervention when appropriate
- ▸ Learn to recognize your teen's nonverbal communication, including signs that he or she may be about to lose control
- ▸ De-escalate situations by ending interactions that get too heated and suggesting a time-out to cool down
- ▸ During a calm period, discuss your teen's anger and help him or her identify ways of staying in control and calming down when upset, including your teen's ideas about what you can do to help
- ▸ Be clear that violent or aggressive behavior is not tolerated, and consistently enforce consequences (e.g., grounding, loss of screen time) for these behaviors
- ▸ Call the police or emergency medical services (911) if a teen is out of control or a situation feels unsafe
- ▸ Design a multifaceted approach to addressing the problem, including possible mix of psychiatric treatment, school-based interventions, involvement in sports or other activities, social skills groups, family therapy, or parent guidance
- ▸ Consider voluntary involvement of social services agencies or the juvenile justice system

---

be aware of this physiological factor and try to de-escalate emotionally intense situations.

While trying to calm things down when they are getting heated makes common sense, in practice many parents do just the opposite. When arguing with a teen about an important issue, parents often become emotional and raise their voices or give nonverbal cues that they are becoming angry. This, of course, can escalate the situation. Parents may be afraid of backing down, fearing that then the teen will not learn an important lesson. Adolescents are better able to absorb a message from parents when the issue is discussed at a time when both sides are calm (and sober). Persisting in an argument when you or your teen is extremely upset is unlikely to lead to a successful resolution of the issue and may tip predisposed teens over into aggression.

To avoid conflicts that result in violence, it helps to recognize your child's warning signals. Many teens demonstrate certain patterns of behavior when they are about to explode. They may pace, suddenly get quiet, clench their jaw, squeeze their fists, and/or breathe rapidly. Being tuned in to these nonverbal signals can help parents know when it is time to let things cool down before continuing the discussion. As a parent, it is also important to be aware of your own physical and emotional reactions. Maintaining a calm voice and continuing to appear relaxed and in control, rather than pacing or gesturing angrily, can help to de-escalate a situation.

When an argument begins to get too heated, it is best to end the discussion and allow you and your teen to calm down. On occasion, teens will recognize when they are becoming too upset and go to their room or elsewhere to calm down. As long as you know they are going somewhere safe, it is best to let them go. If you are the one who needs a cool-down, it is best to say so to your child, rather than simply to walk away. Adolescents may have an intense fear of being abandoned or cut off from their parent. Abruptly ending the conversation or leaving the room may cause them to become more angry or anxious. Instead, say something short, simple, and definitive, such as "I think we're both too upset to have a useful conversation about this right now. Let's take some time to cool down and talk about it later."

When a situation escalates into violent or threatening behavior, parents should do what they need to do to maintain safety. When the aggressive behavior is brief and contained, such as a shove or an object thrown against the wall, it may be best to try to let your teen cool down. Later, appropriate consequences for the behavior should be enforced. In situations that do not feel safe or in which a teen is out of control, it may be necessary to dial 911 or call the police. Understandably, many parents are reluctant to take such actions. They may fear that their child will then have a criminal record; they may not want involvement by the state social services agency. Most of the time, these fears are unfounded. Failing to call emergency services when a teen is out of control can place the family and the teen at risk of serious harm. Furthermore, it can send the message to teens that violence will be tolerated by parents.

If a teen's violent behavior may be related to a psychiatric illness or substance abuse, a psychiatric evaluation at an emergency room may be required. Police or an ambulance should transport adolescents who are not safe to travel with their parents. This evaluation can help determine whether a teen is safe to return home or whether he or she requires psychiatric hospitalization or other forms of intensive treatment to maintain everyone's safety.

At the emergency room, it is important for parents to tell the staff if their child has the potential to become violent or has a history of aggressive behavior. If possible, inform the staff if there are triggers or warning signs for the aggressive behavior.

In certain situations, medications may be given to help your child stay calm and safe. The medication may be sedating, such as diphenhydramine (Benadryl) or a benzodiazepine such as lorazepam (Ativan). For teens who are suffering from bipolar disorder or who are showing signs of psychosis, an atypical antipsychotic medication may be appropriate. Often, the safest and most effective medicine is one that the teen already takes or has taken with good effect in the past.

When the acute situation has passed, focus should be redirected to the prevention of future violent outbursts. Just as violent behavior has many causes, the treatment approach may take many forms. A multifaceted approach is the most effective. This may involve treatment of underlying psychiatric disorders, teaching anger management and problem-solving skills in psychotherapy, addressing school problems through special education programs, family therapy to reduce conflict or offer guidance to parents, and the teen's involvement in positive activities such as sports or community programs. On occasion, voluntary involvement of institutions such as the juvenile justice system or the state department of social services is useful. Appearing before a judge and assigning a probation officer can show aggressive teens that there are potential consequences to their actions, and social services agencies may recognize the need for home-based treatment. Particular attention should be paid to the safety of the home environment for those teens with potential for violence.

Conclusion

Safety is frequently the greatest concern for parents of adolescents suffering from psychiatric illness. Suicidal thoughts and attempts, self-harm, and violence all reach a peak in frequency during the adolescent years, before decreasing in early adulthood. The causes of these behaviors are complex, and therefore, the treatment tends to be multifaceted, with potential interventions involving home, school, the community, and outside agencies or institutions. Although these issues may be frightening, it is important that parents not ignore them in the hope that they will resolve on their own. Rather, by learning about warning signs, listening, staying attuned to a teen's experience, and seeking help when needed, parents can help maintain their families' safety.

References and Additional Reading

Aseltine, R. H., E. A. Schilling, A. James, J. L. Glanovsky, and D. Jacobs. 2009. "Age Variability in the Association between Heavy Episodic Drinking and Adolescent Suicide Attempts: Findings from a Large-Scale, School-Based Screening Program." *Journal of the American Academy of Child and Adolescent Psychiatry* 48: 262–270.

Borowsky, I. W., M. Ireland, and M. D. Resnick. 2001. "Adolescent Suicide Attempts: Risks and Protectors." *Pediatrics* 107: 485–493.

Bridge, J. A., N. L. Day, R. Day, G. A. Richardson, B. Birmaher, and D. A. Brent. 2003. "Major Depressive Disorder in Adolescents Exposed to a Friend's Suicide." *Journal of the American Academy of Child and Adolescent Psychiatry* 42: 1294–1300.

Garofalo, R., C. R. Wolf, L. S. Wissow, E. R. Woods, and E. Goodman. 1999. "Sexual Orientation and Risk of Suicide Attempts among a Representative Sample of Youth." *Archives of Pediatrics and Adolescent Medicine* 153: 487–493.

Klomek, A. B., A. Sourander, S. Niemela, K. Kumpulainen, J. Piha, T. Tamminen, F. Almqvist, and M. Gould. 2009. "Childhood Bullying Behaviors as a Risk for Suicide Attempts and Completed Suicides: A Population-Based Birth Cohort Study." *Journal of the American Academy of Child and Adolescent Psychiatry* 48: 254–261.

Silenzio, V.M.B., J. B. Pena, P. R. Duberstein, J. Cerel, and K. L. Knox. 2007. "Sexual Orientation and Risk Factors for Suicidal Ideation and Suicide Attempts among Adolescents and Young Adults." *American Journal of Public Health* 97: 2017–2019.

20 Autism Spectrum Disorders

Charles Henry, M.D.

In the 1940s, Leo Kanner used the term "infantile autism" to describe a group of children in his psychiatric practice who had trouble with social development, rigid behaviors, and communication delays. Despite considerable research that has occurred since then, Kanner's initial descriptions have remained central to the modern diagnosis of autism. Autism was originally thought to be a rare disorder, with investigations during the 1980s indicating an incidence of about 1 in 2,500 children. More recent studies, however, have raised concern about a potential increase in the number of children suffering from the disorder. Data from the Centers for Disease Control and Prevention note an incidence of autistic disorders of 1 in every 150 individuals. Though most researchers believe that the increase is in large part related to a greater awareness of the disorder, an actual increase in the real numbers of children with autism cannot be excluded as a possibility. What might be causing such an increase has been the source of much controversy and research, making autism a disorder that has captured a significant amount of public attention. Regardless of the controversy, there is overwhelming evidence that autism is a genetic disorder, and though there may be environmental triggers, it is clear that recent suspects such as childhood vaccines or the preservative thimerosal do not cause autism.

While autism has been the cornerstone diagnosis of children afflicted with autistic symptoms, there are five related illnesses that now fall within a broader category of autistic disorders called pervasive developmental disorders (PDD), with autism being the most common illness in the PDD group. Asperger's disorder, though not as common as autism, makes up a significant proportion of children with PDDs. Children with this diagnosis struggle with socialization and behavioral rigidity, like those with autism, but they have relatively little trouble with language. These children may have some impairment in eye-to-eye contact, facial expressions, body postures, or gestures that help to regulate and facilitate social interactions. Childhood disintegrative disorder is a rare illness that occurs in children after several years of normal development; children with the disorder undergo severe regression in social and communicative skills. Rett syndrome usually affects girls, who lose muscle tone, demonstrate repetitive movements, and have disorders of cognition, speech, and socialization. Children who have some milder symptoms of autism but who do not fit into any of the four categories may be given the diagnosis of pervasive developmental disorder not otherwise specified, or PDD-NOS.

Case Presentation

Jack was a fourteen-year-old boy who was diagnosed with autism when he was eighteen months old. When he was one year old, his parents became convinced that he did not respond to his name. He also did not seem interested in making eye contact or pointing at things for his parents to see; he was more curious about inanimate toys and would line up toy cars and trains when playing. When excited, he would frequently flap his hands in a manner that seemed unusual to his parents.

After Jack's pediatrician made the diagnosis, Jack was referred to a pediatric neurologist, who agreed with the diagnosis and made various treatment recommendations. Jack began to receive speech and language therapy, occupational therapy, and a specialized form of behavioral treatment called applied behavioral analysis. He continued in such intensive educational programming throughout elementary and middle school, making significant gains in his language, behavioral flexibility, and social skills. Though he had trouble forming friendships, Jack would at times spontaneously interact with his peers and could engage in some basic conversations around his areas of interest—country music and vacuum cleaners. When greeting new classmates, he would compulsively ask them what model vacuum cleaner they had at home. Despite being instructed to avoid such questions, he had difficulty controlling this obsessive habit.

Jack started ninth grade at his local high school, which had many more children than his prior school did. His class schedule varied daily, and he was required to change rooms on a regular basis. Jack was mainstreamed with the assistance of a part-time aide, and he was receiving pull-out services for academic support in reading and math.

After Jack had fully entered puberty, he became more aware of girls but was awkward in managing interactions with them. Once, and out of character for Jack, he inappropriately touched a girl, who was quite uncomfortable with the incident and reported it to a teacher. Jack's parents were informed about the situation and were quite upset. When this incident was addressed with Jack, he had trouble giving an account of it and became very anxious. He stated that he would never do such a thing again. Despite this statement, he repeated the behavior two weeks later with the same girl. With male peers, Jack had intermittent interactions but was largely isolated. A group of boys picked on him, calling him a freak and making jokes about vacuum cleaners.

Over the past year, Jack had been more anxious and agitated at home. He had always had some trouble with tantrums, particularly when there were unexpected changes in his schedule or his routine. But now that Jack was physically bigger and more intimidating, his parents, especially his mother, were becoming somewhat afraid of him when he was upset. Once, while his mother was trying to take him to an unanticipated appointment with his pediatrician, Jack became agitated and forcefully shoved her. She was quite frightened and yelled at Jack. Jack was initially apologetic, but within an hour, he acted as if nothing had happened. Since this incident, Jack had been obsessively looking up information about violent crimes on the Web.

The family arranged an evaluation by a child psychiatrist, who met with both Jack and his parents. The psychiatrist determined that Jack's current educational program was not appropriate. The doctor recommended a therapeutic classroom setting that specialized in children with PDDs and language disabilities. He also suggested that Jack begin work with a social skills group, with some focus being paid to managing relationships with female peers. His parents received coaching assistance from a behavioral consultant on how to deal with Jack's disruptiveness at home. Regarding his being a victim of bullying, Jack's parents were told to address the situation with the school administration. The doctor discussed medication treatment options, but it was agreed to hold off on this type of therapy while the impact of the other interventions was evaluated.

Children with autism may be affected to variable degrees. Some have severe symptoms, with great trouble functioning socially and academically, and others have much milder symptoms, performing at potentially high levels. These children are often labeled as having high-functioning autism.

Autism and Medical Issues

Although the majority of children and adolescents with autism do not have an associated medical condition, a very small number of children with autistic symptoms may have a chromosomal condition called fragile X syndrome (FSX). This condition is transmitted on the X chromosome; females have milder symptoms than males do. There may be ear or facial physical anomalies in children who have this condition. Physicians may consider evaluation for FXS when they are contemplating the diagnosis of autism; otherwise, no specific medical diagnostic workup is needed.

Some people have theorized a relationship between autism and childhood vaccinations. A number of national organizations including the American Academy of Pediatrics, the Centers for Disease Control, and the Institute of Medicine of the National Academy of Sciences have taken a stand on this issue. Reviews of many scientific studies have shown no evidence of a relationship between childhood vaccines, thimerosal (mercury), and autism. The U.S. Court of Federal Claims found in February 2009 that the scientific evidence is "overwhelmingly contrary" to the theory that the measles, mumps, and rubella vaccine and the vaccine preservative thimerosal are linked to autism. In February 2010, the British medical journal *Lancet* formally retracted a report published in 1998 suggesting a possible relationship between childhood immunizations and autism.

Symptoms and Warning Signs

Autism is generally diagnosed in early childhood, as the symptoms are often striking and evident at a young age (sidebar 20.1). Kanner's triad of symptoms describes the core symptoms of autism. Starting with the socialization difficulties, autistic children have trouble engaging in interactions with others. Nonverbal social functions, such as eye contact and body postures and gestures, are almost always impaired. These children will look off to objects in a room and avoid focusing attention on others who are present. In addition, they do not spontaneously demonstrate a wish to share interests with others; they also seem to have trouble appreciating the internal experiences and feelings of others.

This difficulty that autistic children have in appreciating the perspective of others is sometimes referred to as a theory of mind deficit. With this impair-

---

Sidebar 20.1 | Core Diagnostic Symptom Classes of Autistic Disorders

The diagnosis of autism requires impairments in all three symptom areas, with onset of impaired social interactions, social language, and imaginative play prior to three years of age. Asperger's disorder does not involve serious language delay. The PDD-NOS diagnosis is used when autistic symptoms are present but not enough to give a formal diagnosis of autism or Asperger's disorder (or other related psychiatric disorders). The core symptoms are as follows (not all symptoms in each cluster are necessary for an autistic diagnosis):

1. Impairment in social interaction:
   a. marked difficulty in the use of nonverbal behaviors such as eye to-eye gaze, facial expression, body postures, and gestures that are normally involved in social interaction
   b. failure to develop peer relationships appropriate to developmental level of the child
   c. a lack of spontaneous seeking to share enjoyment, interests, or achievements with other people, such as a lack of showing, bringing, or pointing out objects of interest
   d. lack of social reciprocity, as manifested by not participating in simple social play or preferring solitary activities
2. Impairments in communication (these symptoms are not involved in the diagnosis of Asperger's disorder):
   a. delay in, or total lack of, the development of spoken language, without an attempt to communicate through other means such as gesture or mime
   b. in individuals with adequate speech, marked difficulty in the ability to initiate or sustain a conversation with others
   c. stereotyped, idiosyncratic, or repetitive uses of language that are not directly relevant to the social context
   d. lack of varied, spontaneous make-believe play or social imitative play appropriate to the developmental level of the child
3. Restricted repetitive and stereotyped patterns of behavior, interests, and activities:
   a. preoccupation in stereotyped and restricted interests, with an abnormal intensity or focus such as amassing facts about meteorology or baseball statistics
   b. apparently inflexible adherence to specific routines or rituals that have no clear function
   c. stereotyped and repetitive motor manners such as hand/finger flapping or body rocking
   d. persistent preoccupation with parts of objects such as buttons or parts of the body

Symptom criteria are not included for Rett's disorder and childhood disintegrative disorder.

---

ment, an individual has problems appreciating that others view the world in varying ways. A classic research experiment to test mind abilities involves a social story called the Sally-Anne task. In the illustration, Sally is playing marbles with Anne. While Anne and Sally are still playing together, Sally puts her marble in her own basket and leaves the room. While Sally is away, Anne takes the marble from Sally's basket and puts it in her own basket. Sally then returns to the room. The question for the child is, "Where does Sally think that her marble is?" The correct answer is that Sally thinks the marble is in her own basket because she did not witness the moving of the marble by Anne. Children with autism have trouble with this task, tending to answer that the marble is in Anne's basket, as they have a hard time appreciating that Sally would not have been able to see what Anne was doing. The impairment in performing this task references a fundamental struggle experienced by autistic children. Relating in a social world becomes very difficult when one is not able to see things from the perspectives of other people.

Another core symptom domain of children with autism centers on limitations in their behavioral activities. Children with autism may have a need for sameness, with strong narrow interests, attention to detail, and a tendency to engage in repetitive behaviors. They might obsessively order personal items in an exacting manner or repeatedly watch specific scenes from a recorded video. The 1988 movie *Rain Man,* in which Dustin Hoffman portrays a young adult with autism named Raymond Babbitt, provides many excellent examples of these types of behaviors. In one scene, Ray is at a diner with his brother, played by Tom Cruise. Ray articulates to his brother that Tuesday is pancake day. He goes on to state that along with his pancakes, he needs to have maple syrup and toothpicks. The maple syrup, though, has to come before the pancakes. When it looks as if this expected course is not going to proceed as anticipated, Ray becomes loud, agitated, and disruptive with his brother. Such schedule fixations, with associated anxiety, are commonplace with autism.

Finally, children with autism have significant difficulties with communications and language development. There may be a wide range of language impairment. Some autistic children have severe problems and may only be able to approximate simple words with oral language or may rely on nonverbal signs. Others have only mild communication symptoms that are primarily evident with more abstract and self-referential language. Social conversation flow is generally disjointed and awkward. They may parrot back language that is spoken to them or repeat stereotypic phrases in a manner that is out of context. The development of imaginary play is also delayed. Classically, the autistic child may stare at a spinning fan as opposed to playing with dolls or imitating life with cars or trucks. Of importance, children diagnosed with Asperger's disorder have overall normal function with respect to language and may even have an exaggerated skill in this area.

While the diagnosis of autism is given based on the presence of these core symptoms, autistic children may struggle with other symptoms. For example, these children often have a variety of sensory-motor difficulties. Motor planning and coordination skills are frequently affected. Sensory processing may be peculiar. Occasionally these children will experience sensory stimuli that feel uncomfortable or irritating. Loud noises, unusual food textures, and bright lights may be agitating. On the other hand, the abnormal sensory processing may at times be advantageous to an individual with autism. In Temple Grandin's book

Thinking in Pictures (an obvious reference to sensory processing differences), the author describes how her unique experience of visual information enabled her to problem solve in creative ways during her work with animals.

Due to the ongoing core social difficulties and language impairment struggles of children with autism, they will often have trouble with attention. Attention becomes nearly impossible when social engagement is minimal and language abilities are limited. Nevertheless, there are probably other reasons that also account for the attentional difficulties. In addition, hyperactivity is common in children with autistic disorders. These children may have a great deal of difficulty sitting still and may frequently pace, sometimes with associated hand flapping. Although a separate diagnosis of attention-deficit/hyperactivity disorder (ADHD) is not possible with children who have a PDD diagnosis, recent estimates suggest that approximately 25 percent of children with a PDD diagnosis could also be given a diagnosis of ADHD based on the presence of symptoms.

Anxiety symptoms are also common in children with autistic disorders. Over 40 percent of these children may suffer from significant anxiety symptoms typical of specific anxiety disorders. Frequent causes of anxiety include a change of routine, exposure to new settings, and contact with large groups of people. The anxiety may be severe at times, leading to limitations in functioning and academic underperformance.

As previously noted, autistic children may occasionally become aggressive, with this behavior directed at others or occasionally toward themselves. Most of the time the behavior is mild and short-lived. Simple and straightforward limits are usually able to contain the behavior. Occasionally, the aggression is harder to manage. Parents and school staff may be challenged with this level disruptiveness. Changes in school placement and consultation with a behaviorist may be considered along with the possible use of psychiatric medications.

Finally, children with autism are often classified as intellectually impaired. Studies have estimated that about 75 percent of these children could be classified as having a separate diagnosis of mental retardation. However, it is very difficult to assess autistic children with standard IQ measures. Verbal difficulties can hinder their test performance. It is generally thought that many of these children are very intelligent, but their skills are difficult to access. In some cases, autistic individuals may have exceptionally developed skills in contrast to their overall abilities. The term "savant" or "autistic savant" may be used to describe such individuals. Examples of autistic savants include the accomplished musician Tony DeBlois. He graduated from the Berklee College of Music despite being blind and having severe autistic symptoms. Reportedly, he can play over eight thousand songs from memory. Daniel Tammet, subject of the Science Channel documentary *Brainman*, is a savant with Asperger's disorder who has been blessed with some amazing talents. Perhaps his most well-known feat has been his reciting of the numerical value of pi to over twenty-two thousand digits.

Special Challenges during Adolescence

For autistic children, adolescence can be particularly challenging. Limitations with social relatedness, odd mannerisms and interests, and language difficulties make it hard for them to manage this developmental period. In addition, like all adolescents, they are experiencing changes in their body appearance and an intensification of sexual feelings, as well as potential aggressive tendencies. "Typical" children manage these internal changes as they relate to their peers and develop means of expressing their sexual and aggressive feelings in ways that are socially appropriate. This may be a daunting task for someone with autistic symptoms.

Common problems that may occur as an autistic child moves through adolescence include inappropriate aggressive and sexual actions. As the adolescent has become physically larger and more intimidating, tantrums become more problematic. Further, internal aggressive drives have intensified as part of adolescent development. This combination leads to a not uncommon scenario in which an autistic adolescent is too disruptive for the family or school to handle. At that point, various treatment interventions may be considered, including medication options along with consultation with a behaviorist or a possible change in school placement. Though not the usual case, psychiatric hospitalization may be necessary in order to contain more severe forms of aggression. While there are reports of extreme violence that have taken place in adolescents with PDDs, such incidents are very rare.

Adolescents with autism may express sexual feelings in a way that can cause significant trouble for them. They may make inappropriate gestures or comments to others. Normally these incidents are mild and occur only once or twice. But some autistic adolescents have a hard time controlling this behavior and may even enjoy the reaction from others. Likewise, dating for the autistic adolescent is a rather complicated venture. Despite their social difficulties, higher-functioning autistic children and those with Asperger's disorder will date. Significant support is often necessary, with a focus on sex education, including information on safer sexual practices. These adolescents will also probably need help with the management of emotions during relationships.

With the intensification of aggressive and sexual feelings in autistic adolescents, there may be increased anxiety and impulsive behavior. These teens may be very uncomfortable with such feelings and wrestle with them more internally than externally. They may ruminate about their angry or sexual feelings in a way that is not obvious to those around them. Only upon appropriate questioning will the reason for their elevated anxiety levels become evident.

Although adolescents with autism may have somewhat limited social awareness, high-functioning teens may feel troubled by their social alienation. If such an adolescent has some insight into his or her limitations, these symptoms may be particularly intense. Moreover, the peer struggles that are often elevated during adolescence may affect autistic teens in ways that could cause depressive symptoms. To a more socially interested PDD teen, repeated rejections can take a toll.

Independent of social and psychiatric challenges, it is important to note that children with autism are at risk of developing seizures during adolescence. About 25 percent of children with autism have had some form of seizure. Adolescence represents a time when seizure activity may increase or new onset seizures may emerge. The seizures may be generalized, involving convulsion over the entire body with a loss of mental functioning. Other types of seizures involve limited abnormal motor movements or alteration of sensory experience or awareness.

Treatment

Educational Interventions

Educational interventions and specialized psychosocial therapies are the backbone of treatment for teens with autistic disorders. These treatments should start at the time of diagnosis, which preferably occurs as early as possible—ideally at less than two years of age. Implementing the interventions involves collaborating with the local school district to develop an appropriate educational plan. Under the Individuals with Disabilities Education Act, a school is required to offer a thorough educational evaluation that provides information to create an individualized education program (IEP). The educational plan must be designed to meet the student's unique educational needs. Necessary services must be delivered until an individual reaches age twenty-two. Testing of cognitive and educational achievement, speech and language, and occupational therapy is generally part of the educational assessment. Depending on the student's presentation, other testing may be necessary. Although a school may work to provide an appropriate academic curriculum for the adolescent, in some cases, the program is not adequate to deal with the teen's needs. When this becomes a concern, parents can seek an independent set of neuropsychological testing as well as speech and language and occupational therapy testing. Consultation with an educational advocate or an educational consultant can help facilitate this process. These second opinions can be crucial in drafting an adequate IEP.

Overall, classroom settings may vary significantly. For youth with more severe forms of autism, a substantially separate classroom with a very low student-teacher ratio is advised. Some integration with peers is often important and should be built into the program. Mixed or integrated classrooms with specialized teacher supports are also common and provide adolescents with significant exposure to their peer group. Typically, in such a setting, an individual aide is necessary. Some children are able to manage in a regular classroom, though frequently an aide and modified course work are required. This situation is generally more appropriate for higher-functioning children.

Behavioral Interventions

Applied behavioral analysis (ABA), originally developed in the 1960s, uses methods that involve the implementation of behavioral reinforcers to promote multiple areas of social and educational functioning in autistic children. There is considerable evidence supporting the role of ABA therapies in the treatment of these children. Strict ABA methods are used for adolescents more severely afflicted with autism. Total time per week for such an adolescent should be at least ten hours at school, with a home-based component for another six hours. Broader uses of behavioral interventions, however, are implemented in higher-functioning autistic adolescents. These interventions may target disruptive, aggressive, or obsessive behaviors by using specific reinforcers depending on the behavior of the child. Behavioral techniques may also be used to help desensitize autistic individuals to situations that could cause significant anxiety. Repeated exposures to the anxiety-provoking setting can help to diminish anxiety. Regardless of the type of behavioral therapy or the severity of the adolescent's symptoms, there should be a trained behaviorist who is experienced in working with children with PDDs and who can offer consultation. This consultation should be provided to both the school classroom and to the teen's parents and should occur at least once a week.

Speech and Language Therapy

Children with autism or Asperger's disorder almost always need ongoing speech and language therapy. These therapies should proceed through adolescence. Depending on the child's needs, therapies may focus on basic communication skills and may require assisted communication methods. Such methods include picture-exchange instruments that rely on direct visual forms of communication or more modern computer-related technologies that use both visual and auditory means of communication. With less extreme forms of speech and language interventions, focus may be centered on language pragmatics. These methods are designed primarily for social speech, with an emphasis on such things as turn taking, attending to verbal and nonverbal cues, and improving eye contact. These treatments should occur both individually and in a small group with one other child. Depending on the severity of the symptoms, the interventions should take place from two to five times per week.

Occupational Therapy

Occupational therapy is another important aspect of an educational program for autistic children. These types of therapy should be tailored to the needs of the individual child. Sensory integration therapies that address the sensory needs of the child may be important, particularly in reducing anxiety and agitation.

Sensory-motor therapies may also be relevant in addressing coordination or motor planning skills. Most PDD children require ongoing occupational therapy through adolescence as part of their IEP. Frequency should vary depending on the child's needs. In general, at least one hour per week of direct therapy should be given. Outside activities such as horseback riding, swimming, and biking can further help develop a child's sensory-motor skills.

Social Skills Interventions

Social skills interventions are a key aspect of behavioral programming for adolescents with PDD. The social challenges of adolescence present a time of significant vulnerabilities for those with autistic disorders. A social skills group headed by a trained facilitator should be part of a child's educational program. This intervention should occur at least once a week and preferably two times a week. The responsibilities for social skills interventions may be shared with the speech and language pathologist. If available, after-school social skills groups may supplement school programming.

Vocational Training

For an adolescent, vocational training should be a key part of the academic curriculum. This programming should involve life-skills training, with an emphasis on building independent living skills. Additionally, work experience should be developed. The school program should form alliances with employers in the area to allow adolescents to gain on-site work exposure. To ensure that the child is developing appropriate skills, the school staff should monitor these experiences closely. College may be an option for some people with autistic disorders. Many colleges now offer more specialized support programs that are designed to deal with special populations such as students with autistic symptoms. An educational consultant can be helpful in planning for a college experience.

Psychotherapy

For high-functioning autistic adolescents or those with Asperger's disorder, individual psychotherapy may be a consideration. This intervention can be particularly helpful for those who are struggling with depressive or anxiety symptoms. The treatment can also be useful for social skills development. The therapist should be comfortable in working with PDD adolescents, as their language and social difficulties may complicate the work.

Medications

Medications may be used to treat symptoms related to PDDs. Though these treatments do not significantly address the core symptoms of autistic disorders, medications can help to manage associated symptoms such as anxiety, aggression, or inattention. Before children begin taking medications, it is important to evaluate whether their existing educational programming is adequate. Medications should not be used to substitute for a bad academic curriculum.

For the treatment of autistic disorders, medications from most of the classes of psychiatric medications may be used (table 20.1; see chapter 5 for further information). Though some medications have significant research supporting their effectiveness, only risperidone and aripiprazole have been approved by the FDA for use in autistic children. For those autistic patients with significant irritability, risperidone and aripiprazole have been shown to be quite effective. Despite their potential usefulness, these two medications can have noteworthy side effects: 15 percent or more of children treated with risperidone or aripiprazole experience weight gain. Regular blood testing for evidence of elevated blood sugar and fats is also necessary. Sometimes neurological side effects can occur, including muscle stiffness and, though uncommon, abnormal facial movements. A very serious neurological reaction that involves fever, muscle stiffness, and confusion is a rare side effect but one that can be fatal. Yet, even though these side effects may be quite serious, the benefits typically outweigh the risks, particularly for a child who has serious aggression issues.

Alternative Treatments

There are many alternative treatments available for use in autistic children, but there is little, if any, sound scientific investigation of these methods. Because the disorder can be so severe, parents are often willing to try most anything to improve their child's functioning. Some interventions, such as chelation therapy, can be dangerous; many are quite costly. To assess both the safety of alternative treatments and any potential interactions with prescribed medications, all interventions should be discussed with the managing pediatrician or other physicians caring for the child.

Prognosis

The prognosis for adolescents with autistic disorders depends on the severity of the illness. Early intensive treatment interventions can certainly affect outcome for many children. Some lucky children may ultimately shed their diagnosis of autism. But most continue to struggle with core symptoms. Children with severe symptoms accompanied by apparent cognitive limitations often require ongoing

Table 20.1	**Medications Used for Symptoms of Autism**		
Medication Class	**Representative Medications (Brand Name)**	**Clinical Reason to Prescribe**	**Comments**
Atypical Antipsychotics	Risperidone (Risperdal) Aripiprazole (Abilify) Quetiapine (Seroquel) Olanzapine (Zyprexa) Ziprasidone (Geodon)	Aggression and irritability	Risperidone and aripiprazole are approved by the FDA for treatment in autistic children and adolescents with irritability. Significant side effects include weight gain.
Selective Serotonin Reuptake Inhibitors	Fluoxetine (Prozac) Fluvoxamine (Luvox) Citalopram (Celexa) Escitalopram (Lexapro) Paroxetine (Paxil) Sertraline (Zoloft)	Anxiety and perseverative behaviors	The data are mixed; 50 percent of children may receive significant benefit. Agitation, aggression, and suicidality are potential side effects.
Psychostimulants	Methylphenidate (Ritalin) Dexmethylphenidate (Focalin) Amphetamine salts (Adderall) Dextroamphetamine (Dexedrine)	Hyperactivity, attention, impulsivity	About 50 percent of children receive significant benefit. Side effects are generally mild; there are very rare reports of sudden death.
Alpha-2 Agonists	Guanfacine (Tenex) Clonidine (Catapres)	Hyperactivity, impulsivity	Limited data show benefit to some children. Side effects are mild, with most common being sedation.
Norepinephrine Reuptake Inhibitors	Atomoxetine (Strattera)	Hyperactivity, impulsivity, inattention	May be helpful for these symptoms in some autistic children.

close support through adolescence and beyond. To manage their behavior and provide basic support, such individuals generally need to live in supervised settings such as a group home or assisted independent living with structured day programming. Nevertheless, high school programming is crucial in establishing life skills that can be transferred to later functioning capacities.

Adults with less severe forms of PDDs may be able to live independently or with only loose supervision. Nonsupported employment may certainly be an option, particularly for those with Asperger's disorder. Marriage and family are not common in those with PDDs but may occur in less effected individuals. Their apparent lack of interest in social connections often influences these life choices.

Conclusion

Autism is a serious developmental disorder that is characterized by limitations in social functioning, rigid behaviors, and significant communication delays. Sensory sensitivities, attentional symptoms, disruptive behaviors, intellectual limitations, and anxiety are commonly associated symptoms. Symptom severity can vary significantly. Many children, particularly those with high-functioning autism or Asperger's disorder, have more mild impairments with fewer limitations. Adolescence presents significant challenges for those with PDDs. Sexual and physical development along with the intensification of social demands can be overwhelming for these individuals. Impulsive behavior and disruptiveness may intensify along with a significant worsening of anxiety.

The treatment for autistic children centers on educational interventions and psychosocial therapies. Behavioral treatments form a considerable proportion of the interventions. Speech and language along with occupational therapies are standard. Specialized classrooms settings are often needed. These children should be receiving the assistance of a social skills group, and adolescents in particular require vocational and life-skills training. A medication consultation may be appropriate in managing some of the associated symptoms. Long-term prognosis is highly dependent on the severity of the symptoms. Higher-functioning individuals may be able to live independently, receive educational degrees, and participate in gainful employment.

References and Additional Reading

Deokar, A. M., M.B.G. Huff, and H. A. Omar. 2008. "Clinical Management of Adolescents with Autism." *Pediatric Clinics of North America* 55: 1147–1157.

Foxx, R. M. 2008. "Applied Behavior Analysis Treatment of Autism: The State of the Art." *Child and Adolescent Psychiatry Clinics of North America* 17: 821–834.

King, B. H., and J. Q. Bostic. 2006. "An Update on Psychopharmacologic Treatment for Autism Spectrum Disorders." *Child and Adolescent Psychiatry Clinics of North America* 15: 161–175.

Kuehn, B. M. 2007. "CDC: Autism Spectrum Disorders Common." *JAMA* 297: 940.

Muhle R., S. V. Trentacoste, and I. Rapin. 2004. "The Genetics of Autism." *Pediatrics* 113: e472–e486.

Ospina, M. B., S. J. Krebs, B. Clark, M. Karkhaneh, L. Hartling, L. Tsosvold, B. Vandermeer, and V. Smith. 2008. "Behavioural and Developmental Interventions for Autism Spectrum Disorder: A Clinical Systematic Review." *PLoS ONE* 3: e3755.

21 Conclusion

Psychiatric problems commonly begin during adolescence. Because of the critical developmental processes that are unfolding during this time, these problems have the potential to have lifelong effects, including low self-esteem, occupational underachievement, difficulties with relationships, substance abuse, and unhealthy ways of managing stress. Because adolescents are a work in progress, they tend to be more amenable to change than adults. Intervention during this critical period of development can have profound and lasting effects.

It is often challenging for parents to obtain the help a teen requires. Since adolescence is a time of rapid change, knowing when it is appropriate to seek psychiatric help can be difficult. The changes associated with normal developmental processes can be hard to distinguish from behavioral changes that suggest an emerging mental health problem. When a psychiatric problem is suspected, the mental health system in the United States is confusing to navigate; this is compounded by a shortage of mental health services for children and adolescents.

In this book, we have offered an overview of the major psychiatric disorders that occur during adolescence and an outline of possible treatments. It is our hope that, equipped with this knowledge, parents and those who work with teens will feel better able to recognize potential warning signs and to negotiate the obstacles that stand in the way of obtaining services that a troubled adolescent requires. Although each psychiatric disorder has its own unique pattern of symptoms and the approach to evaluation and treatment should be tailored accordingly, there are a few general principles regarding the identification and management of these disorders.

Adolescence is often a turbulent time, and a major change in teens' behavior that negatively affects their life at home, school, or with friends may be a sign of an emerging psychiatric problem, particularly when these problems persist for more than just a few weeks. Because early intervention can be much more effective than intervention later, it is generally best to err on the side of caution in seeking an evaluation for an adolescent who has symptoms of a mental illness. If parents are uncertain about whether a psychiatric evaluation is truly necessary, the adolescent's pediatrician can be a resource to help understand what is normal teen behavior and what are behaviors that deserve a closer review.

When an evaluation seems to be the best course of action, parents can facilitate the process by coming prepared (see appendix B for an outline of useful information to have with you for an initial psychiatric evaluation). A thorough evaluation of an adolescent should explore aspects of the teen's environment, including family life and school, that may be contributing to the problem. Often, the psychiatrist or mental health clinician performing the evaluation will ask for permission to speak with important people in the teen's life, such as a coach, a teacher, or a school counselor, to obtain a more complete understanding of the teen's behavior. Because psychiatric disorders tend to occur in clusters, meaning that having one disorder increases one's risk of having certain other disorders, a thorough evaluation should involve screening for symptoms of these comorbid problems.

Upon completion of the initial evaluation, the clinician should provide the adolescent and the family with a plan for moving forward. However, many psychiatric problems take time to understand fully, and the diagnosis and treatment recommendations may evolve as a clinician learns more information about the teen. Additional information may be needed to gain a better understanding of the problem. Further testing may include laboratory or other medical tests to evaluate potential medical causes for the teen's symptoms. Cognitive or psychological tests may be required to explore possible difficulties in learning or processing information or to examine symptoms that are difficult to characterize through an interview.

Treatment options should be based on interventions that have had good results, preferably supported by scientific study. That said, every teen is different, and a good treatment plan should also be tailored to fit the specific needs of the adolescent. The treatment options may address family issues, school difficulties, social problems, or other domains. A good plan also involves considering a teen's areas of strength and weakness to elucidate those treatments that will be most successful. For example, adolescents who have language-processing disorders or difficulty with abstract thinking may not respond well to certain treatments such as psychodynamic psychotherapy.

Although a single, straightforward approach to treatment can be effective for some problems, often a multipronged treatment approach is most useful for problems that are complex or difficult to treat. Common components of a treatment plan for adolescents include individual psychotherapy, medications, family therapy, group therapy, skills-based programs such as social skills training, community programs such as sports or camps, and school-based interventions designed to help support a teen's needs. For more severe problems, including those that threaten a teen's safety, intensive treatments such as partial hospital programs, residential programs, or inpatient psychiatric hospitalization may be appropriate.

Unlike certain childhood infections that can be prevented by immunizations, the options for prevention of mental health disorders are not well identified. But some groundwork has been laid by research. For example, there has been substantial research in understanding the underlying factors in adolescents' abuse of alcohol. Adolescents who expect that drinking is fun, believe that the popular kids drink, and have parents who abuse alcohol are at higher risk to begin

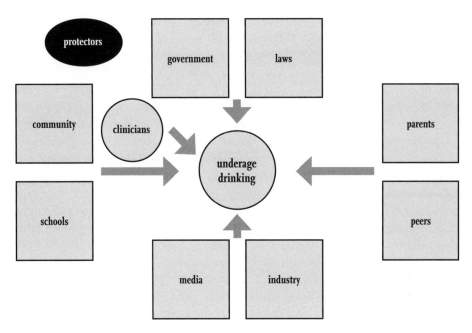

Figure 21.1 Groups that can help to protect an adolescent from underage drinking

drinking alcohol early. A prevention model composed of a coalition of parents and peers, schools and community, government and law, and media and industry can help to offset the prevalence of teenage drinking (see figure 21.1). This effort includes parents as well as the larger environment in which the adolescent lives and interacts.

Data from the Methods for the Epidemiology of Child and Adolescent Mental Disorders study show that the six-month prevalence rate for any mental health disorder among children between the ages of nine and seventeen is 20.9 percent. At least half of all DSM-IV disorders begin by age fourteen. The mental disorders that occur during adolescence have major implications for adolescents' short-term well-being as well as for their adaptation to adult life. Of greatest concern, childhood mood disorders can end in suicide. It is our hope that armed with the information in this book, parents and those who work closely with adolescents will be able to recognize symptoms of mental illness. When mental illness is recognized early and treated appropriately in adolescents, suffering diminishes and outcomes improve.

Unfortunately, there are barriers to the diagnosis and care of adolescents with mental health issues. There are only about sixty-three hundred child psychiatrists in the United States, and this shortage is expected to continue. In addition, mental illness is not covered by health insurance as comprehensively as "medical" illness is. Consequently, children often do not receive mental health care when referred by their pediatricians to mental health clinicians.

In some states, legislation is pending or has been passed requiring the coverage of mental illness in the same way as medical illness. This is termed parity. In addition, there is a growing movement for pediatricians to develop the knowledge and skill sets to diagnose and treat certain types of mental illness in children. And finally, attitudes toward mental illness are changing. Parents are seeking information and referral for their troubled children, medications are more widely prescribed, and there is much more public discussion of mental health issues. With these changes occurring, the outlook is more optimistic that adolescents who have mental health issues will be identified, will obtain appropriate services, and will not feel a stigma about their illness.

As teens with mental health problems transition into adulthood, they will encounter a health care system that no longer has a pediatric orientation. For healthy adolescents, this change should not be a major issue. For those with chronic disease, obstacles can be difficult to surmount. This is especially true for teens with autism, who grow up to discover an adult medical system that does not interact well with them. Autistic adults may not be able to communicate effectively, and they may have odd behaviors. Both may be roadblocks to care from adult providers. As a result, autistic adults may initially stay with their pediatricians, but eventually they do need to have adult providers. Because adult clinicians have little or no experience with autism, autistic adults are at risk for misdiagnosis or no diagnosis of a medical problem. To remedy these issues, Massachusetts General Hospital has initiated a large program to train adult clinicians including nurses and primary care and emergency room physicians in working with autistic adults. It is through these innovative programs that quality medical care will be delivered to autistic adults. In a broader perspective, adult clinicians should also be trained in the care of other mental health disorders that begin in adolescence.

The traditional relationship between an individual and a mental health clinician continues to be the primary method of delivering mental health services to adolescents. Training other health care clinicians in certain aspects of mental health care is an important step forward. In addition, it is important to understand and develop a wider role for community resources in identifying and helping to treat teens with mental illness.

References and Additional Reading

Kutner, L., C. Olson, S. Schlozman, M. Goldstein, D. Warner, and E. Beresin. 2008. "Training Pediatric Residents and Pediatricians about Adolescent Mental Health Problems: A Proof-of-Concept Pilot for a Proposed National Curriculum." *Academic Psychiatry* 32: 429–437.

Monash, B. In press. "Transition of Care." In *Mass General Hospital for Children Adolescent Medicine Handbook,* ed. Mark A. Goldstein, M.D. New York: Springer.

Shaffer, D., P. Fisher, M. Dulcan, M. Davies, J. Piacentini, M. Schwab-Stone, B. Lahey, K. Bourdon, P. Jensen, H. Bird, G. Canino, and D. Regier. 1996. "The NIMH Diagnostic Interview Schedule for Children Version 2.3 (DISC-2.3): Description, Acceptability, Prevalence Rates, and Performance in the MECA Study: Methods for the Epidemiology of Child and Adolescent Mental Disorders Study." *Journal of the American Academy of Child and Adolescent Psychiatry* 35: 865–877.

Appendix A | Resources

Chapter 1: Introduction

Websites

General information on adolescent mental health: http://www.teenmentalhealth.org

Adolescent intellectual development: http://www.massgeneral.org/children/adolescenthealth/ articles/aa_intellectual_development.aspx

Adolescent independence and rebellion: http://www.massgeneral.org/children/adolescenthealth/ articles/aa_independence_and_rebellion.aspx

Screening tools for emotional and behavioral problems in children and adolescents:

Pediatric symptom checklist to be completed by parent: http://www2.massgeneral.org/ allpsych/pediatricsymptomchecklist/psc_english.pdf, http://www2.massgeneral.org/ allpsych/pediatricsymptomchecklist/psc_spanish.pdf

Pediatric symptom checklist to be completed by youth: http://www2.massgeneral.org/allpsych/ pediatricsymptomchecklist/psc_english_y.pdf, http://www2.massgeneral.org/allpsych/ pediatricsymptomchecklist/psc_spanish_y.pdf

Books

Bradley, M. 2003. *Yes, Your Teen Is Crazy: Loving Your Kid without Losing Your Mind.* Gig Harbor, WA: Harbor.

Faber, A., and E. Mazlish. 2005. *How to Talk So Teens Will Listen and Listen So Teens Will Talk.* New York: Avon Books.

Pruitt, D. 1999. *Your Adolescent: Emotional, Behavioral, and Emotional Development from Early Adolescence through the Teen Years.* New York: HarperCollins.

Organizations

American Academy of Pediatrics
141 Northwest Point Blvd
Elk Grove Village, IL 60007
http://www.aap.org

Chapter 2: Introduction to Mental Health Treatment

Websites

Systems of care: http://mentalhealth.samhsa.gov/cmhs/ChildrensCampaign/grantcomm.asp
Mental Health America: http://www.nmha.org/

Chapter 3: Finding Treatment

Websites

National Mental Health Information Center: http://mentalhealth.samhsa.gov/databases/

Finding mental health services: http://mentalhealth.samhsa.gov/publications/allpubs/fastfact2/
default.asp

Video
How to find a mental health professional, from the American Academy of Child and Adolescent Psychiatry: http://www.aacap.org/cs/expert_interviews/mental_health_professionals_
and_insurance

Chapter 4: Psychotherapy

Websites
What is psychotherapy for children and adolescents: http://www.aacap.org/cs/root/facts_for_
families/what_is_psychotherapy_for_children_and_adolescents
How to find help through psychotherapy: http://apahelpcenter.org/articles/article.php?id=52
How to choose a psychotherapist: http://apahelpcenter.org/articles/article.php?id=51

Organizations
American Psychological Association
750 First Street N.E., #605
Washington, DC 20002
http://www.apa.org/

Chapter 5: Psychiatric Medications

Websites
Mental health medications: http://www.nimh.nih.gov/health/publications/mental-health
-medications/index.shtml

Chapter 6: Major Depressive Disorder

Websites
National Library of Medicine, adolescent depression: www.nlm.nih.gov/medlineplus/ency/article/
001518.htm
Antidepressant medications for children and adolescents: http://www.nimh.nih.gov/health/topics/
child-and-adolescent-mental-health/antidepressant-medications-for-children-and-adolescents
-information-for-parents-and-caregivers.shtml

Organizations
American Academy of Child & Adolescent Psychiatry
3615 Wisconsin Avenue N.W.
Washington, D.C. 20016-3007
http://www.aacap.org/

Books

Cobain, B. 2006. *When Nothing Matters Anymore: A Survival Guide for Depressed Teens.* Minneapolis, MN: Free Spirit.

Ginsburg, K., and M. Jablow. 2007. *A Parent's Guide to Building Resilience in Children and Teens: Giving Your Child Roots and Wings.* Elk Grove Village, IL: American Academy of Pediatrics.

Videos

Depression and antidepressants: http://www.aacap.org/cs/expert_interviews/depression_and_antidepressants

Chapter 7: Bipolar Disorder

Websites

National Institute of Mental Health, bipolar disorder: http://www.nimh.nih.gov/health/topics/bipolar-disorder/index.shtml

Organizations

Child & Adolescent Bipolar Foundation
1000 Skokie Blvd, Suite 570
Wilmette, IL 60091
http://www.bpkids.org/

Depression and Bipolar Support Alliance
730 North Franklin Street, Suite 501
Chicago, IL 60610–7224
www.dbsalliance.org

Videos

Definition and treatment: http://www.aacap.org/cs/expert_interviews/bipolar_disorder

Chapter 8: Anxiety Disorders

Websites

Children who will not go to school: http://www.aacap.org/cs/root/facts_for_families/children_who_wont_go_to_school_separation_anxiety

The anxious child: http://www.aacap.org/cs/root/facts_for_families/the_anxious_child

Information from federal agencies: http://mentalhealth.samhsa.gov/publications/allpubs/ca-0007/default.asp, http://www.surgeongeneral.gov/library/mentalhealth/chapter3/sec6.html

Information from the American Academy of Child and Adolescent Psychiatry: http://www.aacap.org/cs/root/publication_store/your_adolescent_anxiety_and_avoidant_disorders

Organizations

Anxiety Disorders Association of America
8730 Georgia Avenue, Suite 600
Silver Spring, MD 20910
http://www.adaa.org/

Chapter 9: Psychotic Disorders

Websites
Schizophrenia: http://www.nimh.nih.gov/health/topics/schizophrenia/index.shtml
National Institute of Mental Health: www.nimh.nih.org

Organizations
American Academy of Child and Adolescent Psychiatry: www.aacap.org
National Alliance on Mental Illness (NAMI): www.nami.org

Chapter 10: School-Related Problems

Websites
Information on individual education plans: http://specialed.about.com/od/iep/Individual_
    Education_Plan.htm
Website produced by Massachusetts General Hospital that provides useful information about
    meeting the educational needs of children and adolescents with a psychiatric disorder: www
    .schoolpsychiatry.org

Organizations
Council of Parent Attorneys and Advocates: www.copaa.org

Chapter 11: Attention-Deficit/Hyperactivity Disorder

Websites
ADHD information: http://www.nimh.nih.gov/health/topics/attention-deficit-hyperactivity
    -disorder-adhd/index.shtml
Conners rating scales for ADHD: www.modern-psychiatry.com/rating_scale1.htm

Organizations
Attention Deficit Disorder Association: http://www.add.org
Children and Adults with Attention Deficit/Hyperactivity Disorder: www.chadd.org

Books
Jensen, P. 2004. *Making the System Work for Your Child with ADHD*. New York: Guilford.
Reiff, M., and S. Tippins. 2004. *ADHD: A Complete and Authoritative Guide*. Elk Grove Village,
    IL: American Academy of Pediatrics.

Chapter 12: Substance Abuse

Organizations
National Institute on Drug Abuse: http://www.nida.nih.gov
Substance Abuse and Mental Health Services Administration: http://www.samhsa.gov
National Clearinghouse for Alcohol and Drug Information: http://www.health.org
National Center on Addiction and Substance Abuse at Columbia University: http://www
    .casacolumbia.org

Books

Califano, J. 2009. *How to Raise a Drug-Free Kid: The Straight Dope for Parents.* New York: Fireside.

Chapter 13: Personality Disorders

Websites

Borderline personality: http://www.nimh.nih.gov/health/publications/borderline-personality
-disorder-fact-sheet/index.shtml

Books

Glass, L., 1995. *Toxic People: 10 Ways of Dealing with People Who Make Your Life Miserable.* New York: Simon & Schuster.

Chapter 14: Behavioral Disorders

Websites

Conduct disorder: http://www.aacap.org/cs/root/facts_for_families/conduct_disorder
Bullying: http://www.aacap.org/cs/root/facts_for_families/bullying

Books

Coloroso, B. 2004. *The Bully, the Bullied, and the Bystander: From Preschool to High School—How Parents and Teachers Can Break the Cycle of Violence.* New York: Harper.
Ludwig, T. 2006. *Just Kidding.* New York: Tricycle.

Chapter 15: Eating Disorders

Websites

Anorexia nervosa: http://www.massgeneral.org/children/adolescenthealth/articles/aa_anorexia.aspx

Organizations

Harris Center for Education and Advocacy in Eating Disorders at Massachusetts General Hospital: http://www.harriscentermgh.org/
The Klarman Eating Disorders Center at McLean Hospital, Belmont, Massachusetts: http://www.mclean.harvard.edu/patient/child/edc.php
National Eating Disorders Association: http://www.nationaleatingdisorders.org/

Books

Herzog, D. B., D. L. Franko, and P. Cable. 2007. *Unlocking the Mysteries of Eating Disorders.* New York: McGraw-Hill.

Chapter 16: Obsessive-Compulsive Disorder and Tic Disorders

Websites

Obsessive-compulsive disorder in children and adolescents: http://www.aacap.org/cs/root/facts_for_families/obsessivecompulsive_disorder_in_children_and_adolescents

Books

Chansky, T. 2001. *Freeing Your Child from Obsessive-Compulsive Disorder: A Powerful, Practical Program for Parents of Children and Adolescents.* New York: Three Rivers.

Chapter 17: Reactions to Stress, Loss, and Illness

Websites

Teen reactions to death of a loved one: http://www.massgeneral.org/children/adolescenthealth/articles/aa_deaths.aspx

Books

Balk, D., and C. Coor. 2009. *Adolescent Encounters with Death, Bereavement, and Coping.* New York: Springer.

Greydanus, D. 2006. *Caring for Your Teenager: The Complete and Authoritative Guide.* Elk Grove Village, IL: American Academy of Pediatrics.

Chapter 18: Reactions to Trauma

Websites

Posttraumatic stress disorder: http://www.aacap.org/cs/root/facts_for_families/posttraumatic_stress_disorder_ptsd

Organizations

National Child Traumatic Stress Network: www.nctsnet.org

Books

Schiraldi, G. 2009. *The Post-Traumatic Stress Disorder Sourcebook: A Guide to Healing, Recovery and Growth.* New York: McGraw-Hill.

Chapter 19: Dangerous Behavior: Suicide, Self-Injury, and Violence

Websites

Teen anger: http://www.massgeneral.org/children/adolescenthealth/articles/aa_anger.aspx

Teen suicide: http://www.teensuicide.us/

Organizations

National Suicide Prevention Lifeline: http://www.suicidepreventionlifeline.org/

Books

Lezine, D., and D. Brent. 2008. *Eight Stories Up: An Adolescent Chooses Hope over Suicide.* New York: Oxford University Press.

Strasburger, V. C., B. J. Wilson, and A. Jordan. 2009. *Children, Adolescents, and the Media.* 2nd ed. Thousand Oaks, CA: Sage.

Chapter 20: Autism Spectrum Disorders

Websites
Autism information center: http://www.cdc.gov/ncbddd/autism/index.htm

Organizations
Autism Society: http://www.autism-society.org

Books
Grandin, T. 2006. *Thinking in Pictures: My Life with Autism.* Expanded ed. New York: Vintage Books.

Grandin, T., and M. Scariano. 1986. *Emergence: Labeled Autistic.* Novato, CA: Arena.

Sicile-Kira, C., and T. Grandin. 2006. *Adolescents on the Autism Spectrum: A Parent's Guide to the Cognitive, Social, Physical, and Transition Needs of Teenagers with Autism Spectrum Disorders.* New York: Berkley.

Williams, D. 1998. *Nobody Nowhere: The Remarkable Autobiography of an Autistic Girl.* London: Jessica Kingsley.

Chapter 21: Conclusion

Websites
"Mental Health: A Report of the Surgeon General": http://www.surgeongeneral.gov/library/mentalhealth/home.html

Articles
American Academy of Pediatrics, Committee on Psychosocial Aspects of Child and Family Health and Task Force on Mental Health. 2009. "The Future of Pediatrics: Mental Health Competencies for Pediatric Primary Care." *Pediatrics* 124: 410–421.

Appendix B | Treatment Organizer

This organizer is provided to help parents keep track of information relevant to their adolescent's psychiatric care. When negotiating the mental health system, it may be helpful to keep key information, including contact numbers, in one place. Bringing this information along for a psychiatric evaluation, be it in an emergency setting or an outpatient visit, can help make the visit more efficient and useful.

Contact Information for Current Treatment Team

	Name	Office Phone	Urgent #	Other #
Psychiatrist				
Therapist				
School Contact				
Other				

Current Medications: Prescription, Over-the-Counter, Alternative

Medication Name	Dose (e.g., 10 mg)	Frequency (e.g., twice daily)	Notes

Allergies or Negative Reactions to Medications

Medication	Reaction

Psychiatric History

When did the problem first appear and what symptoms were present at the time?

_____

_____

When did you first seek treatment?

_____

_____

What diagnosis or diagnoses has/have been given in the past?

_____

_____

What forms of treatment have you tried in the past (e.g., therapy, medication management)?

_____

_____

Past Treatment Providers

Name and Role (e.g., Dr. John Smith, psychiatrist)	Contact Information	Time Period (from when to when)	Notes

Past Psychiatric Hospitalization or Other Treatment Programs

Program	Date	Reason	Notes

Past Medication Trials

Medication Name	Highest Dose	Reason Stopped	Notes

Test Results

Test (e.g., private neuropsychological evalution)	Date	Performed by	Results Summary

Current and Past Medical Problems

Condition (e.g., asthma)	Dates (e.g., diagnosed 9/20/06)	Notes

Primary Care Clinicians and Other Medical Providers

	Name	Contact Information
Pediatrician/family medicine physician, adolescent medicine specialist		
Specialists or other providers (e.g., pulmonologist, physical therapist)		

Other Information

_____

_____

_____

_____

_____

_____

_____

Index

abandonment, adolescent fear of, 291

Abilify. *See* aripiprazole

abstract thinking, difficulty with, 308

academic programs, modification of, 22. *See also* school

acamprosate (Campral), 176

acceptance, as response to stress, 253

"acid." *See* LSD

acid blockers, in anorexia, 222

activation, SSRIs associated with, 93

acute residential treatment (ART), 27–28, 34 table; for substance abuse, 177. *See also* residential treatment programs

acute stress disorder, 262; diagnosis of, 267–268, 271, 275; evaluation for, 270–271; symptoms of, 267–268, 275; treatment for, 271–274

Adderall. *See* amphetamine

addiction, 284; Internet, 8; from methamphetamine abuse, 186. *See also* substance abuse

Addison's disease, bipolar disorder symptoms associated with, 106

ADHD. *See* attention-deficit/hyperactivity disorder

adjustment disorder, 87; anxiety associated with, 119; diagnosis of, 258–259; interventions for, 259

adolescence: changes during, 12; cornerstones of, 37; divorce during, 254; individual identity in, 3; in Internet era, 8; intervention during, 304; normal, 5–8; as transition, 1

adolescents: in ART programs, 27; communicating with, 10–12; decision making of, 4. *See also* communication; teenagers; traumatized adolescents

adrenalin, 251

adults: autistic, 310; bipolar disorder in, 100–101; with Tourette's syndrome, 246

advocacy organizations, 163–164

affect, in schizophrenia, 134

agencies, funding provided by, 23, 25. *See also* state agencies

aggressive behavior, 286; of autistic children, 299, 300; parental reaction to, 291

agitation: in depression, 84; violence and, 288

agoraphobia, panic disorder with, 116

Al-Anon, 176

Alateen, 9, 55, 176, 259

alcohol: and bipolar disorder symptoms, 105; depression associated with, 89; diabetes and, 256; effects of, 178–179; prenatal exposure to, 165

alcohol abuse: depression and, 89–90; incidence of, 178; prevention of, 309, 309 table; underlying factors in, 308–309

Alcoholics Anonymous, 55, 176

alpha-2 agonists, in autistic disorders, 305 table

"alpha-1 agonists," in tic disorders, 245

alprazolam (Xanax), 69; abuse of, 184; for anxiety disorder, 125

American Academy of Pediatrics, 161, 296

American Group Psychotherapy Association, 56

amitriptyline, 68

amotivational syndrome, 180

amphetamine (Adderall, Dexedrine), 70; in ADHD, 159–160; and bipolar disorder symptoms, 105; controlled-release form of, 160; depression associated with, 89; tics triggered by, 243; uses for, 185

anabolic steroids, abuse of, 189–190

Anafranil. *See* clomipramine

"angel dust." *See* PCP

anger: in bipolar disorder, 104; depression and, 91; divorce associated with feelings of, 254; as response to stress, 253

anhedonia, 84

anorexia, 225; case presentation, 213; diagnosis of, 215; medical hospitalization for, 219–220; personality associated with, 217; signs of, 214; symptoms of, 43; treatment options for, 43

anorexia nervosa, 212, 213

Antabuse. *See* disulfiram

antacids, in anorexia, 222

anticonvulsant medications: in bipolar disorder, 107; carbamazepine, 76–77; lamotrigine, 76; oxcarbazine, 76–77; in personality disorders, 200; valproic acid, 75–76

antidepressant medications: in ADHD, 162; for anorexia, 223; buproprion, 67; choosing, 61; mirtazapine, 67–68; monitoring, 94; risks associated with, 67; suicidal ideation and, 93–94; and suicidality, 66–67; tics triggered by, 243. *See also* selective serotonin reuptake inhibitors; tricyclic antidepressants

antihistamines: in anxiety disorder, 126; tics triggered by, 243

antipsychotic medications, 137; for bipolar disorder, 72–73, 74; side effects of, 72, 73; for tic disorders, 245; typical, 72

antipsychotics, atypical, 72–74, 138; in autistic disorders, 305 table; in bipolar disorder, 108; in personality disorders, 200; for tic disorders, 245; in violent behavior, 291

About the Authors

Eric P. Hazen, M.D., is a board-certified child and adolescent psychiatrist and an instructor in psychiatry at Harvard Medical School. A graduate of Brown University and the Yale School of Medicine, he trained in child, adolescent, and adult psychiatry at Massachusetts General and McLean hospitals. He practices at Massachusetts General Hospital and Newton-Wellesley Hospital, where he is the chief of the Division of Child and Adolescent Psychiatry. Dr. Hazen is actively involved in the treatment of many teens with a broad variety of troubles. His professional interests include psychodynamic psychotherapy, the role of mind-body medicine in psychiatry, the psychological development of children and adolescents, and psychiatric issues related to medical illness in the pediatric population.

Mark A. Goldstein, M.D., is the founding chief of the Adolescent and Young Adult Division at Massachusetts General Hospital and an assistant professor of pediatrics at Harvard Medical School. Dr. Goldstein graduated from the Georgetown University School of Medicine, trained in pediatrics at Massachusetts General Hospital, and completed a fellowship in adolescent medicine at Boston Children's Hospital. He is the author of numerous books and articles, including *Your Best Medicine,* and editor of the *Mass General Hospital for Children Adolescent Medicine Handbook.*

Myrna Chandler Goldstein, M.A., is an independent scholar, journalist, and author of numerous books and articles. Her recent works include *Food and Nutrition Controversies Today: A Reference Guide* and *Your Best Medicine.* She recently completed work on *Healthy Foods: Fact versus Fiction,* which was published in 2010.

Charles Henry, M.D., is the director of psychopharmacology in the Lurie Family Autism Center/LADDERS at Massachusetts General Hospital and a clinical instructor in psychiatry at Harvard Medical School.